Vaccinations

A THOUGHTFUL PARENT'S GUIDE

Vaccinations

A THOUGHTFUL PARENT'S GUIDE

How to Make Safe, Sensible Decisions
about the Risks, Benefits, and Alternatives

AVIVA JILL ROMM
C.P.M., Herbalist A.H.G.

Healing Arts Press
Rochester, Vermont

Healing Arts Press
One Park Street
Rochester, Vermont 05767
www.InnerTraditions.com

Healing Arts Press is a division of Inner Traditions International

Note to the reader: This book is intended as an informational guide. The remedies, approaches, and techniques described herein are meant to supplement, and not to be a substitute for, professional medical care or treatment. They should not be used to treat a serious ailment without prior consultation with a qualified health care professional.

Library of Congress Cataloging-in-Publication Data

Romm, Aviva Jill.
    Vaccinations : a thoughtful parent's guide : how to make safe, sensible decisions
about the risks, benefits, and alternatives / Aviva Jill Romm.
        p. cm.
    Includes bibliographical references and index.
    ISBN 978-0-89281-931-7 (paper)
        1. Vaccination of children. 2. Vaccination of children—Complications—Risk
factors. 3. Immunization of children. 4. Vaccines—Health aspects. I. Title.

    RJ240.R65 2001
    614.4'7'083—dc21

                                                    2001024673

Printed and bound in the United States

20 19 18 17 16 15 14 13 12 11 10 9 8

Text design and layout by Priscilla Baker
This book was typeset in Janson, with Arepo as a display face

Contents

Foreword

Vaccinations: A Thoughtful Parent's Guide gives readers a look at the many aspects of this controversial subject, which is a growing concern for today's parents. Many parents struggle with finding the answers to their questions about vaccines, wanting to get the whole picture. Aviva Jill Romm presents readers with the risks and benefits of vaccines, vaccine-preventable diseases, and the most recent research about approaches to immunity and disease prevention. All of this information helps parents make informed choices about immunizing their children.

Choice is a key word, and one that is often not presented to parents. The fact that they can choose whether or not to vaccinate their child is sometimes a new concept and presents some obstacles. Understanding health and disease, learning how to prevent illness when possible, and choosing the treatment with as few risks as possible are the keys to optimal health for our children and families. Freedom of choice in health care includes the choice to vaccinate or not. Parents should question the routine use of vaccines, investigate the subject, ask questions, and read the literature. This does not constitute disagreement, but rather promotes educated decisions. Informed parents can make better choices for their children.

Vaccinations: A Thoughtful Parent's Guide covers another important issue in health care, which is the prevention of disease. The concept of prevention can also be a new one for some parents. Preventing illness by adopting healthier lifestyle changes—including diet; immune support with vitamins, minerals, and herbs; minimal exposure to environmental toxins; and physical activity—can optimize good health and reduce the risk of becoming ill. This book offers parents many ways to incorporate prevention as part of their family's lifestyle. A child with a healthy, strong immune system has better resistance and a vital immune response when needed, minimizing the frequency and severity of illnesses.

Addressing such a controversial subject is not an easy task, and it is one I personally would not have wanted to tackle. The challenge of providing a balanced perspective on the topic in the midst of the overwhelming amount of contradictory information in the literature could not have been an easy one.

Vaccinations: A Thoughtful Parent's Guide does not choose a side. Instead it provides sound information to readers so that they may choose intelligently when making health decisions about their children. Romm refers to the book as a bridge that unites both sides with the common goal of optimal health for all children. This book is such a bridge.

Mary L. Bove, N.D.
Brattleboro Naturopathic Clinic
Brattleboro, Vermont

Acknowledgments

This book has required enormous support, in terms of both time and research effort, to provide you, the reader, with accurate, current, and useful information. I owe ongoing gratitude to my husband, Tracy, who has put up with my countless hours at the computer and more hours of me sprawled across the floor with books and articles piled all around (articles for which he spent many hours searching on-line databases and the medical library), and even more, for his open ear when I talked half with him and half aloud with myself over the many interesting and controversial details, "facts," and opinions I encountered in my research. I'm sure he really didn't want to hear about echinacea, polysaccharides, and macrophages in bed at midnight, but he did listen graciously, even if his eyes were closed.

As a midwife and herbalist, I couldn't ask for a richer group of colleagues and teachers, whom I am also honored to call friends. Over the years this has become quite an array of some of the most colorful, dedicated, humane, humble, caring, intelligent, independent-minded, and pioneering people I have ever met. Each has had time for a question, a piece of information, an insight, a kind word, or a rich discussion. And each makes such a rich contribution to the world that inspires me each day.

A special thanks also goes to my M.D. friends, old and new, and those others of you in pediatrics, family practice, and obstetrics who continue to honor freedom of choice in health care—you know who you are.

Thanks go to Jon Graham of Healing Arts Press for asking me to write this book. Jon, there were times I thought of turning back from this book— away from the complexity and controversy—but your interest in the topic and your support kept me remembering how important this information is and how difficult it is for parents and practitioners to sort through this issue. And to Lee Juvan, for helping me maintain its integrity every step of the way.

I am also thankful to my in-laws, Mendel and Anta Romm, for their emotional support in our move "back home" to Georgia (can you believe it, me, a New Yorker, calling Georgia home!) during the course of writing this book, and to all our friends whose love and encouragement helped it to happen.

I am eternally grateful to all of those families who have invited me into their lives, homes, births, and health care concerns over the past fifteen years.

I know many of you feel you have learned a lot from me. I have also learned so much from you. It is you who can continue to truly make a difference in American health care. Keep your voices strong.

Finally, to my children, whose presence in my life is worth more than words can say. May you be blessed with long lives, much happiness, and great vitality.

Introduction

Primum non nocere—Above all, do no harm

Controversial from the Start

Perhaps there is no topic of greater controversy in medicine today than that of childhood vaccinations. That the topic can even be described as controversial is in itself debatable, as many, indeed most, in the medical and public health professions would argue that it is not controversial and that anything less than universal protection of children by the routine use of vaccinations is a travesty of health care. Yet ever since the modern inception of the use of inoculations in humans, there has been dissent. Even as early as the first half of the nineteenth century in England, there was public outrage and horror over the injection of "filthy material" into humans for the purpose of preventing disease. Indeed, the process of inoculation known as "variolation" was made a felony in England in 1840.[1] Today, however, it is not the government decrying vaccines, it is concerned parents and medical professionals. And though in the past dissenters from contemporary medical mores may have been easily marginalized, today's parents and professionals are prepared to defend themselves with cogent, well-researched arguments. Add the media to the mix and it becomes apparent that with increasing public awareness there is indeed a controversy in our culture regarding the routine and universal administration of vaccinations for children.

New Concerns about Accepted Methods

While vaccine campaigns have received wide public acceptance for the better part of the twentieth century, we enter the new millennium with growing

1

concern from increasing numbers of parents and medical professionals about the safety of vaccinations when compared with the relative risk of disease in our developed Western nation. In the past fifteen years, this voice of concern, particularly from parents, has actually grown into a formidable political force that has had a significant impact on shaping vaccine policies in the United States. In fact, parents such as Barbara Loe Fisher, founder of the National Vaccine Information Center and herself the mother of a vaccine-injured child, have lobbied successfully for new government policies such as the National Childhood Vaccine Injury Act of 1986. This act is a federal vaccine injury compensation program that also includes vaccine safety provisions such as mandatory reporting and documentation of hospitalizations, injuries, and deaths following vaccination.[2] Many of the parents currently active in vaccine politics are themselves parents of vaccine-injured children, all of whom dutifully vaccinated their children before realizing that vaccine reactions were a serious risk. Unfortunately, it is all too often the case that we become aware of the dangers of a procedure only after we experience adverse consequences.

The concerned argue that for many children the risks of adverse reactions to the vaccines outweigh the risks of contracting the diseases in question or the likelihood of injurious consequences from the naturally contracted diseases. Furthermore, they maintain that the rates of vaccine reactions are notably higher than generally reported, and that vaccine consequences may not only take the form of the overtly reportable manifestations such as seizures and death but may also be displayed as the chronic, insidious, and seemingly inexorable health problems that are on the rise in our society, including asthma, allergies, diabetes, learning disabilities, and autoimmune disorders such as multiple sclerosis, lupus erythematosus, arthritis, cancer, and AIDS. Many vaccine opponents add political import to this debate, insisting that there are underlying profit motives on the part of manufacturers and deliberate intent on the part of the medical profession to conceal adverse reactions for fear of litigation.

Vaccine proponents, conversely, argue that while, yes, there are inherent risks to vaccination, these risks are minimal and insignificant compared with the potential risk of "vaccine-preventable diseases," as the diseases for which children are vaccinated are called, and the inevitability of epidemics in the absence of comprehensive vaccination programs. They further contend that vaccine risks appear to be significant only against the current horizon of a society free of periodic outbreaks of life-threatening infectious diseases, a product of long-standing and ubiquitous vaccine programs.

Vaccine naysayers, on the contrary, report, based on historical epidemiological evidence, that disease rates for most infectious diseases were already on the decline prior to the inception of mass vaccination campaigns, attributable to improved hygiene and living conditions, better nutrition, public sanitation measures, clean drinking water, and, secondarily, improved access to medical care.

An Emotional Debate

At times it seems that the arguments on both sides of the vaccine debate are lucid and substantial; at times the arguments seem hysterical and unclear, both sides appearing to take a black or white stand with little room for sensible discussion and mutual respect, and both sides providing emotionally wrenching evidence to support their cases. There is no shortage of stories of the horrors of disease epidemics prior to vaccines, and the number of heartbreaking stories of vaccine-damaged kids is overwhelming. This makes it very hard for most parents to sort through whether, when, and how to vaccinate their children to optimize their health and safety. Many parents understandably find it difficult, if not impossible, to consciously inject disease material into their perfectly healthy and thriving children, knowing that the possibility of adverse reactions is very real even if minimal. As one vaccine activist stated, if the adverse reaction happens to your child, then the risk is 100 percent. On the other hand, parents do feel great concern about the possibility of their healthy children being damaged by potentially preventable diseases.

Political Force versus Personal Freedom

Political force behind the provaccination camp allows healthy disagreement and public discourse between two concerned parties to deteriorate to punitive measures for those unwilling to conform. Reduced WIC vouchers for mothers who do not vaccinate their children, litigation against parents who do not comply with recommended vaccine programs, difficulty enrolling children in school, and even threats of court-ordered vaccination of children against the will of parents are all scenarios familiar to those who hear stories from parents who tried to exercise their freedom of choice in health care. Those who choose not to vaccinate are forced, upon enrolling their children in school, to sign what one mother, a nutritionist and the wife of a physician, described as "bad mommy" forms. These state emphatically that as a parent who chooses not to vaccinate or to selectively vaccinate, you are knowingly subjecting your child to the risk of life-threatening diseases and you accept all responsibility should your child be permanently damaged or die as a result. Parents who openly choose not to vaccinate their children, whether for philosophic, religious, or even minor medical reasons are punished for shunning what has come to be considered the obligation of the decent American citizen. Of course, no doctor or school administrator is ever required to sign a similar form accepting full responsibility should the parent comply with vaccinations and the child be damaged. Nor would they.

Lacking significant political backing, those who oppose vaccine mandates and who want safer vaccine options rely on support groups, information resource groups, and political lobbying to influence parents, physicians, and policy. It has only been in recent years that politicians, such as Representative Dan Burton, whose grandchild was damaged by vaccines and is now autistic, have taken on the vaccine issue as an overt political agenda. Representative Burton, for example, has been a moving force behind the recently completed congressional hearings to investigate possible links between the measles, mumps, and rubella vaccine (MMR) and autism.

What is clear to many is that the question of childhood vaccinations is one that every parent will face, as it is expected that every American child who can be vaccinated, will be vaccinated. Until recently only relatively few parents have even questioned the routine use of vaccinations for their children, but with growing public disclosure of possible connections between vaccinations and such problems as mercury toxicity, cancer, and autism, more parents are taking notice and investigating the issues.

The vaccination controversy is really a twofold debate that extends deeper than just the issue of vaccine safety and efficacy. It is also a question of whether one has the individual right to choose whether to vaccinate. The discussion actually lays wide open the very philosophical foundations of individual freedom on which our country is built. The issue of personal freedom is juxtaposed with public safety. Simply put, the public mandate upon which vaccination campaigns rest is that the individual does not have the freedom to jeopardize public health by choosing not to vaccinate. This premise assumes that it is the nonvaccinated members of a population that threaten the well-being of those who are vaccinated, and that it is the vaccinations themselves that are primarily responsible for promoting health in our society. Implicit in this axiom are many suppositions and assumptions, as well as the seeds for more than a few excellent questions. For example, if vaccinations are so effective, then why does a small nonvaccinating population threaten a well-protected whole? Why has the live polio vaccine been in continued use in spite of the fact that the only incidence of polio in the United States in more than a decade has been a direct result of receipt of a live polio vaccine or exposure to someone who has recently been vaccinated with the live polio? Indeed, vaccination as a biomedical ethics topic has been largely ignored by biomedical ethicists, but it does need to be explored from this vantage point as well. Where do individual freedom and social responsibility begin and end? Even more important, who gets to decide, and based upon what assumptions and evidence?

Seeking Balance

I am conservative on my views regarding vaccination, and as a midwife and health care provider I am a staunch supporter of public health measures. I am not so naive or smug as to assume that alternative medicines and healthy living are always sufficient to prevent or treat disease. Furthermore, having seen what disease can do to the human body, I am humbled by and grateful for medical science. Nonetheless, I am also an ardent advocate of individual freedom in health care, particularly when it comes to injecting the body with substances that are known to cause adverse reactions and that may cause long-term chronic disorders. In my mind, this clearly belongs to the realm of personal choice. As a scientist, I keep my mind open to investigating new possibilities, and as a scientist in the service of humanity, I keep myself open to the first order of medical doctrine: *"primum non nocere,"* first do no harm. Having seen firsthand the increase in chronic childhood health problems over the past several decades, I am concerned about the implications of vaccinations for our continued health as a human species. And having encountered families whose children have been visibly damaged by vaccinations, I question why there isn't more inquiry into vaccine safety. Though serious adverse reactions may be the exception to the rule, they definitely do occur. If there is even a possibility that the increase in childhood learning disabilities or behavioral problems we currently see are related to vaccinations, then I would say more evaluation is necessary. In the meantime I continue to be asked questions about vaccinations on a regular basis, from parents all over the country. They are concerned, want to make the right decisions for their children, and don't know where to find a balanced perspective. Thus, when my publisher approached me with the idea of writing a book on this topic, I accepted.

In writing a controversial book, one inherently takes a risk. On a personal note, a physician colleague of mine, knowing my plans to attend medical school in the next few years, warned me not to mention this book in my medical school interviews, fearing that I would be prejudged for having written a book that admits any problems with vaccines. This did not surprise me, as in the extensive research I did to prepare this book, there is a tone of derision in the medical literature toward any notion of questioning vaccines, and most authors of medical articles go to some lengths to reinforce the importance of continued and noninterrupted vaccine practices in spite of proof that they are associated with numerous health problems. There is also the personal challenge of writing a book that provides a balanced perspective when the literature is rife with seemingly contradictory information. A thorough review of the medical literature, including journal articles and textbooks on medical microbiology, immunology, and epidemiology, provides one with a distinct sense of the benefits of vaccination, with generally little, if any, mention of even well-documented harmful sequelae from vaccines. One must dig deeper for these. Side effects are either considered minor inconveniences or dismissed as "not definitively causal," "necessary risks," or possibly just "coincidental." Studies that clearly elucidate vaccine causality in adverse reactions are frequently referred to as having faulty research methodologies.

Conversely, individuals and groups proclaiming the risks and dangers of vaccinations often appear to do so in an epidemiological vacuum, seemingly ignoring clear evidence of the directly positive impact vaccinations have had on disease reduction and eradication. When referring to epidemiological evidence, both sides seem to highlight selectively or diminish certain aspects of the arguments to reinforce their beliefs. This makes it difficult for even the most discerning reader to come to a clear and definitive conclusion regarding vaccinations. Furthermore, research occurs in such a wide variety of environments and vaccinations are used in such a diversity of populations that what might be true in one environment cannot necessarily be extrapolated to another. Whether to vaccinate for tetanus neonatorum in India may require an entirely different argument than whether to require tetanus vaccines for all children in the United States. Likewise with hepatitis B, pertussis, and Hib (hemophilus influenza type B) vaccines, among others. Indeed, all sides of the argument must be considered individually in order to make appropriate choices.

Another risk one runs in choosing to write about a controversial topic without choosing sides is that neither side feels exonerated by the work, and therefore both sides reject it. But this book is not about choosing sides, nor is it about making one argument wrong and another right. This book actually seeks to be a bridge uniting sides in a common desire to achieve optimal health for all children. In taking a holistic approach to health and disease, this book acknowledges a multiplicity of approaches that are not mutually exclusive.

The Right to an Informed Choice

This book is about helping parents make intelligent health care choices for their children, operating on the premise that the good of the individual and the good of society are not mutually exclusive independent variables but are codependent factors. Mahatma Gandhi said, "Any action that is dictated by fear or coercion of any kind ceases to be moral." Any such actions also cease to promote health. Disease takes many forms, including oppression, and as a culture we must decide which forms we are willing to embrace.

Promoting Optimal Health

As an extension of the vaccine discussion, I explore the nature of health and disease as more than merely a one-dimensional, reductionist phenomenon, though it does address the biologic and physiologic bases of immunity. I offer the reader options for promoting optimal child health through nutrition, hygiene, common sense, stress management, and herbal medicine, whether or not one chooses to vaccinate. This is significant, not just because healthy children are more resistant to infection but because there is some evidence indicating not only that nutritionally well-nourished children may avoid vaccine reactions but also that antibody response to vaccines may be improved in such children, resulting in enhanced vaccine efficacy. Optimal health is the key to a win-win situation, and that is what this book does. We all want what is best for our own children and for all children. It is my hope that this book supports parents and professionals in finding a healthy path through the maze of the vaccine controversy.

ONE

A Curious History

The documented attempts to prevent or reduce disease by means of using infected materials from diseased persons or animals stretch further back in history than one might imagine, to as early as the fifth century B.C.E.[1] Indeed, it is not surprising that conquering illness has been a major human preoccupation for centuries, when considering that epidemics and plagues have decimated entire families in a matter of days and entire communities in a matter of years. In Europe alone, more than 60 million people died of smallpox between the late seventeenth and the late eighteenth centuries—a span of only one hundred years. At the peak of the epidemic during the eighteenth century, Europe lost approximately 15 million people every twenty-five years.[2] Millions of others were left permanently disfigured.[3] In fact, smallpox was an enormous impetus for the original efforts to develop what we now call vaccines.

Early Vaccination Attempts

In the fifth century B.C.E. the notion of immunity first appears in historical medical records. At that time, the Greek historian Thucydides (ca. 460–400 B.C.E.) took note that during a plague in Greece that eliminated nearly one-fourth of the population, some people who were exposed escaped infection, while others became ill and recovered, never again to be infected by that disease.[4] Current vaccine practices are built upon the knowledge that an individual who survives exposure to a disease is subsequently protected from that disease.

Attempts at imparting immunity to disease, particularly smallpox, generally incorporated exudate or scabs from smallpox sores into the treatment protocol. The Chinese allegedly attempted to treat smallpox with inoculation as

8

early as the sixth century B.C.E. However, the first written record of such attempts appeared much later and was entitled *The Correct Treatment of Smallpox*. It is attributed to a Buddhist nun practicing during the reign of Jen Tsung
(1022–1063 C.E.). She purportedly recommended choosing scabs that were
one month old from cases that had only a few pustules, except in hot weather,
when they were to be fifteen to twenty days old. The scabs were dried and
pulverized with specific plants. A silver curled tube was then used to blow the
powder into the nostrils of those not yet ill.[5] Her choice of pustules from a
mild case that had been allowed to develop for some time, past the most virulent stage, indicates that she may have given some thought to the need to
induce a mild reaction rather than a full-blown infection, which might have
occurred from using exudate from badly infected victims. Modern preparations also render infectious material less harmful by weakening them via heat
or through introduction into live animals, known as attenuation.

The Golden Mirror of Medicine, another ancient Chinese medical text, describes four forms of inoculation against smallpox:

1. The nose is plugged with powdered scabs laid on wool.

2. Powdered scabs are blown into the nose.

3. Undergarments of an infected child are put on a healthy child for several
   days.

4. A piece of cotton is spread with the contents of an infected pustule and
   stuffed into the nose.[6]

Attempts to treat smallpox in such a fashion were referred to as "variolation,"
variolus referring to smallpox. Ironically, parents who want their children exposed to childhood illnesses such as chicken pox may to this day recreate method
3 within their families and among playmates. There have even been attempts
to send "infected" clothing through the mail among friends to ensure exposure to childhood illnesses in the early elementary-school years.

The first attempt at oral variolation, referred to as "preventive variolation,"
appears to have been in the early eleventh century, mentioned in a treatise by
Wang Tan, a Chinese prime minister of the Sung emperors.[7] This practice was
also widely exercised by physicians in the Middle East and in India, where
it was practiced at regular intervals by Brahman Hindus in the sixteenth
century.[8] According to Leon Chaitow, isopathic medicine, the attempt to cure
disease by use of its own products, was taught in the Middle Ages by the
physician-teacher Paracelsus, and this method was employed by Druid priests

from ancient Britain and Germany in the Middle Ages.[9] Apparently similar techniques were being utilized in Constantinople in 1672, where an old Circassian woman would cut a cross in the flesh of the "patient" and apply fresh smallpox exudate to the fresh wound.[10] Lady Mary Wortley Montagu of England attempted to introduce this practice into England upon her return from Constantinople in 1721.[11]

JENNER AND SMALLPOX

Smallpox was a disease thought to have been endemic to Africa, Asia, and the Middle East, imported into Europe by the Crusaders and brought to the Americas by slave ships and Spanish conquistadors. It flourished in the overcrowded, unhygienic cities and towns of the early industrial revolution, where there were inadequate food, drinking water, and waste disposal mechanisms.[12] It was from this context that Edward Jenner's work arose.

By the 1700s the concept of immunity from naturally occurring disease was a recognized phenomenon. Families conceived the value of letting a disease run its course through the family so they would not be vulnerable to the next epidemic.[13] The idea of artificially inducing a mild form of the disease was not a far stretch for the imagination and is probably predicated on this observation. The process of variolation became standard among the upper classes in their attempts to ward off disease. It was customary for people to visit the local apothecary's barn, known as an inoculation stable, where the apothecary would "scratch the patient's arms with a knife and cover the wounds with bandages smeared with the dried scabs of smallpox victims."[14] This process may have been preceded by bleedings, starvation, and purging, other common practices of the day.[15] Those who received variolation treatment were usually kept secluded in the barn for two to three weeks, until their fevers subsided and the smallpox scabs dried and fell away. At this point they were no longer considered contagious.

While there were numerous successes from variolation, many who received variolation developed serious cases of smallpox as a direct result and died. Problems in many of those who survived included blindness, scarring, and additional outbreaks of the disease because immunity to it was not guaranteed by this treatment. Furthermore, diseases such as syphilis and tuberculosis were often present in the scabs and exudate drawn from those having these diseases in addition to smallpox, leading to a significant opportunity for such diseases to infect the recipients of variolation. According to Diodati, more than 75 percent of people survived natural smallpox infection, while neither proposed cures nor variolation proved safe means of addressing smallpox.[16]

Jenner (1749–1823), an English physician, often considered the "father of vaccinations," clearly did not invent the process of variolation; he may, however, have been the first to attempt to systematically organize the practice of inoculation.[17] He owes his original insights to a young farmer and cattle breeder named Benjamin Jesty, who became immune to smallpox after contracting cowpox from his cattle. Jesty intentionally inoculated his wife and two young children with cowpox to protect them from susceptibility to a smallpox epidemic. Jesty's family remained immune for fifteen years. In 1776 Jenner pronounced that dairymaids who contracted cowpox, a relatively minor disease, could not contract smallpox. He attempted to prove this by taking infected material from the hand of dairymaid Sara Nelms and injecting it into the arm of a healthy eight-year-old boy named James Phipps. Forty-eight days later Jenner injected smallpox into Phipps and it had no effect. He concluded that the boy had been successfully vaccinated, the term *vaccine* being derived from the Latin word *vacca*, meaning "cow." Jenner went on to promote his vaccine publicly. It wasn't until years after his own successful experiments had been published that Jenner acknowledged Jesty's contribution to his own knowledge and understanding.[18] As was typical of the male-dominated profession of science of the day, Lady Montagu's earlier attempted contribution was not duly recognized.

It wasn't long, however, before Jenner's colleagues disputed his claim, and Jenner himself had to admit that there were ample cases of dairy hands who caught smallpox in spite of previous infection with cowpox disease. In response, in 1798 Jenner created a new vaccine using "horse-grease," insisting that men who handled horse-grease, a puslike, greasy, rancid secretion from infected horse hooves, prior to milking cows were unable to contract smallpox. He now postulated that children could be protected from smallpox if they were injected with cowpox from cows who had been infected with horse-grease. Jenner called this "horse-grease cowpox" and began to publish on the subject. He even began to inoculate people using secretions directly from the horses. The public was revolted by his suggestions, and every attempt to verify his recommendations led to failure.[19]

However, in 1806, when Dr. Robert Willan, an esteemed physician of the time, published a treatise on vaccinations and mentioned only the cowpox vaccine, it was "exalted as the true prophylactic" and the public readily accepted it.[20] Shortly after, Parliament granted Jenner large sums of money to promote his vaccines. It quickly became common practice throughout Europe to give it to all infants. However, there were numerous reported cases of smallpox among the vaccinated. At first the cases were denied, and then it was said that when cases occurred among the vaccinated they were milder. When it became apparent that people were dying even after having been vaccinated, these cases were said to be a result of what was called "spurious cowpox." Explanation after explanation was given for vaccine failures. One proposed solution was to give multiple vaccinations in one treatment, each on a different place on the body. Revaccination was also suggested.

Fortunately, most epidemics of smallpox were self-limiting and regionally contained. According to Neil Miller,[21] prior to the compulsory vaccine laws of 1853, the highest death rate from this disease for any two-year period in England was only two thousand cases. It was realized, though, that those who were vaccinated easily transmitted the disease to others; vaccination prevented the disease from spreading only if everyone was vaccinated against it. Thus, in the early 1800s compulsory mass vaccination laws were born, with Bavaria being the first country to initiate such regulations in 1807.[22] However, the most devastating epidemics occurred after the institution of compulsory vaccination laws. Between 1870 and 1872 in Germany, more than a million people had the disease, of which 120,000 died. Ninety-six percent of these had been vaccinated.[23] This was after fifteen years of compulsory vaccinations. Eventually, after disastrous outbreaks of smallpox in Europe, Jenner's methods were prohibited, though smallpox vaccination continued until 1979, when the World Health Organization (WHO) declared smallpox to be eradicated worldwide.[24] Currently, general compulsory vaccination requirements vary from country to country, from certain countries in South America requiring compulsory vaccination en masse several times annually for all children within a certain age range, to routine compulsory vaccines given by a private physician or clinic, to countries in western Europe that do not have compulsory vaccination laws, making vaccinations voluntary.

The Dawn of a New Vaccine Era: Pasteur to Present

During the eighty-seven years between Jenner and Pasteur, new ideas were germinating and being explored, particularly those of attenuation, defined as "a particular change in the culture mode" that can "diminish the virulence of the infectious microbe," and passage of infectious materials through animals to reduce their virulence in people.[25] Louis Pasteur, a research chemist, developing ideas based on Jenner's methods peppered with advances in scientific understanding, set out to address the issue of animal disease. He developed vaccines to prevent chicken cholera as well as sheep and bovine anthrax. He recognized the need to replace person-to-person vaccination with something safer and less likely to transmit other diseases.

By now the ideas of attenuation and virulence were well developed, and Pasteur was able to reduce the infectivity of bacteria so that they could be administered with less risk of actually causing the disease while still conferring immunity. The significance of this is that he did so using material derived from isolated specific bacteria. Microscopes were not yet powerful enough to detect viruses. Thus was born the germ theory—his understanding that different organisms cause different diseases. This idea has become a bedrock of modern bacteriology, immunology, and medicine. While Pasteur was unable to isolate the rabies virus, he recognized that this infection was transmitted through saliva. He attenuated the organism by injecting infected dog saliva into the spinal cord of a rabbit. He subsequently harvested the spinal cord, dried it, and used this as the basis for his rabies vaccine. The opportunity to give his injection to a human being came in the summer of 1885, when he was presented with a young boy named Joseph Meister, who had been bitten by a rabid dog. Given that there was no known cure for rabies at the time, the experiment seemed only reasonable. After receiving a series of injections, each more virulent than the last, over a ten-day period, Meister was still alive, becoming the first person known to have survived the bite of a rabid animal.[26]

NOT ALL POPULARITY

Pasteur's work was not received with pure acclaim. In fact, many of his contemporaries claimed that his rabies vaccine killed more people than it cured.[27] "Pasteur's critics noted that it was often the case that the same suspect animal had bitten more than one individual and those that did not receive Pasteur's vaccine fared just as well, if not better, than those receiving the rabies vaccine. In some cases the untreated animal survived whereas the treated patient died."[28] Indeed, the vaccine was extremely reactive and caused numerous deaths. At the time, there was tremendous public outcry against vaccination practices for humans. Plotkin and Mortimer describe these as "vitriolic protests against any type of vaccination."

Pasteur, however, was as savvy as he was smart, and he used his skills to establish himself as an international vaccine authority, setting up the Pasteur Institute to further his mission. However, accusations against Pasteur go further. It has been suggested that many of his cures may have been contrived.[29]

In 1905 Paul Remlinger, a military physician who had trained at the Pasteur Institute and for five years supervised antirabies practices in Constantinople, divulged that the institute had quietly concealed a high incidence of paralysis and other neurological disorders from the rabies vaccine in order to avoid adverse publicity.[30]

There is further question about Pasteur's integrity and the originality of his work. For example, in 1887 Pasteur's laboratory published a paper on the successful development of a killed cholera vaccine, claiming credit for the discovery, in spite of the fact that a paper to this effect had been published sixteen months earlier by scientists Edmund Salmon and Theobald Smith of the United States.[31] Salmon and Smith were working for the U.S. Department of Agriculture at the time of their discovery of killed cholera vaccine, and their acclaim was nowhere near as great as Pasteur's. Nonetheless, the U.S. government and the Pasteur Institute were engaged in a dispute over discovery rights for several years. Interestingly, the Pasteur vaccine was in use until 1953, and there is scant mention of his questionable principles in history or medical books.

Pasteur's contemporaries and colleagues were also starting to make significant discoveries about immunity and pathogens. In 1882 Élie Metchinkoff discovered phagocytes, the white blood cells that destroy invading organisms; Paul Ehrlich demonstrated passive acquired immunity, the ability of female mammals to confer immunity to their young via breast milk, and he also made important discoveries about antibodies. In Paris, Pierre Roux and Alexandre Yersin demonstrated that it was diphtheria toxin that led to the clinical symptoms of diphtheria. And in Germany, Emil von Behring discovered the basis for the diphtheria vaccine: antitoxin. Unfortunately, these preparations were often lethal to humans. It was Ehrlich who discovered the dosing strategy for diphtheria toxin, which is still followed today.[32]

DO MICROORGANISMS CAUSE DISEASE?

The simple notion that bacteria (and, we now recognize, viruses) cause disease fits very smoothly into the increasingly mechanistic worldview of the late nineteenth century. The theory went something like this: There are microorganisms in our environment, they get into us and make us sick, we kill them with powerful substances, and we recover. Or we prevent them from making us sick with different powerful substances (vaccines) and we do not become ill. Beginning. End. But not all scientists of the late nineteenth century were satisfied with this simple mechanistic perspective.

Pierre Jacque Antoine Bechamp, a contemporary of Pasteur and a scientist whose work has all but fallen into obscurity, was assiduously working toward a greater understanding of microorganisms and disease. Actually, it is reasonably suggested that much of Pasteur's work was built on Bechamp's discoveries of the influence of microorganisms on fermentation, and that Pasteur may have plagiarized Bechamp's work to some degree.[33]

Bechamp did not believe that microorganisms cause disease but that they arose and multiplied in diseased states, being the mature forms of organisms called microzymas, which naturally inhabit our cells. This belief that bacteria could not exist without a supportive environment or medium was shared by Eclectic physicians (medical doctors who incorporated botanical, homeopathic, and nutritional therapies into their practices) of the late 1800s and 1900s, who viewed "morbid matter" as disease-producing material that provided a medium for bacterial growth. In fact, the bacteria were seen as organisms capable of breaking down the morbid matter and "cleaning it up."[34] Lindlahr, who was such a physician and the author of the book *Nature Cure*, viewed chronic and acute illness as manifestations of decreased vitality that allowed waste matter and toxins to accumulate in the body and form breeding grounds for disease. Alcoholic beverages and narcotic stimulants, drugs, vaccines, antitoxins, accidental poisoning, and suppression of acute diseases (nature's cleansing and healing efforts) were considered contributing factors to diminished vitality.[35]

The contrast of the two views can be compared to contemporary allopathic views versus holistic views of health and disease. In the former, disease is caused by organisms outside the body that randomly invade the body. In the latter, it is believed that a healthy body can resist the generation of disease, whereas weak or sick tissue provides ample breeding ground for infections. In the former view, the human being is unable to exert any influence over infection, being entirely vulnerable to the environment. In the latter, the individual is able to affect health through nutrition and other practices that promote health and allow for individual empowerment.

This contrast, which may seem just a quaint bit of history, actually provides fertile ground for arguments on both philosophical and physiological grounds both for and against vaccination. As vaccine critic Leon Chaitow puts it, "This divergence of views is fundamental to the understanding of alternatives to standard immunization procedures," with the alternative argument reinforced by the reality that not all of those exposed to infectious agents become sick with the disease associated with those particular organisms.[36]

By the end of the nineteenth century, modern medicine was well on its way to an almost single-minded battle against infectious organisms. There existed two human virus vaccines, the Jenner variola vaccine and Pasteur's vaccine for rabies, both live vaccines. There were also three human bacterial vaccines: cholera, plague, and typhoid, all of which used killed bacteria. The foundational theories of immunology and vaccinology were laid, and while they have been elaborated and refined, they continue to form the basis of these sciences today.

THE MODERN VACCINES

New vaccines are constantly being researched and developed in the effort to eliminate or eradicate diseases such as HIV and cancer, as well as other "problems" of human existence—even pregnancy in the form of contraceptives delivered with vaccine-based vectors. The time between the early 1900s and early 1970s was one of rapid vaccine development and refinement, yielding most of the common childhood vaccines currently used. Investigations are also under way to find methods of administering vaccines in developing nations to reduce problems that arise from lack of cold storage and adequate access to sterile needles for injectable inoculations. Foods, for example, are currently being genetically engineered to contain measles, in order to have a simple and recognizable method of widely providing a vaccination against this disease, which is still a major cause of mortality and morbidity in developing nations.

The first pertussis vaccine was developed in 1912 by Jules Bordet and Octave Gengou, who sought to halt the spread of whooping cough in Tunisia. The bacteria were grown in large pots and killed with heat, and formaldehyde was added as a preservative. This mixture was injected into children, though it was known to contain impurities, because it was unknown how to separate the antigens (the protective mechanism) from the impurities. It was considered a crude vaccine. Ironically, a very similar vaccine, the whole-cell pertussis vaccine, was still in use in the United States until just a few years ago. Attempts to purify and improve the pertussis vaccine were ongoing, creating such confusion on the European and American markets that in 1931 the American Medical Association (AMA) deleted the pertussis vaccine from its approved drugs list.[37] It was discovered in the 1940s that adding an "adjuvant" to the vaccine, a substance that enhances the vaccine's stimulation of antibody production, could improve the vaccine's effectiveness while allowing fewer bacteria to be used. In 1943 Pearl Kendrick, a U.S. researcher who had, in 1932, devoted her life's work to pertussis vaccine research, documented that alum, or aluminum-based substances, could serve this purpose. These were then added to the pertussis vaccine. Many vaccines still include aluminum-based substances to this day (for better or worse, as we shall see in chapter 3). It was this same researcher who, thinking of the discomfort of children in receiving multiple injections, was responsible for having pertussis combined with diphtheria and tetanus, to yield the DPT vaccine. As we shall see later, of all the vaccines, pertussis has been implicated in the greatest number of vaccine reactions, which has been a problem since the beginning of its use. Several years ago U.S. physicians began offering parents the option of using the acellular pertussis vaccine, made with the least reactive parts of the pertussis bacterium. This has long been used in Japan, which touts a significantly lower vaccine reaction rate than the United States. However, the Japanese also do not immunize for pertussis until after the second year of life, and this may be partially responsible for the decreased incidence of problems. In some studies acellular pertussis does appear to be less reactive; in others, however, similar reactions as with the whole-cell vaccine have been noted. See chapter 5 for a complete discussion of possible vaccination reactions and side effects.

The contagious nature of measles was first demonstrated in 1911, when researchers Goldberger and Anderson passed human measles infection on to monkeys. It wasn't until 1954, when new technology was made available, that Enders and Peebles successfully isolated the virus in monkey and human kidney tissue. Adapting the virus to chicken embryos, and the subsequent cultivation of the virus in chicken embryo tissue, led to the development and licensure of the measles vaccine in 1963.[38]

Mumps has rarely been considered a serious or dangerous disease; nonetheless, the vaccine was developed to prevent the rare complications that can occur in adolescent males who contract mumps, and the rarer problems associated with mumps in childhood. Researchers Johnson and Goodpasture identified the mumps virus in 1934 as being the causative agent involved in this illness, when saliva from infected human patients injected into monkeys produced parotitis, a swelling of the parotid glands and a symptom characteristic of mumps. Subsequent propagation of the mumps virus in embryonated chicken eggs led to the development of the vaccine.[39]

Rubella, nearly always a nonserious disease in children (sometimes entirely asymptomatic, in fact) can be detrimental to the unborn baby of a pregnant woman, particularly when contracted during the first trimester, but also in later trimesters. It can lead to what is known as congenital rubella syndrome (CRS), which includes blindness, deafness, heart disease, mental retardation, and other serious birth defects as well as fetal death. The association between rubella and congenital problems was first noticed by Norman McAlister Gregg, an Australian ophthalmologist who related it to congenital cataracts. He began to notice an inordinate number of babies brought to him with this problem and found that their mothers had been exposed to rubella during an outbreak in 1940. Epidemiologists and teratologists from Australia, Sweden, the United States, and Great Britain confirmed his findings. For the next two decades efforts were ongoing to isolate the infectious agent and gather statistical information on CRS. In 1962 the rubella virus was isolated by a group of scientists in Boston and another in Washington, D.C. This time experimentation was being done with African green monkeys. A pandemic of rubella beginning in Europe in 1962–63 and reaching the United States by 1964 led to thousands of pregnancy terminations for fear of CRS, as well as a trail of CRS babies. This caused a tremendous push in the medical and scientific communities for the development of a vaccine. By 1965–67 several strains of attenuated rubella were being prepared for clinical trials, and in 1969–70 the rubella vaccine was available on the commercial market, later to have a tremendous impact on the reduction of the epidemiology of both CRS and rubella.[40]

Poliomyelitis is a disease that has been in the human population for centuries but, until the first half of this century, never posed a problem. It wasn't even described as a clinical entity until the late eighteenth and early nineteenth centuries.[41] After this time, increasingly serious epidemics arose, leading to increased interest in the development of a vaccine against polio. "By 1953, the incidence of paralytic poliomyelitis in the United States was more than 20 per 100,000 population. Although not a particularly high rate compared with other diseases, such as measles, it generated tremendous public concern because of its mysterious seasonal incidence (an attribute that is still not adequately explained by conventional medicine), its disfiguring nature, and its propensity for paralyzing the respiratory muscles."[42]

Early work in 1912 led to the discovery that polio viruses can be present in the digestive tract and could spread from asymptomatic persons, but this discovery was virtually ignored. The route of poliovirus transmission was not definitively determined until nearly thirty years later. The first human trials with poliovirus were done using material derived from infected monkey tissue. This was used in children in 1936 in independently conducted field trials, in spite of the fact that "appropriate tests for safety and efficacy were lacking, and there seems to have been little concern for known risk attendant with the injection of central nervous system tissue. . . . Thousands of subjects received these vaccines, some of whom developed paralysis soon after inoculation, often in the inoculated limb."[43] About a decade later it was demonstrated that it

18

was possible to use a formaldehyde suspension of central nervous system (CNS) tissue from monkeys to induce antibody formation. These were considered to be noninfectious preparations. Later the virus was propagated in monkey tissue and treated with formalin to make it more immunogenic. Massive field trials were conducted in 1954, and shortly after, in April 1955, the Salk vaccine, a noninfectious poliovirus vaccine invented by Jonas Salk, was introduced in the United States. Soon after, the Sabin virus, a live virus developed by Albert Sabin, was introduced, and based on several beliefs it became the vaccine of choice for polio. These beliefs include the confidence that live poliovirus (LPV), also commonly referred to as oral poliovirus (OPV), could be given without risk of paralysis; only OPV could be expected to have a significant impact on preventing naturally occurring poliovirus in the community; and the OPV was expected to confer more permanent and complete immunity than the killed poliovirus (KPV, now referred to as IPV, or inactivated poliovirus).[44]

By 1964 OPV was used almost exclusively, and in that year the American Academy of Pediatrics (AAP) clearly emphasized a preference for this vaccine. The U.S.S.R. had made a similar decision, while Sweden, Finland, and Holland chose to use the IPV. Until recently the practice of administering four doses of OPV to children had persisted, but recently, in light of the fact that all cases of poliomyelitis are a result of the vaccination, the Centers for Disease Control (CDC) recommended giving two doses of IPV, followed by two of OPV; the CDC has now revised that recommendation to the exclusive use of IPV.

The 1980s and 1990s have seen the development of several new vaccines for children—including hepatitis B vaccine, Hib (hemophilus influenza type B) vaccine, varicella (chicken pox) vaccine, and rotavirus vaccine—as well as consequences associated with each.

COMPULSORY VACCINATIONS

Mandatory mass vaccine programs apparently emanated from the smallpox epidemics of the nineteenth century. During the 1800s it was realized that vaccinations weren't always effective at preventing infection; in order to be so, the entire population had to be vaccinated. One would think that either vaccines work or they don't, but physicians of the time realized that the only way even to remotely guarantee the ability of vaccines to do what was promised was to ensure that the infectious organisms could not find any susceptible host in the human population. This is the premise from which we derive the concept of "herd immunity." Herd immunity is the threshold level that vaccine coverage must reach for a population to be protected from a certain disease. Different diseases have specific levels at which herd immunity occurs. For example, herd immunity to pertussis occurs when 92 to 95 percent of the population is vaccinated; polio requires 80 to 85 percent vaccine coverage, and measles 88 to 95 percent coverage.[45] Compulsory immunization laws required full compliance with vaccination requirements or the facing of legal consequences.[46]

MASS VACCINATION, COMPULSORY VACCINATION, AND ROUTINE VACCINATION

It should be noted that mass vaccination, compulsory vaccination, and routine vaccination are three distinct entities, though they can be combined. In mass vaccinations at-risk populations are targeted (for example, children, pregnant women, homosexuals), and vaccines are given en masse at various predetermined sites within a specific time frame. They are generally administered by public health nurses and physicians, or those specially trained to carry out the inoculation procedures. An example of a mass vaccination campaign is the practice of some South and Central American countries to vaccinate all children under two years old biannually for childhood diseases, regardless of their previous vaccination history or immunity status. These are generally done as broadscale campaigns mandated by the government and public health officials to prevent or limit an epidemic in a susceptible population. Vaccine recipients are generally not screened for allergies, previous reactions, current illness, or other contraindicating factors.[47]

Routine immunization is the practice with which most parents are familiar—taking the child to the doctor or clinic for regular visits at which the child is vaccinated. Arguably, routine vaccinations are a part of long-term mass vaccination campaigns, in which populations are targeted and attempts are made to vaccinate as many as possible in that sector.[48]

Compulsory, or mandatory, vaccinations are those that are required by a jurisdiction as a legal matter and for which there are consequences for noncompliance. Currently in the United States, legislation varies from state to state, with individual states having certain vaccine requirements for rights such as school attendance to be granted. Each state has its own set of exemptions as well, whether these be medical, religious, philosophical, or a combination. Chapter 6, "Personal Choices and Public Policies," provides a comprehensive look at specific vaccination policies and state exemptions.

TWO

Declining Disease Rates and Vaccine Efficacy

Vaccines have played an important role in keeping certain diseases under control, but it is evident from epidemiological and historical records that other factors such as hygiene, nutrition, and living conditions are also responsible for reducing disease incidence. It is unclear, however, whether vaccines or improvements in nutrition, hygiene, sanitation, water quality, and living conditions had a greater impact on disease reduction in the first half of the twentieth century. This chapter is not intended to discredit the value of vaccines but to illustrate that vaccinations may be secondary factors in protecting us from disease. It is by becoming aware of both the importance of vaccines and their limitations that we can make the most informed and effective decisions for our children's health and the health of our society as a whole.

The Decline of Infectious Diseases

While many medical references do briefly mention the role that social changes and nonmedical public health interventions played in disease reduction, few deviate even slightly from the belief that disease declines can be attributed primarily to vaccinations. Indeed, it appears to be fully accepted by vaccine proponents that without vaccines we would again have rampant epidemics of pertussis, diphtheria, measles, and so on. Such opinions are not hard to find in the plethora of information on the benefits of vaccines that is easily accessible through the pediatrician's office, the county health clinic, and medical Web sites.

According to the *World Health Statistics Annual*, 1973–1976, volume 2, "There has been a steady decline of infectious diseases (for example, smallpox, diphtheria, whooping cough and scarlet fever) in most developing countries regardless of the percentage of immunizations administered in these countries. Improved conditions are largely responsible as well as improved nutrition, as the primary determinants in the decline in death rates."[1] Medical historian and social critic Ivan Illich illustrates this point:

> The infections which prevailed at the outset of the industrial age can illustrate how medicine came by its reputation. Tuberculosis, for instance, reached its peak over two generations. In New York the death rate was certainly very high indeed in 1812, and declined to 37 per thousand by 1892, when Koch cultured and stained the first bacillus.[2]
>
> The rate was down to 180 per 10,000 when the first sanatorium was opened in 1910, even though "consumption" still held second place in mortality tables. After World War II, before antibiotics came into (general) use, it had slipped to eleventh place with a rate of 48. Cholera, dysentery and typhoid similarly peaked and dwindled outside medical control. By the time the etiology was understood, or their therapy had become specific, they had lost much of their relevance. The combined death rate for scarlet fever, diphtheria, whooping cough and measles from 1860 to 1965, for children up to 15, shows that nearly 90 percent of the total decline in death rate over this period had occurred before the introduction of antibiotics and wide-spread immunization against diphtheria.[3]

It is further argued that smallpox epidemics were much more likely to occur in communities where wide-scale vaccination campaigns were practiced. By 1810 Jenner himself knew that his vaccine did not confer lifelong immunity.[4] Nonetheless, Jenner's work, which preceded Pasteur's first human vaccine against rabies by only about ninety years, was the beginning of the modern fury of vaccine research, mass vaccination campaigns, and compulsory vaccinations.

Dr. Richard Moskowitz, a Harvard University graduate with a medical degree from New York University and a long-time family-practice physician, remarks, "There is widespread agreement that the time period since the common vaccines were introduced has seen a remarkable decline in the incidence and severity of corresponding natural infections. But the customary assumption that the decline is *attributable* to the vaccines remains unproved, and continues to be questioned by eminent authorities in the field."[5] He goes on to say that the incidence and severity of pertussis, for example, had already begun to decline precipitously long before the introduction of the pertussis vaccine. Moskowitz emphasizes this point, quoting epidemiologist C. C. Dauer, who in 1943 stated: "If mortality from pertussis continues to decline at the same rate during the next 15 years, it will be extremely difficult to show statistically that [pertussis immunization] had any effect in reducing mortality from whooping cough."[6]

Determining Efficacy

Delineating the primary causative factor in the history of the decline of infectious diseases by using statistical evidence is not a simple or straightforward matter for the following reasons:

1. Hidden underlying factors may obscure information. For example, there may have been significant underreporting of infectious diseases, particularly when cases were mild, self-limiting, and required only minimal treatment (statisticians refer to such factors as "confounding variables").

2. Data and statistics can be manipulated to support opposing sides. This is common to both vaccine advocates and vaccine opponents.

3. In at least a few cases it seems that after the introduction of certain vaccines, diseases were redefined or reclassified with new criteria, making statistics seriously flawed (referred to as "massaging the statistics").

4. Physicians, often with the honest but spurious belief that once a person has been vaccinated for a certain disease he or she is not able to contract that disease, misdiagnosed conditions such as polio in previously vaccinated patients, diagnosing it as aseptic meningitis, also skewing statistics.

5. Certain diseases, such as pertussis, can be very difficult to diagnose, making underreporting likely.

6. There is often not a clear statistical differentiation of the vaccine status, health status, socioeconomic status, or other factors that might influence disease prevalence or likelihood.[7]

Dr. Alan Hinman, former director of the Division of Immunization, Center for Preventative Medicine of the CDC, makes the telling comment that "the very nature of epidemiological data has contributed to the controversy, since there is virtually no epidemiological study with absolutely incontrovertible results that allow only one interpretation." Antimicrobial drugs cannot even be given certain credit for declines in these diseases once they were available, as Swedish studies document that declining death rates from infectious disease after the introduction of antibiotics parallel the rates of decline prior to the introduction. "It may well be that other unknown factors, such as nutrition, changes in socio-economic and educational status, and the like have contributed to the decline in mortality observed in the United States since the turn of the century." This is not to dismiss the value or contribution of vaccines and antibiotics but to say that "in the true perspective of the natural history of the diseases mentioned [diphtheria, measles, scarlet fever, and pertussis], they have played but a small part."[8]

Edward Mortimer, a staunch vaccine advocate, states in his article "Immunization Against Infectious Disease": "Clearly there are multiple reasons for the decline in mortality due to infectious disease in the United States in this century, and in many instances it is impossible to determine the relative contribution of different factors. There is little question that the natural history of some infectious diseases has changed spontaneously over the years for reasons not entirely clear."[9] We find corroboration of this fact by Moskowitz when he discusses the work of the celebrated microbiologist Rene Dubos. Dubos observed that "microbial diseases have their own natural history, independent of drugs and vaccines, in which asymptomatic infection and symbiosis are far more common than overt disease."[10] Part of the variation in the natural history of disease is the virulence of microorganisms, which can change over time. We have seen this clearly with the increased prescription of antibiotics over the past fifty years and the consequential increases in antibiotic resistance, leading to more-virulent strains of bacteria. Microorganisms can also lose virulence, and humans can develop resistance to disease. In the late nineteenth century, scarlet fever was such a serious matter that isolation hospitals evolved to contain outbreaks. It is now recognized that the "evolution of the microorganisms to a milder form has resulted in the condition now being of minor importance only."[11]

Would these declines in mortality have continued to the point that disease incidences would eventually have become as low as they are now without vaccines ultimately being introduced? Or did the vaccines enhance and then maintain the decline? Unfortunately, these are questions that are difficult to answer in a highly vaccinated population, and it is difficult to match cohorts exactly with other nations. However, indications from other developed Western nations that lack compulsory vaccination programs suggest that diseases would indeed have continued to decline, with potential for minor periodic outbreaks to occur. Outbreaks of some diseases do continue to occur, even in vaccinated populations.

Furthermore, underlying the supposition that vaccines were primarily responsible for reducing infectious diseases in this country is the unquestioned assumption that vaccines are always effective. This chapter looks at the individual factors that skew accurate assessment of vaccine efficacy and looks at the efficacy rates of many common vaccines. It should not be dismissed that vaccines have an appropriate place in modern public health and disease control. They are particularly important as a preventive measure in developing nations that lack the public health advantages to which disease decline in developed nations is attributed. Indeed, developing nations continue to suffer terribly from disease, owing to lack of many of the advantages we have, in spite of mass immunization programs.[12] Perhaps we need to focus more attention on the ingredients that promote health rather than just trying to control disease.

Determining Vaccine Efficacy

Vaccine efficacy is typically determined in one of two ways. The first is the ability of the vaccine to induce antibodies known to be protective, and the second is the ability of the vaccine to provide protection in the face of exposure.[13] It is known that the vaccines in use today do stimulate protective antibodies in most of the population that receives them. There are several problems with using this method for analysis of vaccine efficacy, however. For one, children are not routinely screened for the presence of antibodies. We have very little idea of how many children develop antibodies from routine vaccination, and broadscale evaluation of this is impractical and cost prohibitive. Therefore, we do not really know what portion of the vaccinated population is actually immune—we only know how many are vaccinated. We do know, however, that vaccinations do not always seroconvert—that is, not everyone who receives them develops the protective antibodies.

A curious former client of mine took her recently vaccinated child to the pediatrician and had his antibody levels checked for a particular disease against which he'd been fully vaccinated. His antibody level did not show immunity to the disease. However, this does not mean he is not immune. A second problem with using antibody levels as determinants of immunity is the well-established fact that a child with a high antibody titre can still contract the disease, and a child who shows no evidence of immunity based on serologic testing can be immune.[14]

The most effective technique for evaluating vaccine efficacy appears to be tracking disease incidence in vaccinated and nonvaccinated populations over a

25

long period of time, and in comparing disease incidence as well as mortality during the prevaccine era with the vaccine era. Again, this does not take into account confounding variables such as whether children were breast-fed, whether they had decreased immunity and therefore greater susceptibility to infection, whether they had mild or serious cases of infection, or their nutritional and socioeconomic status, factors well known to contribute to disease incidence. It also does not account for underreporting, misdiagnosis, and other similar considerations that can substantially distort statistics. Nor does it take into account the difficulty of interpreting confusing statistics. Here is an example from a 1978 article in *Science* by Edward Mortimer, entitled "Immunization Against Infectious Disease: Active Immunization Programs Are Endangered by Complacency and Litigation," in which the author takes the position that lack of prevalence of infectious diseases owing to vaccine programs has led to decreased diligence by professionals and the public in maintaining high vaccine rates.

> The lack of visibility of vaccine-preventable diseases in the United States has also resulted in a certain amount of complacency in both health professionals and the public. In 1975 only 116 deaths were reported from diseases against which children are routinely immunized. This has resulted in less than the optimum number of children being immunized. For example, in 1975 only 64.8 percent of 1- to 4-year-old children had received three or more doses of poliomyelitis vaccine, compared to 73.9 percent in 1965. The low was 1973 with 60.4 percent. Only 75.2 percent of 1- to 4-year-olds had received three or more doses of diphtheria and tetanus toxoids and pertussis vaccine, and 65.5 percent measles vaccine. This latter deficit resulted in localized outbreaks of measles with more than 41,000 cases in 1976.[15]

The text above leads to numerous questions. Between 1965 and 1975 had polio rates gone up even though vaccine rates had gone down? How many of the children had received one or more doses, and how much immunity is conferred from incomplete vaccination? If vaccine rates had gone down so much, why were there not outbreaks of infectious diseases? And finally, how much can disease protection be attributed to vaccine coverage when less than 65 percent of the population is adequately vaccinated, especially when considering that there is often as much as a 10 to 20 percent failure rate of vaccines, potentially leaving less than 50 percent of the population actually protected? One can see the difficulty in relying upon such statistical reporting, and the ease with which statistics can be molded to fit the needs of the researcher. As one colleague, an international vaccine specialist with the Centers for Disease

Control (CDC), put it, vaccine statistics are a bit like the tobacco industry statistics—the tobacco industry could amass mounds of statistical evidence "proving" that cigarettes don't cause cancer, simply by selectively choosing statistics that represent their cause.

There is a strong tendency in our society to stress both the benefits of vaccines and the harmful outcomes associated with not vaccinating, making it likely that more emphasis is placed on reporting disease incidence in the nonvaccinated than vaccine failures in the vaccinated. However, statistics often cited by vaccine critics evidencing that higher percentages of vaccinated children than nonvaccinated children contract diseases during an outbreak is also a limited factor to look at. In any instance of an outbreak in a highly vaccinated population, it is virtually inevitable that the number of vaccinated children who contract the disease will be equal to or greater than the number of unvaccinated children who contract the disease. That is because the number of vaccinated children vastly outweighs the number of those unvaccinated. Here is a decent explanation of this phenomenon, described by the U.S. Department of Health and Human Services and the CDC in a jointly created booklet entitled *Six Common Misconceptions about Vaccination and How to Respond to Them*, an otherwise highly propagandist work with no references or citations to verify its claims:

> In a high school of 1,000 students, none has ever had measles. All but 5 of the students have had two doses of measles vaccine and so are fully immunized. The entire student body is exposed to measles, and every susceptible student becomes infected. The 5 unvaccinated children will be infected, of course. But of the 995 who have been vaccinated, we would expect several not to respond to the vaccine. The efficacy rate for two doses of measles vaccine can be as high as >99% effective. In this class, 7 students did not respond, and they, too, became infected. Therefore, 7 of 12, or about 58%, of the cases occur in students who have been fully vaccinated.[16]

Of course, there are many assumptions here, as well as missing information that could be relevant. For example, 100 percent of people in a population who are susceptible do not necessarily contract a disease. Second, stating "The 5 unvaccinated children will be infected, of course" is a gross and propagandist assumption and use of syntax and psychology. Just because a child is unvaccinated doesn't mean he will contract a disease. And further, but perhaps most important, what was the outcome of the infection? Did the vaccinated children who contracted the disease fare better than their unvaccinated cohorts? Do they have chronic health problems such as a 50 percent greater incidence of allergies than their nonvaccinated classmates, as is common in vaccinated populations? Statistical evaluations are not simple or unbiased.

Nonetheless, this is the best method that we have, and the one I will use to illustrate that while vaccines may be an important part of disease control, they may not protect us as completely as we are led to believe.

Statistical Evidence and Specific Diseases

The late and renowned pediatrician Dr. Robert Mendelsohn asks, in his typically direct and commonsense manner, "If immunisations were responsible for the disappearance of these diseases in the United States, one must ask why they disappeared simultaneously in Europe, where mass immunisations did not take place."[17] Moskowitz asserts that many diseases, including smallpox, diphtheria, tetanus, tuberculosis, cholera, and typhoid, all began to disappear near the end of the nineteenth century, "long before antibiotics, vaccines, or any specific measures designed to eradicate them."[18] Mortimer attributes such declines to human intervention in areas such as sanitary control of water supplies and refuse, and improved food handling, as well as quarantine measures (as with tuberculosis, mortality from which declined dramatically by 1945, prior to the development of effective antituberculosis drugs).[19]

Having discussed smallpox in chapter 1, let's now take a look at the disease incidence and outbreaks from the nineteenth century to the present of many of the previously common childhood diseases.

PERTUSSIS

Pertussis was prevalent and reached a peak incidence of mortality and morbidity in the nineteenth century, when it was common to find families huddled together in cramped environments in the cities of both Europe and America, "where backyard privies, unclean water from public wells, and inadequate nutrition were commonplace."[20] There is no doubt that for millions this was a dread disease, especially when one considers that the popular treatments of medical doctors of the day included bleeding, purging, and practically poisoning the patient with cathartics made from mercury.[21]

Mortality and morbidity from pertussis declined continually in western Europe and the United States from the mid–nineteenth to the mid–twentieth centuries. Deaths from pertussis declined from 210 per million in the 1870s to 21 per million in 1940, though few Americans had by then received the pertussis vaccine, which had only recently been developed. Pertussis, or whooping cough, exhibited a mortality rate of 12.2 per 100,000 population in the United States in 1900. By the late 1930s, prior to widespread immunization against pertussis, the mortality rates had decreased to approximately 2 per 100,000. In England 1 of every 1,000 children under the age of fifteen died of pertussis in the late nineteenth century; by 1940 this rate was down by 90 percent. In Sweden and Germany declines in pertussis mortality rates were comparable and significant.[22]

The whole-cell pertussis vaccine has the greatest reputation for inducing severe reactions, including a variety of permanent neurological sequelae, and death. In fact, it was because of this that Great Britain decided not to require children to receive the pertussis vaccine, and thus vaccine rates for pertussis decreased dramatically. This provides us with an interesting basis for comparison, as well as the opportunity to see what has happened to mortality rates due to pertussis. Not surprisingly, pertussis incidence has risen, but what is striking is that in spite of this, most cases are mild and no fatalities have been associated with the disease. Dr. J. Strom notes that since around 1967, pertussis has manifested as "increasingly mild, abortive forms with a corresponding reduction of the severe, clinically typical cases."[23] John Tanager, in a letter to the *Lancet* in 1982, wrote, "Due to the ineffective vaccine and the present mild clinical course of pertussis in Sweden the vaccination was stopped in 1979." He reports that in the years 1977–1979 there were nineteen thousand cases with not a single death.[24] Such reports are typical from western European nations. Doctors have reported little difference in the intensity and duration of cases in vaccinated and unvaccinated children.

Estimates for the efficacy of pertussis vaccine vary. The earlier pertussis vaccines used in England were considered to be between 20 and 60 percent effective; this vaccine was made stronger and is now considered to be 80 percent reliable.[25] According to Edward Mortimer, data indicate the vaccine to be between 70 and 90 percent effective, though he adds that measuring effectiveness is complicated by the fact that it is difficult to diagnose the disease, which is generally underdiagnosed in vaccinated populations, especially among adults, who are assumed to be immune.[26]

Resurgences of pertussis have occurred as epidemics in the United States in spite of a high rate of pertussis vaccination. In 1993 there was an outbreak of pertussis in the greater Cincinnati area, with 6,335 cases reported. The conclusion from an article in the *New England Journal of Medicine* was: "Since the 1993 pertussis epidemic in Cincinnati occurred primarily among children who had been appropriately vaccinated, it is clear that the whole-cell pertussis

vaccine failed to give full protection against the disease."[27] In some age categories the vaccination rate was as high as 82 percent for those who had received
three or more doses, and 74 percent had received four or five doses.[28] Serious
complications of pneumonia or atelectasis occurred in a small group of infants. There were no deaths.

A 1989 article in the *Journal of Pediatrics* reveals that "pertussis remains a
significant health problem in Nova Scotia, despite nearly universal vaccination."[29] Of those who contracted pertussis, 91 percent had been fully vaccinated, and 96 percent of those had been vaccinated appropriately for their age,
leading to an estimation of 45 percent vaccine efficacy. The authors add that
"the reported incidence of pertussis is likely to be an underestimate of the true
incidence of the disease because the disease is frequently under diagnosed."[30]

It is inevitable that with high vaccination rates in any given population,
and the certainty that there will always be some vaccine failures, most children
who contract such a disease will have been vaccinated. The question then becomes: Does a 45 percent efficacy rate justify the risk of the vaccine if the
disease itself is typically mild and self-limiting?

Yet the debate continues, with vaccine proponents insisting the vaccine
has a high efficacy rate and a low rate of complications compared with the
risks associated with the disease. It seems that the "incontrovertible evidence"
presented by both vaccine proponents and detractors is anything but absolute.
In an article by Drs. Alan Hinman and Jeffrey Koplan, for example, they elaborate on the high rates of complications one might expect in the absence of a
pertussis vaccine, estimating that it is more prudent to use the current vaccine,
in spite of associated complications. They cite the pertussis vaccine as having
an 80 to 90 percent efficacy rate, higher than that suggested by other articles
and evidence from epidemics.[31] Rebutting such information from an earlier
article of Dr. Koplan's in the *New England Journal of Medicine*, Dr. Gordon
Stewart of the University of Glasgow comments:

> First of all, they assumed that if there were no vaccination program, the inci-
> dence, complications, and death rate from whooping cough would now be what
> they were in Massachusetts from 1940–1950. This is surely untrue of any infec-
> tious disease. Secondly, they assumed the vaccine gives 70 percent protection.
> This figure overlooks recent reports from North America and from Australia
> and the United Kingdom that 30 to 50 percent of cases occur in vaccinated
> children. Thirdly, they indicated that they were using the most pessimistic ap-
> proximations of toxicity of pertussis vaccine. This is not so. Recent reports
> from the United States indicate much higher frequencies of toxicity. . . . What
> is surprising is that they went so far as to predict that the absence of their pro-

gram would lead to a 71-fold increase in cases of whooping cough and an almost fourfold increase in deaths. In making such a prediction, they ignored verifiable information that this has not happened in West Germany, the United Kingdom, or other countries where pertussis vaccine has been withheld on a massive scale for some years or has been unavailable.[32]

Pertussis vaccine may also have waning efficacy, with immunity to whooping cough not being sustained. Susceptibility may be as high as 95 percent twelve years after full vaccination.[33] It is well established that the disease does not manifest with classical symptoms in adults, more often appearing only as a mild persistent cough. These adults are frequently unsuspecting carriers of pertussis and are generally not diagnosed as so, because they are assumed to be immune based on their positive vaccine history. According to Randall Neustaedter's research, the most dependable studies of vaccine efficacy encompass those children living in a house with someone who had contracted the disease. Such studies show a variable vaccine efficacy of 63 to 91 percent.[34] As for declining efficacy, one study showed an efficacy rate of 80 percent after the last dose, 50 percent between four and seven years, and none after twelve years.[35]

MEASLES

Mortimer gives comparable evidence regarding the decline in the incidence of measles, which went from 13.3 per 100,000 population in 1900 to 0.3 per 100,000 in 1955 prior to the introduction of the measles vaccine. Miller asserts that between 1915 and 1958, a 97.7 percent drop in measles-related mortality had occurred, and was consistent even when measles peaked in incidence, as it periodically did.[36] This decrease in mortality is associated with two significant factors: decreases in family size, which were dramatic between 1915 and 1935, and the natural history of the disease.[37] As measles mortality was twenty times greater among poor families, the decrease in family size naturally led to a decrease in the overall incidence.

Natural selection of measles appears to have involved increased tolerance to the disease over successive generations owing to repeated exposure. Over time this made contracting the disease safer. In the absence of vaccinations, most of the population contracted the disease and developed natural antibodies that conferred lifelong immunity. Women with immunity passed this immunity on to their offspring through pregnancy (transplacentally) and through breast milk. This passive immunity generally protected children well through their first year of life. As with other microorganisms, it also appears that the organism lost some of its virulence over time.[38]

31

Introduction of the measles vaccine coincided with a continuing dramatic decrease in incidence. However, it must be remembered that even by as late as the early 1970s less than one-fourth of all children had been vaccinated, making it hard to attribute such a reduction to the vaccine.[39] In fact, the killed vaccine that was introduced in 1963 was found not only to have limited effectiveness but to lead to "atypical measles," a very dangerous form of the disease. Its use was discontinued in 1969.

Measles vaccine does not confer certain or indefinite immunity. In a 1978 survey of thirty states, more than half the children who contracted measles had been adequately vaccinated.[40] "Reports of epidemics in fully vaccinated populations have appeared periodically and consistently since the vaccine's introduction."[41] Also, reporting to vaccination surveillance systems may be inadequate, distorting the actual incidence of measles in vaccinated children. For example, in 1974 the CDC determined there were 36 cases of measles in Georgia, whereas the Georgia state surveillance system reported 660 cases in that same year. A survey of New York City pediatricians found that only 3.2 percent actually reported measles cases to the health department.[42]

Measles epidemics commonly occur in highly vaccinated populations. Of all reported cases of the measles in the United States in 1984, more than 58 percent of the school-age children who contracted measles were adequately vaccinated. In an outbreak in 1985, in a reported case group of 1,984 people, 80 percent had been appropriately vaccinated. A review of measles outbreaks in the United States demonstrated that approximately 60 percent of cases were among school-age children.[43] Canadian studies yield similar results. Again, higher vaccine levels in a community along with anticipated vaccine failures inevitably lead to such statistics. Therefore, the real focus must examine the risk of the disease versus the risk of an adverse reaction from the vaccine, and the likelihood of either occurring.

A recent measles epidemic at a major California university, whose student body was 92 percent vaccinated, led to the nationwide recognition that measles can and does occur in "protected" young adults and may be especially problematic in such older populations. Hence it is now recommended that revaccination occur for college-age students. This is reinforced by many colleges that now require proof of revaccination before matriculation is permitted. It should be noted that while many consider the problem of susceptibility to measles in those who are vaccinated to be one of waning immunity, there are those who believe it is related to primary vaccine failure.[44]

The measles vaccine has led to a dramatic shift in the epidemiology of the disease—that is, which population the disease typically affects. Prior to the vaccine era, the disease was most common in early childhood, particularly in four- to five-year-olds. It was very rare in infants, who almost universally acquired passive immunity from their mothers. By 1993, more than 25 percent of all measles cases were in babies less than a year old. CDC officials attribute this to the fact that those women who were vaccinated for measles as girls in the 1960s, 1970s, and 1980s could not confer passive immunity on their offspring, as only the naturally occurring disease stimulates an adequate antibody level for doing so.[45] The vaccine is not given to children in this age group, leaving babies vulnerable to infection from which they would naturally have been protected.

The disease itself was likely to cause a mild, nonthreatening illness, rarely causing mortality or long-term sequelae, and it conferred lifelong immunity. Adolescents and adults, who often experience more of the serious consequences of measles illness, were less likely to contract the disease. Currently, however, we are seeing a shift in the average age of infection toward higher-risk categories. Statistics from 1995 indicated that measles infection occurs most frequently among ten- to fourteen-year-olds, followed by those five to nine years old and fifteen to nineteen years old.[46] It is also known that when measles occurs in those outside the pediatric range or in those previously immunized, it may appear in the atypical form, a serious complication. Catherine Diodati, biomedical ethicist and author of *Immunizations: History, Ethics, Law, and Health*, discusses atypical measles as follows:

> The following signs have been noted with atypical presentations of measles: the absence of Koplik's spots, abnormal measles rash, persistent high fevers necessitating hospitalization, hypoxia (lack of oxygen at the cellular level affecting heart and respiratory functions and causing mental confusion), and giant-cell pneumonia. . . . An atypical or absent rash during infection indicates that the immune response is only partially effective and that the virus may linger and become manifest at a later date. . . . Missed measles rash . . . has been associated with various immunoreactive diseases (e.g. arthritis), sebaceous skin diseases (for example, seborrheic dermatitis), degenerative disease of the bone and cartilage . . . and certain tumors.[47]

Indeed, it is very likely that in a population where there is no longer any passive immunity and revaccination is occurring during young adulthood, the disease will once again shift epidemiologically and find a new host in the adult and elderly populations. The only solution to the vulnerability of contracting measles by those previously vaccinated is continual revaccination.

POLIO

Polio is another example of a disease whose incidence had begun to decline prior to the introduction of the vaccine. The killed polio vaccine developed by Salk was introduced in 1955, and in 1959 Sabin's live poliovirus was introduced. Both are still in use in the United States today, though until 1998, the live vaccine was the preferred method. Vaccine advocates rest all credit for reduction in the polio epidemics of the 1950s on mass vaccination campaigns. However, epidemiological evidence paints a conflicting picture. For example, from 1923 to 1953, prior to the introduction of the Salk vaccine, the polio death rates in the United States and England had decreased by 47 percent and 55 percent, respectively. Other European countries share similar statistics. In Great Britain the disease had already declined by 82 percent by 1956, just at the beginning of the vaccine campaign.[48] Epidemics ended even in countries that refused mandatory and systematic vaccination programs.[49]

What is interesting about the decline in polio is that unlike other diseases, the decline cannot be attributed to improvements in sanitation, improved water supplies, and the like. It is, in fact, a disease that had its origins in developed nations.[50] It is suspected that the poliovirus can become less virulent over time and the human host more resistant, allowing declining mortality even in the continued presence of the microorganism.[51] The shift in the disease from endemic to epidemic first occurred in societies with advancements in hygiene and sanitation, such as the industrialized, urban environments of the United States and Europe early in the twentieth century.[52] As developing nations improve their infrastructure, the disease increases in prevalence.

Polio vaccines were developed in the hope of preventing paralytic cases, yet even during major epidemics of poliomyelitis, more than 90 percent of all those exposed will remain asymptomatic, and most others will experience symptoms no more severe than the common cold. Paralytic cases are infrequent, occurring in less than 1 percent of all exposures to the disease.[53] Bear in mind, however, that even 0.5 percent in a population of 10 million is still an alarmingly high rate of paralytic cases. In underdeveloped nations where sanitation is poor, the virus is widespread, and nearly all children have antibodies due to infection during infancy.

It has become well established that the only new cases of polio in the United States since 1980, aside from a very few imported cases, are the direct result of vaccination or result indirectly from exposure to shed virus from one who has recently been vaccinated.[54] Since 1973 the number of annual cases of polio due to wild virus is exceeded by those resulting from the vaccine

(vaccine-associated paralytic poliomyelitis, or VAPP).[55] In 1976 Salk testified that the live virus vaccine, which has been used almost exclusively since early in the 1960s, was "the principle cause if not sole cause" of all reported polio cases in the United States since 1961.[56]

Of all the diseases for which one might try to establish the efficacy of the vaccine, polio is the most challenging because of changes that were made in disease classification after the introduction of the vaccine. This is an example of the difficulty of establishing evidence and reliable statistics in cases where there are confounding variables. Prior to the introduction of the live poliovirus, a polio epidemic was defined as 20 cases per 100,000. After its introduction, the new definition of an epidemic was established to be 35 cases per 100,000.[57] This made it much more difficult to classify polio outbreaks as epidemics. Furthermore, the diagnostic criteria for polio changed. Prior to the introduction of the live vaccine, a diagnosis of paralytic polio could be made if the patient evidenced paralytic symptoms for twenty-four hours. Since at least 1969, however, the CDC definition of paralytic polio has required that a diagnosis of paralytic polio could not be made unless the patient exhibited neurological symptoms that persisted for at least sixty days after the onset of symptoms, or the patient died.[58] This significantly reduced the number of cases that qualified as poliomyelitis, enhancing the appearance of vaccine efficacy.

Mislabeling of the disease may have been another common phenomenon leading to the appearance of a disproportionately low incidence of poliomyelitis as compared with the prevaccine era. Prior to the introduction of the polio vaccines, cases of aseptic meningitis were not typically differentiated from polio, as their clinical manifestations are so similar. During the 1950s, cases of polio were diagnosed six times more often as aseptic meningitis. However, we see a startling trend occurring in the 1960s with reported cases of aseptic meningitis on the rise while reported cases of polio were on the wane. Here are some figures from the *Los Angeles County Health Index: Morbidity and Mortality Report, Reportable Diseases:*[59]

Date	Viral or Aseptic Meningitis	Polio
July 1955	50	273
July 1961	161	65
July 1963	151	31
September 1966	256	5

Looking at the first and last sets of numbers together we get a startling picture of the inverse relationship between the disease incidence during the years prior to the change in frequency of diagnoses and after.

As discussed earlier, many doctors had such confidence in the vaccines that they naturally assumed that the presence of polio-like symptoms in a previously vaccinated patient could not be interpreted as polio but must be another disease. Unfortunately, such reinterpretations of polio make it exceptionally difficult to assess the impact of the vaccine on disease incidence.

RUBELLA

Rubella is a mild virus that may appear as a rash and slight fever but is often asymptomatic. Children are vaccinated against rubella not for their own protection but to protect pregnant women from being exposed to the disease. Rubella virus in the pregnant woman can lead to severe congenital problems in the fetus, a problem known as congenital rubella syndrome (CRS). Prior to the use of the vaccine, rubella epidemics spiked every six to nine years, with 100 to 500 cases per 100,000. Thousands of babies could be affected by CRS in a rubella outbreak. After the vaccine was introduced in 1969, the cases dropped to fewer than 10 per 100,000.[60] The use of the vaccine appears to have dramatically reduced the incidence of CRS. However, a number of articles on the efficacy of the rubella vaccine in providing lasting immunity have appeared in the medical literature since the early 1980s. The problem therein is that prior to use of the vaccine, most girls reached womanhood immune to rubella owing to natural exposure to the disease. Currently, most women in the United States have not had rubella or been naturally exposed to it but have been vaccinated against rubella. It is thought that the vaccine protection wanes over time, thereby leaving women who think they are protected susceptible at a time when they are the most likely to become pregnant.

According to a study done through the Department of Pediatrics at the Bowman Gray School of Medicine, the overall susceptibility rate of sixth graders was 15 percent, a rate that researchers say is similar to that of the prevaccine era.[61] They suggest that additional measures are required to reduce the risk of CRS. The method suggested is to target populations of preadolescent girls, at approximately twelve years of age, and revaccinate, as has been done in several western European countries. In one study by Dr. Stanley Plotkin, then professor of pediatrics at the University of Pennsylvania School of Medicine, 36 percent of adolescent girls who had been vaccinated as babies against rubella lacked any serologic evidence of being immune.[62]

Interestingly, the 1980 study reveals that lower-income students were less susceptible than upper-income students, 10.2 percent susceptibility versus 16.5 percent susceptibility. The authors suggest that this may be due to a greater opportunity for natural exposure among the lower-income population.[63] Greater immunity means less likelihood of CRS among childbearing women, raising significant questions about switching the epidemiology of the illness to a potentially more vulnerable age group.[64]

SCARLET FEVER AND INFLUENZA

Between 1900 and 1910 mortality from both scarlet fever and streptococcal sore throat was more than 10 per 100,000 population, declining to 0.5 per 100,000 before the advent of interventions with antimicrobial drugs.[65] This is significant to look at in relationship to the issue of vaccinations, as no vaccine was developed for scarlet fever, in spite of the death toll associated with it at one time. In this case antibiotics are credited with the decline. While scarlet fever is not feared today, it should be remembered that it was once a dreaded disease with a high fatality rate. So was the flu (influenza) a feared disease that occurred in epidemics and took many lives. We have developed vaccines for it, including the disastrous swine flu vaccine that continues to haunt recipients with long-term adverse effects, including severe degenerative diseases. Yet most healthy people experience only a few days of discomfort and no adverse effects.

DIPHTHERIA

Diphtheria is no longer considered a threat in the United States, where widespread vaccination is credited with its eradication. It continues to be a problem in developing nations. The following information appears in *Beyond the Magic Bullet*, by Bernard Dixon:

> Immunization against diphtheria, introduced on a large scale around 1940, appears to have had a dramatic effect on the incidence of disease. The number of cases in Britain fell by between fifty and sixty thousand each year, until 1955, since when there have been only sporadic outbreaks. However, if we take a longer time scale over the past century, and alter the criteria, we see a different picture. Diphtheria deaths in children went down continuously from 1300 per year in 1860, to under 300 per year in 1940, with a particularly large drop around 1900, the year when antitoxin was first used. Yet the steepest decline was between 1865 and 1875—before the diphtheria bacillus had even been isolated.[66]

While diphtheria could be a terrible disease for those who experienced the worst of cases, most people did not succumb to the disease or its potentially devastating sequelae and they gained permanent immunity, generally by late childhood.

Diphtheria vaccine may also be associated with failure to protect adequately against the illness. In Germany, for example, where compulsory vaccination was the rule, there was a great increase in cases in 1945, from 40,000 cases to more than 250,000 cases. Neustaedter summarizes this as a 17 percent increase in the number of cases and a 600 percent increase in deaths from diphtheria.[67] Parisians saw a 30 percent increase in 1944 despite compulsory vaccination, and similarly in Hungary, where vaccines were also required, there was a 35 percent increase in cases over two years. In the latter case, compulsory vaccines had been standard since 1938. There was a threefold increase in Geneva, Switzerland, between 1941 and 1943, though there had been a mandatory vaccine policy since 1933.[68] In Norway during this time vaccines were not compulsory, yet there were only fifteen cases of diphtheria on record.[69]

At the end of World War II, the vaccine was discontinued and there was a dramatic decline in disease incidence in spite of postwar poverty and inadequate nutrition.[70] In Chicago in 1969 there was a diphtheria outbreak, in which 25 percent of those who contracted the disease had been fully vaccinated and another 12 percent had received less than their full series of vaccines but showed serologic evidence of immunity.[71]

A 1975 report on diphtheria from the FDA Bureau of Biologics determined that diphtheria toxoid is not as effective as anticipated, and the provision of permanent immunity is not certain.[72]

It is clear that vaccines have contributed to disease reduction. Unfortunately, it is difficult to determine the extent to which vaccines have reduced disease incidence or whether their natural continued reduction would have occurred in their absence. And if vaccines are responsible for the reduction, at what cost has this triumph been won? We must consider the prices: our loss of natural immunity to certain diseases, the disruption of the natural history of the disease (which might have resulted in reduced disease virulence over time), and long-term consequences that are just becoming evident, such as increasing levels of chronic health problems that may be vaccine related. We will explore these issues in subsequent chapters, but first, a look at the amazing immune system.

THREE

The Marvelous Immune System

Perhaps one of the most fascinating aspects of our human existence is the functioning of the immune system—the physiologic actions of which are intended to maintain clear boundaries between "self" and "other." It is our immune system that is responsible for protecting us from invading microorganisms, whether they are bacteria, viruses, or larger parasites, and that also allows us to integrate some of these into our systems in mutualistic (mutually beneficial) relationships. Indeed, this amazing system has probably appeared in the media more in the past fifteen years than at any other time, with the widespread prevalence of HIV and AIDS, conditions that lay bare the significance of a healthy immune system for protecting human life. Yet for many the immune system is an abstract concept or the image of a military defense complex prepared to strike all enemy invaders on the home front. But this is to miss the richness and intricacy of this highly developed cascade of chemicals and blood cells that begins to develop in utero and continues to meet new challenges throughout our lives, with a seeming intelligence. While it would be impossible to do full justice to the immune system in anything less than several textbooks and illustrative commentaries, this chapter will elucidate the basics of how our bodies respond to invading organisms. We will also take a look at how vaccines work, what effects they have on immunity, and finally, what vaccines are composed of. In chapter 7, "Natural Approaches to Health and Immunity," we will discuss many factors, such as nutrition and stress management, that go into the optimal functioning of this system.

New Frontiers in Immunity

Lest the science in this chapter appear reductionist, it is important to choose a perspective on the immune system that is holistic from the start. Francisco Varela puts it quite succinctly when he says that new views on immunology "suggest that the immune system is more accurately thought of as a cognitive network analogous to the brain and nervous system," however, lacking "spatially located sensory organs."[1] The immune system is an independent network whose principal purpose is to establish and preserve molecular identity. In this way it can be thought of as a proactive network rather than simply a reactive, defensive mechanism. As Walene James writes, quoting Varela: "Seeing the body as a flowing system of interconnected, reciprocal networks continually interacting in a molecular bio-dance is part of the newer contextual thinking," allowing the "mutual dance between immune system and body . . . to have a changing and plastic identity throughout its life and multiple encounters."[2]

We can step further outside the limitations of physical science by acknowledging the tremendous impact mind and emotions have on immunity. Seeing ourselves as intelligent beings with sentient cells that are but a microcosm of the macrocosm of each of us, we realize that there is a delicate chemical interplay between all of our various systems. This is apparent in the inverse relationship between stress and immunity—stress increases and eventually immune function decreases. Neuropeptides, our chemical messengers of emotion and our links between emotional and physical experience, may be part of the mechanism. Further, our adrenal hormones, for example, epinephrine (adrenaline) and norepinephrine (noradrenaline), may also provide us with clues to the connections between our emotional wellness and the efficiency and success of our immune response, as they are influenced by one and influence the other. The emerging field of psychoneuroimmunology, which literally links the experience of the psyche—the mind or the soul—to that of our immune system, exists to study such connections, the importance of which will be elaborated on in chapter 7. What is important to bear in mind now is that the sensitivity of the immune system is enormous and incredibly effective to have allowed the human organism to evolve in environments where billions of microorganisms are a constant and given fact. Vaccination seeks to instigate our immune system to a state of heightened responsiveness to potentially pathogenic organisms while bypassing certain aspects of natural exposure to disease. While this can indeed be a critical factor in disease prevention, the long-term costs to the optimal functioning of the human organism may be greater than previously expected.

Because vaccines confer artificial immunity rather than natural immunity, many writers prefer to use the term *vaccination* rather than *immunization* when referring to inoculations.[3] I have chosen to follow this convention throughout this book.

The ABCs of Immunity

The human body has evolved remarkable physical mechanisms for maintaining the integrity of its "space." The following sections will discuss the nature of viruses and bacteria, and the various mechanisms our bodies have evolved to live with them in our shared world.

BACTERIA, VIRUSES, AND PARASITES

We share our environment with a multitude of microorganisms—many of which seek us, quite literally, as their hosts. These microorganisms fall within the categories of viruses, bacteria, fungi, and worms. It is only the first two categories that we will discuss, other than when necessary for illustrative purposes, as it is for these two groups of organisms that vaccines are given.

Bacteria are microscopically small, single-celled organisms that inhabit nearly every corner of our planet in vast numbers, ranging from the upper atmosphere and the polar ice caps to the deepest reaches of animal bodies and the ocean. Few surfaces, other than those that are extremely acid, very hot, or very dry, lack bacterial colonization. Some scientists believe that their mass outweighs that of all plant and animal life on earth, combined.[4] Some bacteria are autotrophic (they can produce their own food, as do plants), while others are not, relying on nutrients from other living beings. There are also those that live on material that is no longer living, such as unprotected food. This latter class is known as decomposers, and they also serve important functions in the environment. Most bacteria require oxygen for survival, but some, such as those in the genus *Clostridium*, of which tetanus (*Clostridium tetani)* is a member, thrive in anaerobic environments, such as deep in the soil or in puncture wounds where there is little oxygen.

Bacteria are generally one of three shapes: rod-shaped (bacillus), round (coccus), and spiral-shaped (spirillum), though it is now believed that they can adapt their shapes, and possibly even transmutate into other forms of bacteria, a concept known as pleomorphism.[5] Interestingly, emerging thought in microbiology draws upon theories of great thinkers such as Pierre Bechamp and Wilhelm Reich, some of whose works have been previously discredited by scientists of their day.

Many bacteria live in a commensal relationship with the human species; that is, they live in or on us without causing us harm—at least, as long as our bodies keep their growth in balance and their numbers do not overwhelm our systems, and also as long as they inhabit only certain parts of the body. *Escherichia coli* is an example: as long as its colonies stay within the intestinal system and they do not proliferate out of control, no harm is done.

Other bacteria live in mutualistic relationships with us—we benefit them and they benefit us. Such a reciprocal arrangement exists in the presence of some bacteria that do us no harm and actually prevent the colonization of other more pathogenic organisms. For example, certain strains of bacteria that inhabit our intestines allow us to synthesize vitamin B_{12}.

Antibacterial agents are often used in the treatment of bacterial infections. While they are ineffective against viruses, they are commonly prescribed during viral infections in order to prevent secondary bacterial infection. The overuse of antibiotics can have negative consequences for humans. Antibiotics reduce the population of beneficial bacteria that we harbor, which can lead to proliferation of other harmful organisms, such as yeasts, leading to yeast infections. Second, bacteria can evolve to become resistant to antibiotics; therefore, we create increasingly resistant strains of microorganisms against which we have no medication and possibly limited immune resistance.[6]

Examples of bacteria for which vaccinations are given include tetanus, diphtheria *(Corynebacterium diphtheriae)*, and pertussis *(Bordetella pertussis)*. Interestingly, it is the endotoxins (a toxin produced within the bacteria that is released when the bacteria are broken down) produced by these bacteria, rather than the organisms themselves, that cause the harmful consequences of the diseases with which they are associated.

VIRUSES

Viruses are peculiar little organisms that scientists are constantly working to understand. They are basically infectious, submicroscopic particles consisting of a core of RNA or DNA, surrounded by a protein coat. Though they are biologically active while within living organisms, they are inert outside of living organisms. In fact, they cannot function at all or reproduce unless using the host's cell to do so, making them easy to classify as parasitic. And much like other spores, some can become quite hardy (they take a crystallized form), remaining inactive for indefinite periods of time. Many scientists question whether viruses are living things at all, or whether they are merely fragments of genetic material existing in our environment.

Once inside the host, viruses rely on what is typically referred to as our "cellular machinery" to carry out their genetic instructions. Virtually all forms of life are susceptible to viruses, and viruses are the source of many of the worst epidemics humankind has faced, including rabies, smallpox, polio, and yellow fever. Most of the vaccines given for childhood diseases are for those caused by viruses, including measles, polio, mumps, rubella, hepatitis B, and varicella (chicken pox). Viruses may also be involved in cancers and autoimmune diseases. Viruses are constantly mutating, so that new versions of old viruses, or even new viruses, can arise at any time, presenting challenges to the immune system as well as sometimes making current treatments and prophylactic measures ineffective.

INNATE AND ADAPTIVE IMMUNITY

The body has two distinct lines of defense against invading microorganisms, the innate defenses and the adaptive defenses. The innate defenses include the physical barriers of the body that deter unwanted or unrecognized microorganisms from entering, as well as chemical and white blood cell responses. They are generally quite efficient and sufficient for the task. However, should these mechanisms fall short of deterring pathogens, the adaptive immune response comes into play. Adaptive immunity differs from innate immunity primarily in that the adaptive immune response includes a specific memory for previously encountered organisms, so should reinfection occur, the body is able to respond to that infection rapidly and directly. Antibodies and T-cells are facets of the adaptive response. It is upon such a response that vaccinations rely for efficacy.

PHYSICAL BARRIERS TO INFECTION

It really never ceases to amaze me how perfectly designed we are, even in ways that we are mostly unaware of, down to the chemical composition of our skin. Yet it is these subtle nuances that allow us to continue to survive, enjoy life, and evolve along with our environment. The chemical and physical barriers of the body that prevent the penetration of potentially pathogenic microorganisms provide perfect examples of our wonderful human architecture.

The skin is the ideal place to begin. Few bacteria can survive for any length of time on the skin, as the lactic acid and fatty acids of which our sweat and sebaceous secretions are composed create too low a pH for them to tolerate. This is why skin loss, as from burns or trauma, can leave the path open for infection—a major barrier to the inner body has been removed. The inner membranes of the body also have a protective barrier—the mucus they secrete. Mucus prevents bacteria from sticking to the cells that line the body (epithelial cells). This epithelial layer also heals itself very quickly, often within twenty-four hours, making it a reliable barrier if there has been local trauma.

Once microorganisms get caught in this sticky mucus, they can then be expelled by mechanical efforts such as coughing and sneezing, or through tears, saliva, and urine, other fluid mediums that protect the body's surfaces. Furthermore, some of the body's fluids also contain chemicals that are actually antimicrobial.

As mentioned earlier, bacterial flora support us in a mutualistic relationship by inhibiting the growth of harmful bacteria and fungi, especially on the surfaces lining the body. They do this either by competing for essential nutrients, by nature of their occupancy utilizing available space, or by producing substances that inhibit the growth of competing microorganisms.

"CELL EATERS"

Though we have evolved elaborate systems of protection in the form of physical barriers to infectious agents, sometimes these defenses are weakened, whether through trauma, dietary changes affecting pH, or stress affecting our biochemical composition. When microorganisms enter into our personal space, they meet the next protective mechanisms of the body, the phagocytes, which literally translates as "cell eaters." The cells that have the main protective responsibility are called "professional phagocytes," perhaps emphasizing our cultural preference for hiring experts to do a job (no amateurs here, thank you). The phagocytes, a group of leukocytes (white blood cells), consist of two primary families of cells, the macrophages ("large eaters"), and the smaller macrophages called polymorphonuclear phagocytes (also known as polymorphs, neutrophils, and PMNs). Both have their origin in the bone marrow, but when they are mature they become prevalent throughout the body. White blood cells are the main mediators of the entire immune response.

The macrophages are especially concentrated in certain areas of the body, including the basement membranes of the small blood vessels, connective tissue, and the lungs, liver, brain, kidneys, and lining of the lymph system and spleen. Here they are particularly beneficial for removing waste and foreign matter. The PMNs are short-lived cells found predominantly in the bloodstream and are able to function in anaerobic, inflammatory conditions. The macrophages are generally involved in infections where the organisms live with the human cell; the PMNs are primarily involved when there is pus-forming bacteria.

44

Phagocytosis begins when the phagocyte adheres itself to the microbe, usually by recognizing some of the carbohydrates on its surface. This then activates a contractile mechanism in the phagocyte that allows it to extend armlike projections around the microbe until it is fully engulfed by the phagocyte. The phagocyte then releases a variety of chemicals, including forms of highly reactive oxygen, that break down the microorganism, thus killing it. Some phagocytes are also partially responsible for repair of body tissue, for example, by helping to dissolve or prevent blood clots.

So how do these phagocytes know when an organism has penetrated the body's protective defenses? A process called chemotaxis occurs, in which chemicals produced by bacteria attract phagocytes to them. Because this is a weak method, however, we have evolved a more complex means of drawing assistance to damaged tissue. This is known as the complement system.

Complement is a delicately orchestrated and highly complex series of reactions of protein enzymes that collectively, and in an effective cascade of stimulus and response, cause the target microorganisms to be more susceptible to engulfment by phagocytes, increase the inflammatory response, and allow microbes to be destroyed. The advantage of the increased inflammatory response, which involves degranulation of the mast cells (cells involved in the inflammatory response) and consequent release of such chemicals as histamine, heparin, and platelet-activating factor, is the increased flow of blood and plasma, and thus phagocytes, to the damaged, invaded, or infected area of the body.

In addition to these incredible feats of immunity, our bodies produce additional substances that maintain our health and integrity. Interferon is an example of such a substance. Interferons are proteins formed by our cells when they are exposed to viruses. When noninfected cells are exposed to the interferon, they become protected against viral infection. When one cell becomes infected, it produces interferon to which all the cells around the infected cell(s) react, becoming protected from that virus. It does this by causing the cells to produce enzymes that interfere with viral replication. This effectively serves to contain the virus and inhibit its spread. Natural killer (NK) cells take the task one step further and destroy the virally infected cells. They are able to differentiate the infected from the healthy cells by recognizing substances on the surfaces of the virally infected cells. By releasing chemicals that damage the infected cell, they protect us from viral spread.

All of these processes fall into the category of humoral immunity. These efforts are the primary attempts of the immune system to maintain the fine line between our bodies and other organisms with which we live. Sometimes, however, more extensive means are required to protect these boundaries.

ADAPTIVE (CELLULAR) IMMUNITY

Much as we have evolved elaborate means to protect ourselves from infections, so too have microorganisms evolved elaborate means to avoid our immune systems. Many have found ways to mutate to forms that evade the detection of our innate immunity. For example, some bacteria do not trigger the complement pathways, while others do so only at their flagella, so that the main body of the bacterium avoids all damage—quite clever indeed! Other cells may not be vulnerable to the chemical agents our bodies deploy for their destruction and our protection. We have therefore by necessity evolved even more complex means of immunity, known as adaptive immunity or cellular immunity, which are able to recognize, identify, and remember specific organisms and develop specific immune responses to each. These specific immune responses, known as antibodies, are what vaccines are designed to stimulate our bodies to produce, conferring the type of immunity provided by natural infections that trigger cellular immune responses.

Vaccines work on the principal that injecting a small amount of antigen into the system will trigger an initial immune response and a second injection of the vaccine will enhance the reaction with further antibody formation, creating a specific memory of that organism. Future exposure to the organism should then allow the body to quickly recognize and mount a full-scale response to the organism, without vulnerability to the disease to which the body is theoretically immune. Since such immunity is developed over time, adaptive immunity is also referred to as acquired immunity.

ANTIBODIES TO THE RESCUE

Antibodies are produced by our B-lymphocytes (thus named because they mature in our bone marrow) when they encounter a foreign protein—called an antigen. Every antibody has on its surface a recognition site, able to distinguish individual antigens when they are next encountered. These antibodies bind microorganisms that have evaded the innate immune mechanisms, and sites on the antibody then stimulate the complement system to become activated. As with innate immunity, complement immunity facilitates the destruction of unwanted microorganisms. The complement pathway activated by the innate system is known as the alternate complement pathway; when activated by the adaptive immune response, it is the classical pathway. Though each complement pathway differs slightly in how it is activated, the net results are the same. Antibodies are also able to interfere with the functioning of antigenic microorganisms in a variety of ways, including preventing the antigen from binding to cells, blocking microorganisms from picking up essential nutrients, and finally, preventing damage to cells by bacterial toxins.

Antibodies may be present in the body as a result of past infection or unknown exposure to an infectious agent, by transplacental transfer from mother to fetus during pregnancy, or through vaccination. They belong to a group of proteins known as immunoglobulins (Ig) found in the serum portion of the blood. Each B-lymphocyte is a highly complex cell with approximately 100,000 immunoglobulins on its surface, which identify only specific antigens. Different immunoglobulins have specialized functions within the body. There are five major immunoglobulins: immunoglobulin gamma A (IgA), immunoglobulin gamma D (IgD), immunoglobulin gamma E (IgE), immunoglobulin gamma G (IgG), and immunoglobulin gamma M (IgM).

IgA is found primarily in the fluid secretions of the body, such as saliva, tears, intestinal mucus, and respiratory mucus, and it serves to protect the mucus membranes from invasion by viruses and bacteria. IgD is found in small quantities in normal human serum, and its functions are unknown. IgE is produced by the lining of the respiratory and intestinal tract. IgE binds specifically to the mast cells, which, as mentioned earlier, are involved in the inflammatory response. When antigens bind to IgE, mast cell activity is stimulated. High levels of IgE are found in those with allergy-related diseases. IgG, also known as gamma-globulin, is the most abundant antibody found in the human body. IgG is capable of crossing the placenta and is therefore the principal immunoglobulin involved in stimulating immunity in the baby prior to birth. It is also the main antibody for bacteria, viruses, and antitoxins. IgM, or macroglobulin, is the initial antibody found after infection and vaccination, being formed in the initial stages of most immune reactions. The life span of most antibodies is anywhere from several weeks to many years.

In addition to B-lymphocytes, there are T-lymphocytes (T-cells), so called because they mature in the thymus gland. Viruses and certain species of microorganisms live within our cells. When they die, the proteins from these organisms are taken up into vacuoles in our cells and are bound with a substance known as major histocompatibility complex (MHC). The T-lymphocyte is able to recognize these fragments of antigens in our cells, and it possesses a receptor for binding with MHC. When it spots the MHC-antigen combination, it binds itself to the infected cell and becomes activated. There are three main types of T-cells: T-helper (TH) cells, which induce antibody formation by B-lymphocytes; cytotoxic T-cells (TC), which kill microorganisms in cells and are also responsible for the rejection of skin grafts; and T-suppressor cells, which inhibit the production of antibody-forming cells for the B-lymphocytes. Generally 60 percent of T-cells are helper cells, and 20 to 30 percent are suppressor cells. An imbalance in this ratio can indicate a compromised immune system. The TH and TC cells are capable of releasing interferon, and this improves the functioning of the NK cells, reminding us of the integration and cooperation of the various aspects of the human organism.

ARTIFICIAL IMMUNITY

When one is exposed to an infectious agent through natural exposure or illness, and the body is required to respond with an adaptive immune response, as just described in detail, permanent immunity is often acquired. Such immunity is termed natural immunity. This is in contrast to immunity conferred via vaccinations, referred to as artificial immunity. Artificial immunity can be either *passive* or *active*, as described below.

PASSIVE IMMUNITY

Passive immunization, which is less commonly employed in recent decades since the development of more effective active vaccines, was relied upon heavily in the past. It is used after exposure to known pathogens and involves the administration of antibodies derived from the blood of a person or animal (generally horses) recovering from the specific disease infecting the person. The recovering person or animal will have large amounts of circulating antibodies; these increased antibodies, when introduced into the sick person—generally given as an injection or occasionally intravenously—assist the body simply by quickly raising the antibody levels.

Passive immunity usually lasts for several weeks, at most a few months, after the administration of the antibodies; this method does not confer lasting immunity.[7] It is typically used only during known epidemics to protect those who are vulnerable or who have recently been exposed but have not yet manifested disease symptoms. The technique either prevents the disease entirely or reduces its severity. Natural passive immunity, as discussed earlier, is the type of immunity conferred upon the fetus by the mother, through the transplacental transmission of antibodies, and to the newborn and nursing baby through the breast milk, which is notably high in antibodies. Natural passive immunity generally confers varying levels of immunity for at least the first six to twelve months of life, and possibly significantly longer if the breast-feeding relationship is extended.

Tetanus, diphtheria, and measles are a few examples of diseases for which immunoglobulin therapy is administered. Because of the high level of reactions (allergic, anaphylactic) from horse serum, human immunoglobulin is preferable and is generally used. Natural passive immunity to tetanus rarely occurs.

ACTIVE IMMUNITY

Vaccinations are designed to emulate the natural process of active acquired immunity by stimulating an antibody response that is intended to be permanent. In natural infection, most microbial agents enter the body via the mucosal surfaces (respiratory passages or intestinal surfaces), stimulating an IgA response (recall that IgA is an antibody associated with protection at the level of the secretory membranes), to be followed later by IgG and IgM antibodies. Most vaccines enter the body via the bloodstream, having been administered in the form of an injection. Oral poliovirus vaccine is the only one to enter the body through the typical natural route, orally, from where it then acts upon the intestinal mucosal lining.[8] Most vaccines, therefore, do not stimulate IgA antibodies initially; rather, they stimulate IgG first.[9] Research is being conducted on the development of such products as intranasal vaccine sprays for several viruses, including measles, rubella, and other viral infections, in order to initially stimulate the IgA antibodies and more closely imitate natural immunity. The hope is that this will confer permanent immunity similar to that seen after natural infections.[10] Indeed, it has been demonstrated that "the most effective vaccines are those that most closely simulate the recovery or protective mechanisms seen following convalescence from the natural disease."[11] Furthermore, immunity is rarely induced after one vaccination, thereby necessitating numerous shots to stimulate the full antibody response, and boosters for when antibody responses begin to wane. Unfortunately, vaccine adverse reaction incidence frequently increases with increasing numbers of injections.

LIVE VERSUS KILLED VACCINES

The status of the antigen itself is another important aspect of vaccinations. Vaccines can contain either *live* or *killed* immunogenic material. Those that contain live attenuated agents are more virulent and capable of inducing both stronger immunity and stronger adverse reactions than the killed counterpart. Their conferred immunity tends to be long-lasting, and both humoral and cell-mediated.[12] Live vaccines are also capable of replication and have a tendency to revert to wild strains, which can be highly infectious, virulent, and able to cause the disease for which the vaccination is being given in the recipient.

Killed vaccines, on the other hand, tend to be less reactive than live vaccines and are incapable of either replication or reversion to wild strains. They are therefore much safer than live vaccines. However, they are thought to induce shorter periods of immunity, leading to the need for "booster" shots.

Poliovirus vaccines are an excellent example in the controversy of live versus killed vaccine. It had been thought since shortly after the introduction of the polio vaccine that the live vaccine, given orally, was preferable, because it entered the body via its natural portal and conferred the most complete immunity. However, it has also been known since then that poliomyelitis can be caused by the vaccine itself. Most European countries administer only the killed vaccine for this reason. The American Academy of Pediatrics and the Centers for Disease Control have recently recognized the dangers inherent in the live virus and have issued recommendations that only the killed virus be used in most circumstances. It has been found that the killed virus confers immunity effectively with fewer side effects and without the ability to revert to wild-type virus.

Vaccine Production and Components

Now more than ever there is growing awareness about the things we put into our bodies. Organic foods, natural body products, and natural medicines have seen a rising popularity in the past decade, as people have grown increasingly concerned about the possible harmful effects of pesticides, additives, and genetically engineered components on our health. It might therefore be appalling to consider the components of our medicines, particularly those that are given when people are well.

Over the past hundred or so years, painstaking research has gone into the safest and most effective mediums on which to grow the microorganisms for vaccines, as well as the products with which to attenuate and preserve them. The following is a sampling of the various components of the common vaccines administered to our children. The information is taken directly from package inserts from major vaccine manufacturers.[13]

Measles, mumps, and rubella vaccine is a live virus vaccine derived from live measles virus grown in chick embryo cell culture, live mumps virus propagated in chick embryo cell culture, and live rubella virus grown in human lung cells (diploid lung fibroblasts). The measles and mumps viruses are grown in a medium made of salt solution with amino acids, vitamins, and fetal bovine serum, with sucrose phosphate, glutamate, and human protein (albumin), collectively referred to as SPGA, as a stabilizer. Neomycin antibiotic is also added.

Rubella is grown similarly, with sorbitol and gelatin also added.

Diphtheria, tetanus, and acellular pertussis vaccine is a sterile combination of diphtheria and tetanus toxoids and inactivated pertussis antigens adsorbed onto an aluminum hydroxide base. They are generally cultivated on bovine extracts with various chemical mediators such as barium chloride used to extract the vital antigenic components. Formaldehyde and glutaraldehyde are used to detoxify the resulting components. A chemical preservative, 2-phenyoxyethanol, and another substance, polysorbate-80 (Tween 80), are in the final product as well.

Inactivated poliovirus vaccine cells are incubated in cultures of monkey kidney cells from a continuous line. The cells are grown in a medium that contains newborn calf serum, originating from countries free of bovine spongiform encephalopathy. It contains 2-phenyloxyethanol and formaldehyde as preservatives, and also contains streptomycin, neomycin, and polymyxin.

Varicella vaccine, the live virus vaccine used to prevent chicken pox, has been controversially accepted by various religious groups, as it is based on human embryonic lung tissue. These cell-line cultures originated from tissue obtained from legal abortions in the 1960s. However, new fetal tissue is not used to produce the vaccines. Vaccine manufacturers use human cell lines from FDA-certified cell banks.[14] The virus was obtained from a child with natural chicken pox and was then introduced onto the embryonic tissue. This was then transferred to and propagated in embryonic guinea pig cell cultures, and finally generated in human diploid cell culture. Sucrose, phosphate, monosodium L-glutamate, gelatin, potassium phosphate, potassium chloride, residual components of DNA and protein, EDTA, neomycin, and fetal bovine serum are also found in varying amounts in the final product.

Very little research has been done into the long-term effects of the aluminum found in vaccines. However, there is a great deal of speculation and concern that it may have deleterious effects on our cerebral and neurological tissues.[15] It is unknown what quantities of aluminum in the blood may lead to long-term problems, including motor paralysis, liver and kidney degeneration, learning disabilities, and dementia.[16]

It is known that the gelatin, chick embryo, and neomycin can make certain vaccines problematic for children with sensitivities to these substances (egg allergies triggered by the chick embryo component). It is also in question whether injecting children with these antigenic substances early in life, and during the formative stages of their immune systems, in fact creates a susceptibility to allergies. It is medically well established that vaccines increase allergies.[17] Furthermore, vaccines increase the likelihood of inflammatory bowel disorders.[18] Allergies are often found in cases of inflammatory bowel disease, as the irritated lining of the bowel mucosa allows for greater entrance of antigens into the general circulation, increasing allergic, inflammatory responses systemically.

Formaldehyde, also known as formalin, has been used to reduce the toxicity of microbial toxins since very early in the history of vaccine production. Toxoids, such as for diphtheria and tetanus, must be detoxified by a substance such as formaldehyde lest they be lethal upon injection. Toxoids are powerful substances even in minute quantities. Formaldehyde is a known carcinogen if ingested, and its ability to fully reduce the virulence of infectious agents is questionable, thereby causing vaccine critics to question its cost-benefit value in vaccine manufacturing and the safety of vaccines in which it is included.

The presence of thimerosal (trade name is Merthiolate), a mercury derivative, in the hepatitis B vaccine led to the discontinuation of administration of hepatitis B vaccine to infants for a brief period in 1999. There was significant concern that its inclusion in the vaccine may cause safe blood level limits of mercury to be exceeded, endangering the health and safety of newborns and children, who may already be exposed to toxic amounts of mercury from foods and the environment, even prenatally. Even as I write, the National Academy of Science is convening meetings to research the problem of mercury contamination in our environment. One piece of their study was the review of mercury levels in newborns based on fish consumption by pregnant mothers. It was found to correlate at alarmingly high rates. Indeed, recent recommendations that I have become aware of include not serving tuna fish to school-age children more than once weekly because of high mercury levels. Nonetheless, because of the expense and relative scarcity of thimerosal-free hepatitis B vaccine, it is now policy to give the mercury-free product only to children under six months of age, and to give the thimerosal-containing product when the other product is not available.[19] The concern appears to have been very short-lived, and hepatitis B vaccine is once again being given to neonates in most hospitals, despite the fact that most are not born to mothers that test positive for hepatitis B.

New concerns are arising regarding the safety of vaccine ingredients along with increasing concern over mad cow disease. While vaccine manufacturers are asserting that there is no risk of contracting the disease from vaccine made on bovine culture mediums, vaccine batches made from European bovine materials may be destroyed as a precaution. Thus far, no connections have been established between vaccines and the disease, but the issue is only recently coming to the attention of the public in the United States.

THE BIG PICTURE

Differing views on vaccination and immunity yield different ideas of what "the big picture" really is. Some see the importance of preventing childhood diseases as so great that occasional severe adverse effects are considered necessary casualties, "sacrifices" for the greater benefit of humankind. Common reactions such as fever, screaming, appetite loss, swelling, and inflammation are considered just par for the course. Others, however, see a gray area between the black and white of frequent mild reactions and rare severe reactions. They see these manifesting in the form of chronic autoimmune problems, behavioral problems, respiratory problems, and other chronic health problems, which are increasingly prevalent in our society. Some consider vaccines to be miraculous medicines that can relieve humanity of burdensome diseases. Others see vaccines as overwhelming to young and developing immune systems, leading to increases in diseases that severely reduce the quality of human life with their degenerative and chronic natures. It is indeed rare for children to be exposed naturally to a plethora of diseases and chemical challenges all at once, as is the case with, for example, trivalent vaccines such as the DPT or MMR vaccines. We are only now realizing the effects of environmental pollution on our planet and bodies. Have small groups of parents and professionals become overly hysterical about the potential harm from vaccines, forgetting the magnitude of problems associated with childhood diseases, or are they sounding the alarm just in time before we reach a level of chronic disease in our society that is just as problematic as disease epidemics, if not more so?

FOUR

The Childhood Illnesses and "Vaccine-Preventable Diseases"

Health care decisions can be made intelligently only if one is well informed about the issues and options involved in each of the circumstances one faces. To make a truly informed choice regarding vaccinations requires a thorough knowledge of each illness that your child might face, including symptoms and consequences, as well as the pros and cons of each vaccine. Thus educated, you are also accepting responsibility for your decision and the outcome, prepared to respond to a problem should the need arise. While many families who rely primarily on natural medicines may adopt the belief that they will simply trust in nature and the integrity of the immune system, forgoing vaccines with no further thought, I strongly believe this to be a facile approach to health care. Nature, while extremely beneficent, is also dispassionately harsh, sparing no sentiment in obliterating entire communities with typhoons, volcanic eruptions, and disease scourges. Ask any doctor over sixty years old about the polio outbreaks of the 1950s, or what it was like watching a patient succumb to diphtheria, and one is quickly reminded of nature's force and, at times, fury. Modern periodic outbreaks of disease can be sobering reminders of times when most families knew someone who died of one of the diseases for which we now vaccinate.

Nonetheless, this does not invalidate the decision not to vaccinate or to vaccinate selectively. It all comes down to individual informed choice and responsibility. At best one can consider vaccination policies to be mass campaigns intended for the good of all. However, such policies do not consider individual needs, health status, and immune system predilection. Choosing to accept the risks associated with a disease is not better or worse than choosing to accept the risks of a particular vaccine. Both require thoughtfulness, careful consideration, and a weighing of risk versus benefit. It is unlikely that most children will ever experience a severe reaction to a vaccine. It is also unlikely that most children will ever be exposed to a life-threatening infection. However, it is likely that most children will have mild reactions to most vaccines, and perhaps subclinical moderate reactions that can lead to chronic health problems. It is also true that children do have some risk of exposure to serious infectious diseases to which they may be vulnerable. Certain factors, such as day care centers or travel, increase their risk of exposure. We each have to choose the risk we can live with and make choices appropriate to our children's needs and circumstances. In chapter 6 we will explore the vaccine decision-making process, and later chapters will also address vaccine-related risks. Now let's take a look at the actual diseases for which children are vaccinated.

The Recommended Vaccine Schedule

The recommended vaccine schedule tells physicians and parents which vaccines to give to children and when. It is based on several factors, including the age at which vaccines are considered the safest to administer, at what ages children require protection from certain diseases, and convenience in giving vaccines. The latter primarily influences the number of shots given in any one doctor's appointment, with the goal of giving as many shots in one visit as possible to avoid inconvenience to the parents, who would otherwise require numerous office visits, and it influences the trend of giving multiple vaccines in one dose to minimize the number of injections needed, thus reducing the child's discomfort. The recommended schedule is reviewed each year by the CDC Advisory Committee on Immunization Practices (ACIP) to ensure that it "remains current with changes in manufacturers' vaccine formulations, revisions in recommendations for the use of licensed vaccines, and recommendations for newly licensed vaccines."[1]

Current vaccine recommendations call for giving fifteen to nineteen injections by age six, twelve of which are given by eighteen months of age.[2] The recommendations for specific vaccines, as developed and approved by the CDC and the American Academy of Pediatrics, are as follows:

DTP or DTaP (diphtheria, tetanus, whole-cell pertussis or acellular pertussis)

2, 4, 6, and 18 months and 4 to 6 years

Until recently, the DTaP was recommended only in the fourth and fifth doses but now is approved for all five doses (provider/user choice).

DT (diphtheria, tetanus)

2, 4, 6, 18 months

For children who can't receive the pertussis component of the vaccine.

Tetanus

Booster 10 years after the last tetanus dose, and every 10 years thereafter.

MMR (measles, mumps, rubella)

15 months and 4 to 6 years or 11 to 12 years

Polio

Inactivated poliovirus (IPV) at 2 and 4 months and between ages 6 and 18 months and between ages 4 and 6 years.[3]

Hepatitis B

6 months (or at birth if mother is positive for the disease), plus two more doses—there should be a minimum of 4 weeks between the first and second doses and a minimum of 4 months between the second and third doses.

Hib (Hemophilus influenza type B)

2, 4, 6, and 12 to 15 months

Shots should be given at least 2 months apart.

Some states don't require this vaccine.

Varicella zoster (chicken pox)

12 to 18 months

Some states don't require this vaccine.

Parents wishing for updates on this list can visit the CDC Web site at www.cdc.com. You can check this site periodically for the most current information because vaccine protocols do change. It has only been in the past five or so years that our country has switched to acellular pertussis and inactivated polio vaccines. Similarly, vaccines have been discontinued or retracted from the market, and physicians aren't always aware of the changes. In 1975 it was estimated that 12.6 percent of children under five years of age were still receiving the smallpox vaccine though the Public Health Service had recommended against its use in 1971.[4] Another example is the rotavirus, which on October 22, 1999, ACIP recommended be removed from the vaccine schedule after the vaccine was strongly associated with intussusception of the bowel in at least twenty infants.[5] (After its withdrawal from the market, reports of at least one hundred additional cases were made.)

Preventing extraimmunization is another reason for gaining an awareness of what vaccines your child is supposed to receive and when. Extraimmunization is a phenomenon that might occur "considerably more than previously appreciated."[6] According to Robert Davis, M.D., M.P.H., extraimmunization rates varied for each vaccine, being about 2.5 percent for measles-containing vaccine (which this author assumes to be MMR), to more than 14 percent for poliovirus vaccine (IPV or OPV not specified). Overall, a study by Suzanne Feikema and her colleagues found that 17 percent of children were extraimmunized for at least one vaccine. Interestingly, 27 percent were underimmunized for at least one vaccine. Sometimes extra- and underimmunization occurred in the same child, but for different vaccines. The authors of this study state that "little is known about the effects of receiving extra doses. The Advisory Committee on Immunization Practices (ACIP) recommends that children not receive more than 6 doses each of diphtheria and tetanus toxoids before the age of 7 years because extra doses may cause local or systemic effects. . . . It has been postulated that extra doses [of the other vaccines] are more likely to induce hypersensitivity to vaccine components."[7] (Conversely, inadequate vaccination may not confer the expected protection.) The authors speculate whether changes in immunization schedules confuse physicians, who may therefore accidentally administer too many or too few vaccines. It is up to parents who choose to vaccinate to be aware of the routine and make certain that the physician is well informed of changes in the schedule.

Robert Davis, in an editorial about that article, comments that concerns over extraimmunization should not cause parents to abandon vaccination programs and that the risk of "withholding vaccinations still far outweighs concerns about cost or the small added risk of adverse events associated with extraimmunization."[8] This may be true, but considering there has been little research done on the matter and the authors of the original article state that "little is known about the effects," I am left to wonder: From where did he draw this conclusion?

The "Vaccine-Preventable Diseases"

What follows is a discussion of the routes of exposure, symptoms, risks, and conventional prevention and treatment for what are known in the public health and medical worlds as the vaccine-preventable diseases. Alternative medical approaches to these diseases can be found in chapter 8, "Botanical Medicine, Immunity, and Illness."

MEASLES

The written history of measles can be tracked back to the writings of Persian physician Rhazes of the tenth century, and even earlier to a Hebrew physician, Al Yehudi.[9] *Rubeola* and *morbilli* were terms that first appeared in the Middle Ages, *morbilli* stemming from the Latin word for disease, *morbus*. While it was considered a minor disease, the term *measles* seems to have sprung from the Latin root *miser*, meaning miserable. The disease is caused by a spherical, single-stranded RNA virus of the morbillivirus strain, in the Paramyxoviridae family, closely related to the canine distemper virus. Prior to vaccinations it is thought that anywhere from 400,000 to 4 million cases of measles occurred annually in the United States, with approximately 450 deaths.[10] In addition there were thought to be up to 11,000 cases with seizure disorders or encephalitis, up to 25 percent of these involving permanent brain damage or deafness. By 1976 the disease incidence declined to about 30,000 cases per year with approximately 30 deaths, with about 67 percent of the population vaccinated against the disease. By 1992 there were 2,237 cases reported in the United States, with 4 deaths.[11] Disease rates have remained relatively low, with periodic epidemics occurring among both vaccinated and unvaccinated populations.

Symptoms

Measles is a highly infectious seasonal disease, appearing most commonly in late winter and early spring. It affects nearly all those who are susceptible who come in contact with it. Peak incidence is in the late winter and early spring.

Measles is transmitted person to person via large respiratory droplets and by airborne routes such as aerosol droplets; in other words, through coughing and sneezing. The interval between exposure and symptoms is nine to fourteen days. It is most contagious during the prodromal (initial) stages of the disease and is generally considered to be contagious for two to four days before the onset of the rash and for four days after the rash appears.

The prodromal stage, which lasts for about two to four days, has symptoms comparable to those of other typical upper respiratory infections, with fever, malaise, runny nose, cough, and conjunctivitis. The fever normally stays in the range or 101 to 103 degrees Fahrenheit at this stage.

Koplik's spots, distinctive small white spots that appear on the insides of the cheeks, appear about two days before rash onset and persist for one to two more days after the rash is noticeable, during which time the fever may get as high as 105 degrees Fahrenheit. The measles rash appears fourteen days after exposure, beginning at the head (over the face, forehead, hairline, ears, and neck) and spreading from there to the extremities over the next three to four days. Initially the rash blanches on pressure, but after a few days it turns into a contiguous brownish rash that does not blanch. The rash may itch considerably. There is also likely to be appetite loss, diarrhea, and generalized swelling of the lymph nodes, as well as a cough and extreme sensitivity to light (photophobia). Typically the fever subsides as the rash fades, taking up to four or five days. This leaves the child feeling much more comfortable. The disease generally runs its course in ten days; hence it was often referred to as "ten-day measles."

Atypical measles is a form of the diease that can occur in those previously vaccinated with killed measles virus, no longer in use in the United States. It is a severe form of the disease that generally presents with fever, headache, and stomach pain and an unusual rash that appears at the extremities and progresses toward the head. Severe complications, especially pneumonia, may result, and fatality is much higher in atypical cases.

Risks and Complications

The complications associated with measles are otitis media, pneumonia, postinfection encephalitis, hearing loss (generally unilateral but can be bilateral), subsclerosing panencephalitis (SSPE, which occurs seven years after a measles infection), and death. Encephalitis is a serious complication, and though rare, it results in a death rate of one in eight who develop it, and 50 percent of those with encephalitis suffer some permanent central nervous system damage.

The remainder, however, recover completely. SSPE is a rare (less than 1 in 100,000 cases) degenerative disease of the central nervous system caused by a defective version of the measles virus that causes persistent measles infection. It will be discussed further in the chapter on vaccines and adverse reactions. Pneumonia is more likely to occur in young children, whereas acute encephalitis is more common in adults. Swelling of the trachea and glottis are also possible. In recent national outbreaks, measles morbidity requiring hospitalization approached 30 percent of all cases, which is quite high. Permanent damage was low, however, and most of the morbidity was for ear infections and respiratory infections.

Figures vary on how many children are expected to experience serious complications in a measles outbreak, and most are based on prevaccine numbers or statistics from developing nations, the latter of which are likely to be significantly higher than in the United States or other developed nations. Today, improved medical care significantly reduces the likelihood of incurring permanent damage from measles infection.

While the disease may be considered devastating in developing nations, where it carries a mortality rate as high as 10 percent, it is generally a mild disease in developed nations, with complications being more the exception than the rule, particularly in healthy children. In developed nations, "while serious complications occur, they are relatively rare compared with the situation in developing nations. . . . Malnutrition is also an important factor leading to the marked severity of measles in the developing areas of the world because of defects in cellular, and possibly humoral, immunity."[12] Furthermore, "crowding, with exposure to an increased dose of virus, may be the most significant and important factor, determinant of the severity of infection."[13]

Experiencing natural measles nearly always confers permanent immunity to the disease. James Cherry, a pediatrics professor and prolific author of provaccine articles, sums up quite nicely the risks of measles for those susceptible: "As long as they stay in this country, these susceptibles will be relatively safe—probably increasingly so as more and more children are immunized."[14] The risk for these children, he says, is in travel to areas with endemic or epidemic measles, where they themselves might contract it, or they might expose others to it upon return from their journey.

Conventional Treatment

Typical measles treatment consists primarily of keeping the child comfortable, maintaining bed rest, and providing quiet activities to help pass the time. Plenty of rest and fluids are very important. For children with photophobia, their room should be kept only dimly lit. Eye secretions from conjunctivitis should be cleansed with warm water (or saline), and tepid baths and agents to reduce fever are often given. Medication for itching can be applied to the skin, and a humidifier can be used to reduce cough and nasal congestion. Of course, complications must be treated as needed, and in such cases hospitalization may be required.

Antibiotics are not effective against measles, as it is a viral infection; however, physicians may prescribe antibiotics in the event of a secondary infection. Acetaminophen (for example, Tylenol) or ibuprofen (for example, Advil) may be given to control fever, but aspirin should never be given to children suspected of having measles, as it can lead to a serious complication known as Reye's syndrome.

Food for Thought

In the prevaccine era, measles was expected to affect nearly every member of the population before the end of childhood. It was very rare in children under a year, as they maintained passive immunity from their time in utero and from breast-feeding. With the advent of vaccines, the epidemiology of the disease shifted so that more cases occurred in late adolescence, when the disease is more likely to have devastating effects. Clinical surveys show that prior to the vaccine era, at least 95 percent of Americans had measles by age fifteen, and serological studies of young adults entering military service showed that 99 percent previously had measles. In the prevaccine era the highest incidence of disease was among five- to nine-year-olds, and the next highest was in those under five. Fewer than 10 percent of cases occurred in children over age ten, and 3 percent in those over age fifteen.[15]

In 1933 A. W. Hedrich published a major study on patterns of measles in Baltimore, Maryland, from 1900 to 1931, concluding that when 68 percent of the population under fifteen years of age was immune to measles, epidemics didn't occur.[16] In measles outbreaks in 1976 and 1977, however, as many as 60 percent of cases occurred in children over age ten, and 26 percent of cases occurred in those over age fifteen, demonstrating a clear epidemiological shift in the disease.[17] A combination of a partially unvaccinated population along with primary vaccine failure and waning immunity contribute to susceptibility in older populations.[18]

Measles Today

National Public Radio recently (June 30, 2000) broadcast the news that measles is no longer endemic in the United States. *Endemic*, according to *Taber's*

Cyclopedic Medical Dictionary (fifteenth edition), means "A disease that occurs in a particular population, but has low mortality, *as measles*" (emphasis mine). Interesting that measles would be the example given. Okay, so measles is no longer endemic, nor epidemic. Indeed, according to public radio spokespersons, new cases are a result of exposure to imported measles, meaning someone returning from travel abroad or emigrating to the United States brought measles with them. So what does this mean for routine measles vaccinations?

This change in disease status is considered tremendous progress in medicine, attributable to a long-term and successful vaccine campaign against measles virus, which might now allow us to discontinue this routine medical practice, as we eventually did with smallpox vaccine (thirty years after the disease was eradicated!). But this is not the case, and indeed we are told we must be sure to maintain high levels of measles vaccinations. Looking at the definition of endemic, then, I wonder at the logic of creating the need to vaccinate forever against a disease that is given as the example of one that has low mortality and is no longer considered a menacing presence in our society. Granted, there can be severe consequences to measles virus infection, especially in those who contract it post–elementary school age. But these are rare, and it has been the use of the vaccine that has raised the incidence of disease in the most at-risk populations while decreasing it in the lowest-risk populations. Conversely, in a population where measles occurs periodically it usually does little lasting damage and confers permanent immunity long before puberty. Now women who have been vaccinated can no longer confer natural immunity against measles virus to their babies, and college students must be revaccinated. If nobody gets the measles naturally anymore, we may be summoning a future measles disaster, as none of our population will have natural immunity. If the disease is truly no longer endemic, then must we continue to vaccinate children against the possibility of imported cases? It was emphasized in the NPR report that now we must keep vaccination rates consistently high in order to prevent measles from reemerging.

MUMPS

Mumps is an acute, contagious viral infection affecting the salivary glands, caused by a member of the paramyxovirus family. Humans are the only known host for this organism. Mumps was first described by Hippocrates in the fifth century B.C.E., and the name "mumps" is thought to have been derived from the Old English verb, which meant to grimace or mumble, perhaps describing the patient's facial expression or efforts to talk with a swollen jaw.[19] Generally there is painful swelling in one or both of the parotid glands (the disease is also known as parotitis), the salivary glands located on the jaw beneath the ear.

Mumps is spread by contact with infected saliva and respiratory secretions. The incubation period is twelve to twenty-five days, though usually eighteen days, and a child is contagious for approximately a week before symptoms begin until about nine days after the glands have become swollen. It most commonly occurs in children ages five through fifteen and is more frequent in boys.

Symptoms

The onset of mumps is gradual, with the initial symptoms being chills, fever, malaise, headache, appetite loss, and aching muscles. Pain beneath the ears and under the jaw begins about twenty-four hours after these other symptoms, after which the salivary glands can become extremely sore and swollen. Often the swelling in one gland begins to subside just as the other begins to swell. The earlobe may be pushed forward owing to the swelling, and the surrounding area may be quite distorted from the swelling. Jaw movement may be extremely painful, making eating and drinking difficult. Salivation may be increased or diminished. In one-third of all cases, no parotid swelling occurs. Swelling generally lasts for about a week or just under. Fever is moderate, ranging between 101 and 102 degrees Fahrenheit (38.3 to 38.9 degrees Celsius), though it may occasionally become higher than this. Approximately 30 percent of all mumps infections are asymptomatic and unapparent by serological testing.

Risks and Complications

Mumps is considered to be a mild disease of childhood, with mumps-related complications being rare.[20] Though it is well recognized that mumps is generally harmless and that natural infection confers permanent immunity, the occasional severe complication led to the use of the mumps vaccine. Complications that may occur as a result of mumps infection include deafness, myocarditis, pericarditis, arthritis, postinfectious encephalitis, mastitis, nephritis, hepatitis, thyroiditis, and thrombocytopenia. It is remotely suspected that there may be a connection between mumps infection and diabetes mellitus, testicular and ovarian tumors, Guillain-Barré syndrome, and several other unusual conditions; however, such associations are not definitive.

Encephalitis, meningitis, and meningoencephalitis occurred at a rate of 2 to 4 cases per 1,000 mumps cases between 1960 and 1968, as reported to the CDC; however, distinction is rarely made between the dangerous forms of meningitis and the disease known as aseptic meningitis, which is generally self-limiting and rarely leaves permanent damage. In most cases where there is central nervous system involvement, the outcome is excellent. Possible permanent problems can include deafness (usually in one ear only), facial paralysis, transverse myelitis, and psychomotor dysfunction.

About 20 percent of males that contract mumps past puberty will develop orchitis, inflammation of a testis. It is almost always unilateral and rarely leads to sterility problems.[21] Orchitis has also been detected in children as young as three years old. Symptoms of orchitis include swelling and severe pain of the testis. Approximately a third to half of patients with orchitis will have some degree of testicular atrophy, but even this does not automatically mean that sterility will be the consequence. Females with mumps may develop inflamed ovaries, but no connection has been found between this and impairment of fertility.

Conventional Treatment
Treatment simply consists of bed rest, a soft diet, and medications for headaches and general discomfort. Local cold packs are applied to control swelling of the testicles if necessary. Complications, of course, are treated as appropriate.

Food for Thought
Mumps is rarely a serious disease, with 30 percent of all cases being asymptomatic, yet we routinely vaccinate all children for it. As with measles, though to a lesser extent, mumps infection has shifted from a disease of early childhood to a greater incidence in children over ten, when complications, if they are going to occur, are most likely.

RUBELLA

Rubella virus, a cubical, medium-sized lipid-enveloped virus with an RNA genome belonging to the togavirus family, was discovered in the late 1700s but didn't gain in importance until the 1940s. The term *rubella* means "little red" and the disease was named thus by a British physician describing an outbreak in a boy's school in India in 1841.[22]

It is primarily spread through the respiratory tract, particularly the nose and throat. It is likely that some people shed the virus in greater quantity than others and are thus highly infectious. Prior to vaccinations, rubella was both endemic and epidemic, occurring primarily in the spring among children six to ten years old and occasionally in older children. There were also major epidemics every seven years. Unlike measles virus, which will cause infection in most susceptible individuals, many individuals will not contract rubella in an epidemic and will therefore remain susceptible. However, in crowded environments and close quarters (for example, day care centers, army barracks) most of the susceptible population will become infected.

The significance of rubella is not in its effects in the childhood population but in its potential to cause congenital rubella syndrome (CRS) in unborn babies whose mothers are exposed during pregnancy. CRS can lead to a number of serious birth defects—particularly if the mother was exposed during her first trimester—including, but not limited to, mental retardation, deafness, blindness, cataracts, autism, cardiac anomalies, and intrauterine growth retardation. Rubella vaccination has played a tremendous role in decreasing the incidence of CRS in the population since the 1960s. In 1969 there were 57,686 cases of rubella reported in the United States (the highest number recorded in one year); this number was down to 160 cases with one death by 1992. However, in 1994 there were more than 200 cases, with 75 percent of these occurring in adults over twenty years old.[23]

Symptoms

The incubation period for rubella is fourteen to twenty-one days. It causes a mild generalized infection with symptoms such as slight fever, sore throat, mild conjunctivitis, and drowsiness. The superficial glands of the neck and behind the ear may be slightly enlarged. The rash erupts on the first or second day and may possess either a pale red, scarcely elevated appearance or a bright red appearance. The rash begins on the face and spreads quickly over the whole body. The rash also fades so quickly that the face may no longer have a rash by the time the extremities do. It may be difficult even to detect the rash other than when the child has just been in a hot bath or shower. The skin may peel slightly, but this is not always the case. The entire illness lasts only three to five days. Childhood infection with rubella is often asymptomatic and therefore likely to go unnoticed.

Risks and Complications

Arthralgia and arthritis are commonly observed in adults who contract rubella. Rarely, thrombocytopenia and encephalitis may occur as complications. The greatest risk is to nonimmune pregnant women who transmit the disease transplacentally to the fetus. This may result in a first-trimester miscarriage, or the pregnancy may continue, and in most cases some degree of CRS results. After the first trimester, exposure results in no other complications than deafness. In 1964 to 1965 an outbreak occurred with an estimated 12.5 million cases. Five thousand women had surgical abortions, 6,250 had miscarriages,

2,100 infants died at birth, and 20,000 babies who survived had CRS. Prior to vaccine use, 5 percent of the population was involved in epidemics, with approximately 60 babies in a nonepidemic year sustaining CRS damage.

Conventional Treatment

As rubella is generally so mild an infection, there is no specific treatment for normal cases of rubella in children other than to control the itching associated with the rash, provide fluids, encourage rest, and give tepid sponge baths.

Food for Thought

The reduction in CRS as a result of the rubella vaccine seems evident. However, it is readily acknowledged that the rubella vaccine provides a quickly waning immunity. Thus, the susceptibility rates of women of childbearing age to the virus may be comparable to rates from prevaccine years.[24] The improvement, therefore, is not in increased immunity in the childbearing population but in decreased incidence in children, lessening opportunities for exposure of pregnant women. However, waning immunity can also mean that women, having never contracted rubella as children because they were vaccinated, enter their childbearing years with no protection from the vaccine and without natural immunity to the virus. This is a problem that has led to recommendations in many countries for the revaccination of preadolescent females. Furthermore, it has been recommended that all hospital personnel in regular contact with pregnant women (for example, obstetricians, obstetric nurses) be revaccinated so that they are not carriers of rubella. Most obstetricians, however, refuse to be revaccinated for rubella, in spite of low serologic evidence of immunity.[25]

DIPHTHERIA

Diphtheria is now a rare disease in the United States. It is caused by a toxin produced by the bacterium *Corynebacterium diphtheriae*, a gram-positive bacillus, and not the bacteria itself. The disease was described by Hippocrates in the fifth century B.C.E., who documented what may have been the first recognized case.[26] After this time, only isolated reports of the disease appear until the seventeenth century, at which time it became a traumatic illness that occurred in outbreaks throughout southwestern Europe. These outbreaks occurred every twelve years well into the eighteenth century. The disease was first noted in the United States in New York in 1771. In temperate climates the disease can occur year-round, but it is most common in the autumn and winter months.

It is now virtually eliminated in the United States, with only eighteen cases reported between 1980 and 1986, and four cases in the United States in 1992.[27] Before 1900 in the United States, the most comprehensive epidemiological data on the incidence of diphtheria comes from Massachusetts, where between 1860 and 1897 the mortality rates from the disease were between approximately 50 and 200 per 100,000 annually. A significant decrease in the incidence of diphtheria was occurring between 1900 and 1930, with a 90 percent reduction.[28]

By 1900, prior to the introduction of the vaccine, the death rate was down to 20 to 25 per 100,000 annually. Some say this is attributable to improved hygiene and sanitation, others attribute it to the introduction of the diphtheria antitoxin. Prior to the use of the antitoxin, case fatality rates were around 50 percent and by World War I were down to approximately 15 percent. However, the greatest drop recorded occurred between 1865 and 1875, prior even to the isolation of the diphtheria bacillus.[29]

Humans are the only host, and the bacteria are spread person to person via direct physical contact and exposure to contaminated articles belonging to an infected person. Coughing and sneezing can also spread the disease, and the disease can be carried by a person who appears entirely healthy. The organism is hardy for several hours outside the respiratory tract, but indirect contact does not appear to lead to infection.

Some researchers claim that after the introduction of the compulsory diphtheria vaccine in Germany and France, the incidence of the disease skyrocketed.[30] Norway, which refused the compulsory vaccine campaign, had only 50 cases in 1943, while nearby Germany had 150,000 cases and France experienced 47,000 cases.

Symptoms

Diphtheria causes an inflammation of the membranes of the upper respiratory tract, particularly the pharynx, larynx, trachea, and posterior nasal passages. A form of diphtheria can also affect the skin. The symptoms of classic diphtheria begin after an incubation period of one to five days. The initial symptoms are mild, with slight fever rarely rising above 101.3 degrees Fahrenheit (38.5 degrees Celsius) throughout the course of the disease, and a headache and sore throat often occurring at the outset. Children typically display malaise and irritability. About a day after the fever begins, small patches of pus appear on the back of the throat, and within two to three days this spreads, forming a contiguous membrane that may cover a significant area. This yellowish or grayish membrane is firmly attached; the lymph nodes at the front of the neck become enlarged, and a "bull-neck" appearance arises from swelling and inflammation. In cases of diphtheria in which only the area behind the nasal passages is infected by a false membrane, the predominant symptom is fever. There may be a strong, putrid odor of the breath. The membrane begins to slough off approximately a week after the onset of symptoms. This may occur in pieces or as a whole membrane. At this point the acute symptoms begin to abate, but there is danger of aspiration of the membrane.

Pharyngeal diphtheria is the most common form of this disease in unvaccinated groups, occurring in 75 percent of all cases. The other 25 percent of cases lead to laryngeal involvement. In a very small number of cases (2 percent) there is involvement of the skin, ear canal, vagina, or conjunctiva. Laryngeal cases are the most dangerous, as death can occur from obstruction of the respiratory passages.

Because diphtheria is so uncommon in the United States, its diagnosis could easily be missed, leading to delay in important early treatment. Therefore it is essential, particularly if your child is unvaccinated, that you be aware of the symptoms of diphtheria and raise this possible diagnosis to a physician should you ever suspect that your child has this disease.

Risks and Complications

The acute phase of diphtheria is generally uneventful, mostly being very unpleasant, though local acute damage can occur. The risks are by far the greatest in relation to damage caused by the toxin in other areas of the body, which can lead to serious damage to the cardiovascular and nervous systems. Damage to the nervous system might not become evident until as much as three to ten weeks after the infection began. Organ damage can result in mortality, but neuropathy generally resolves itself spontaneously, as does myocarditis, when the patient survives the disease. Death is most common in the very old and very young, though the disease rarely occurs in children under one year of age. Without medical treatment, the incidence of nervous system damage and death is high. Complications and death rates are directly related to the speed at which diagnosis is made and treatment is begun.

Conventional Treatment

The general treatment calls for strict bed rest during both the acute and the convalescent stages of the illness—keeping in mind that complications can occur many weeks after the acute stage. When there is myocardial involvement, bed rest is critical to positive outcome and may be as significant as early antitoxin therapy.[31] The diet must be very soft, with as much of it as possible liquid, and should consist of nourishing broth, water, and fruit juices. Medical treatment includes the administration of diphtheria toxoid and erythromycin or penicillin for prophylaxis, while then keeping the patient under close watch for seven days. Diphtheria antitoxin is given when the patient cannot be kept under observation.

If diphtheria is suspected, diphtheria antitoxin should be administered as soon as possible, preferably even before waiting for the results of throat cultures to return. The membrane that has formed should not be disturbed, as this could lead to unnecessary damage and bleeding. Gargling should not be done, though the mouth may be rinsed and nasal discharges may be suctioned.

Surgical intervention may be necessary in the case of laryngeal diphtheria, and intubation or tracheotomy may need to be performed. Medications for complicated cardiac arrhythmias may need to be used if this occurs.

Food for Thought

Because diphtheria toxoid was introduced before the days of clinical trials, and its benefits seemed so evident, diphtheria toxoid has never been subjected to controlled clinical trials that would be acceptable by contemporary standards.[32] The disease is considered milder with fewer complications when it occurs in those who are partially or completely vaccinated; however, according to Plotkin and Mortimer, "in the past in the absence of vaccination, most acquired immunity to the disease without experiencing clinical diphtheria." Antitoxin immunity is present at birth owing to maternal antibodies and diminishes by six to twelve months of age. In nonvaccinated populations, 75 percent or more of the population is again immune by late childhood, owing to the commonness of subclinical infection.[33] The diphtheria vaccine is considered 87 percent effective in conferring immunity.[34]

PERTUSSIS (WHOOPING COUGH)

Pertussis, also known as whooping cough because of the characteristic cough that develops in the middle stage of this infection, is caused by *Bordetella pertussis*, a small, gram-negative bacillus. The disease is generally caused by close respiratory contact rather than airborne exposure. It was once a major cause of morbidity and mortality in childhood, with more than 250,000 cases and 7,518 fatalities in the United States in 1934. The reported number of cases began to decline dramatically by 1930, prior to the introduction of the vaccine, and this was accelerated after the vaccine's introduction in the 1940s.[35] The rates of pertussis in the United States are currently 3,000 to 7,000 cases annually, with 5 to 20 fatalities. It is thought, however, that the incidence of whooping cough may be grossly underreported, which may primarily be due to poor detection.[36] While the disease is rarely fatal anymore, it can be serious or even life-threatening in those under six months old. The epidemiology of the disease has changed since the introduction of the vaccine, with the highest occurrence previously being among one- to four-year-olds but with infants under one year having the highest incidence now.[37] Pertussis is an endemic disease that causes outbreaks every three to five years. "Widespread immunisation of children does not appear to have altered these intervals."[38] Immunity from vaccination is less dependable than that from natural disease. Adolescents and adults may be frequent and unwitting carriers of the disease, passing it on unsuspectingly to younger children.[39]

Symptoms

The incubation period for pertussis is nine to twenty days, with initial symptoms being no more dramatic than those of a simple upper respiratory infection. In fact, the initial symptoms may be no more than a persistent dry cough that leads the parents to think the child simply has an allergy.[40] The illness is typically divided into three stages as follows:

Stage 1: One to two weeks: there is difficulty breathing, cough, and sometimes fever.

Stage 2: Two to three weeks: severe paroxysmal coughing attacks; this is the most severe and potentially dangerous stage.

Stage 3: Coughing begins to diminish and recovery commences.

Complete recovery from whooping cough can take two to three months, leading it to be referred to as "the hundred-days illness." Traditional Chinese medicine terms this disease "the cough of enlightenment."

During the full-blown stage of the disease, the paroxysmal coughing can be quite dramatic, occurring as frequently as thirty times in a day and causing the child to appear as if he or she will collapse from lack of breath. The face may turn red or blue, and the child may vomit at the end of the coughing fits. The characteristic whooping sound is caused by air being forced through the glottis, which becomes narrowed from inflammation. The child is likely to be exhausted by coughing fits, though in milder cases the child may simply resume activities as before the coughing fit. Some children, however, are fine for most of the day and appear normal between coughing bouts. For many children, the coughing fits are worst at night, preventing both the child and the parents from getting much-needed sleep. Dehydration can occur from frequent vomiting and prolonged fever, and lack of nutrition is common owing to difficulty with eating. The coughing may be so severe and the mucus so thick and abundant that the child may appear to be drowning during coughing episodes.

Risks and Complications

The complications associated with pertussis in well-nourished, generally healthy populations are infrequent. Minor complications that can occur include subconjunctival hemorrhages and nosebleeds that result from coughing fits. Facial swelling, ulcers under the tongue, and otitis media may also occur. Serious complications, which may lead to fatality, include those of the pulmonary system, such as bronchopneumonia, plus encephalitis, seizures, and nutritional problems because of difficulty eating solid foods. Eating generally leads to coughing, and this is followed by vomiting, severely compromising nutrition. Encephalitis complications and seizures can lead to death or permanent brain damage. Such complications are most common, though not exclusive, to those under four years of age who contract the disease. While encephalopathy was thought to occur in only 47 of 6,002 cases of whooping cough between the years 1932 and 1946, it is thought that approximately one-third of cases of encephalopathy will lead to fatality and one-third will lead to permanent damage. The others will recover without residual damage.

Conventional Treatment

There is evidence that giving antibiotics in the initial stages of the disease may prevent infection or reduce its severity, and this is therefore the treatment of choice if pertussis is recognized early. Once the coughing has set in, antibiotic therapy does not reduce the disease, as the paroxysms are caused not by the bacteria but by a toxin produced by the bacteria that causes the irritation. Once into this stage, comfort measures to reduce coughing, aid in the expectoration of phlegm, and maintainence of general immunity and nutrition are all that can be done.

Should complications arise, appropriate medical treatment should be initiated.

Food for Thought

Pertussis has become a generally self-limiting disease that causes discomfort and inconvenience but little damage in a well-nourished, healthy population. It also confers permanent immunity. More than any other vaccine, the whole-cell pertussis vaccine is associated with serious side effects and consequences, and the acellular vaccine recently put into use in the United States may not be entirely safe either. There are divergent opinions on the current use of pertussis vaccine as represented by the opposing sentiments reflected in Edward Mortimer's chapter on the pertussis vaccine in *Vaccines:*

> There is no question that the development and widespread use of the pertussis vaccine in developed countries have been associated with a remarkable decline in morbidity and mortality from the disease. However, it is also clear that in several of these countries, mortality rates from pertussis were declining even before the advent of the vaccine. Indeed, in the United States, infant mortality from pertussis declined 70% from 1900–04 to 1935–39. In England and Wales infant mortality from pertussis declined approximately 90% from 1918 to 1948 before widespread use of the vaccine. . . . The explanation for this decrease in case-mortality rates is not clear but may include such factors as improved social and economic conditions; better nutrition; decline in other debilitating conditions of childhood such as diarrhea; . . . quarantine measures and lower birth rates. . . . The decline in pertussis-related mortality prior to the institution of widespread immunization has led some researchers to argue that pertussis vaccine is currently superfluous and that it should be abandoned except for high-risk groups.[41]

In direct opposition to this view is evidence that in developed nations that called a moratorium on the use of pertussis vaccine owing to the frequency and potential severity of side effects, pertussis rates—and mortalities—increased. In Japan, England and Wales, and Sweden, rates of pertussis that had been as low as 400 cases with 10 fatalities climbed to as high as 10,000 cases with as may as 113 fatalities in Japan, and 40 fatalities in Britain.[42] Clearly, the vaccine confers some measure of protection against the disease, but some researchers question at what cost.

TETANUS

Tetanus infection is caused by the agent *Clostridium tetani*, a gram-positive, spore-forming, anaerobic bacillus that produces one of the most potent neurotoxins known. Tetanus was first described in the medical writings of Hippocrates, but the cause was not recognized until the late nineteenth century. It is a strict anaerobe, meaning it cannot multiply in oxygen-containing environments. The spores are extremely hardy and may persist in the soil for months—even years. They can survive boiling and many disinfectant treatments.[43] The manure of horses and other mammalian farm animals, as well as dogs, guinea pigs, and even some smaller animals, is contaminated by tetanus, which lives in the intestines and mouths of these animals. The proverbial "rusty nail" associated with causing tetanus likely refers to nails used to shoe horses, which were commonly found in horse pastures, where they may have become contaminated (anyone who keeps horses knows how regularly they lose their shoes). However, rusty nails do not automatically transmit tetanus, though they can cause nasty puncture wounds that could be suspect. Puncture wounds, because they are difficult to clean and expose to air, can easily harbor tetanus infection and therefore require special attention.

Tetanus spores have been found in samples of street dust and in hospital operating rooms and can be present in products that are soil based, such as clay.[44] Indeed, in 1999 two babies born in the United States who had green clay applied to the umbilicus as a natural treatment after birth developed tetanus. Both recovered and suffered no permanent damage, though hospitalization and medication were required. In the United States, tetanus has been primarily a disease prevalent in the Southeast, but spores have been located across the nation, with no specific pattern. Tetanus appears to have a propensity for nutrient-rich soils with an alkaline pH, in warm, moist climates.

Tetanus infection can occur with even mild wounds that go unnoticed, such as a cut while gardening or a slight splinter (up to 50 percent of cases); it is considered more likely to occur when there has been acute trauma, especially puncture wounds or lacerations, leading to anaerobic conditions that allow the spores to grow and the organism to reproduce.[45] The bacillus produces a toxin known as tetanospasmin, which acts on the central nervous system and leads to muscle rigidity and paralysis. In developing nations, tetanus neonatorum, tetanus infection in the newborn, is still a leading cause of death in children under one year. It is caused by traditional treatments generally containing animal dung, which are applied to the umbilicus of the newborn.

Broadscale use of tetanus vaccine among American soldiers in 1941 led to significant declines in wartime cases of tetanus as compared with rates from World War I. World War I rates were 700 cases per 520,000 wounded; World War II rates were 12 cases per 2.73 million wounded. The British military showed a similar decline in cases.[46] In both countries, however, rates were thought to be declining significantly long before the introduction of vaccines, because of improved hygiene and wound care. In fact, proper hygiene and wound care are very important in reducing the likelihood of tetanus infection.

Symptoms

Incubation can be from one day to several weeks, generally occurring between the third day and third week after exposure to the spores. The closer the injury is to the central nervous system, the quicker the disease manifests and the more severe it tends to be. Therefore, head, neck, and face injuries tend to manifest within a week and may be the most devastating. Wounds may or may not be accompanied by visible signs of infection or tissue damage. Wounds that develop tetanus tend to be severe; however, even minor punctures such as a splinter can lead to tetanus infection. There seems to be some relationship between the length of time between inoculation with the spores and appearance of symptoms and the severity of the disease. In other words, the longer the incubation period, the less severe the disease tends to be, though survival rates are not necessarily increased.[47]

The most common initial symptom of tetanus is lockjaw, a tightening or spasming of the muscles that control chewing, present in more than 50 percent of all cases. Fever may be present, and there may also be headache, irritability, and chills. A spasming of the facial muscles may then occur, leading to a peculiar expression with raised eyebrows, tightly shut eyelids, wrinkled forehead, and extended corners of the mouth (known as risus sardonicus).

Other muscles may also be involved, causing changes in posture, with rigidity of the back, extremities, and abdominal muscles. Seizures, during which there may be slightly elevated temperature, may be triggered by sudden sounds, movements, or changes in lighting. Mental functioning, however, is not altered. Spasm of the respiratory muscles can cause sudden death from asphyxia.

In newborns, symptoms generally begin two to fourteen days after the birth and include poor sucking and excessive crying, with other previously described symptoms following to some extent.

The disease typically remains acute for between one and four weeks, then gradually diminishes. Death rates vary from 25 percent to 70 percent, but with high-quality medical care, mortality can be as low as 10 to 20 percent.[48] Most of the cases of tetanus in the United States occur in those over fifty years old, and predominantly in women, presumably because of waning immunity or lack of vaccination.

Risks and Complications

While tetanus infection is currently rare in the United States, when infection occurs it carries a high mortality rate on an individual case basis. According to Neustaedter, however, during 1982 to 1984, when a total of six cases occurred in the United States in children and adolescents, there were no fatalities.[49] One U.S. physician, an early believer in alternative and complementary medicine, remarked to me in the mid-1980s that he drew his line of radicalism at tetanus vaccination, which he considered crucial. He told me that one of the worst experiences he ever had as a medical student was observing a patient

74

with tetanus. It is considered, even by many vaccine critics, to be the most benign of vaccines, though complications have been known to occur. Reactions are typically mild and of short duration.

Conventional Treatment

Treatment for tetanus infection is aggressive and intense, consisting of giving the patient a dose of Tetanus Human Immune Globulin (THIG), debriding the wound (removing any tissue in the vicinity of the injury that might be damaged or infected), and giving muscle relaxants to control spasms. The environment must be kept calm, with no sudden sounds, changes in lighting, or sudden movements that might trigger spasms. Assisted ventilation may be necessary if there is involvement of the respiratory muscles. Appropriate nutrition must also be maintained.

Horse serum THIG is best avoided if possible, as it is associated with a much higher rate of reactions than the human THIG. Neither THIG nor tetanus infection confers future immunity.

Food for Thought

Tetanus vaccine spores are present in the environment, and the disease attacks healthy children. Parents will have to weigh the unlikely risk of contracting this disease against the unlikely risk of a vaccine reaction, keeping in mind the very serious nature of this illness. Because children play outside and regularly sustain cuts and scrapes, this can potentially be a great source of anxiety for the parents of unvaccinated children. Subsequent chapters will look at vaccine risks and wound care. In any case, recognizing the symptoms of tetanus and seeking medical care immediately should this condition be suspected is critical to your child's well-being.

POLIO

Poliomyelitis can be caused by one of three infectious strains of the poliovirus, and it is an acute infectious disease that takes its toll on the central nervous system. It is transmitted person to person through respiratory and fecal-oral contamination routes, in the latter case including contamination from changing the soiled diapers of a baby who has recently been vaccinated with the live oral polio vaccine (OPV). Outbreaks have historically occurred primarily during the summer and early autumn in the Northern Hemisphere, and primarily in industrialized nations. Winter outbreaks there are extremely rare, but outbreaks occur year-round in tropical areas.

The disease affects all age groups, but children are more vulnerable. It is thought that adults are more likely to have acquired some measure of immunity. Passive immunity may be strong until six months of age from maternal antibodies acquired prenatally. As discussed in previous chapters, it was not considered problematic until the late eighteenth and early nineteenth centuries.[50] Even during massive epidemics, however, most cases remained subclinical, with fewer than 1 percent of the population evidencing paralytic forms.

As with other infectious diseases, rates of polio were fast declining prior to the introduction of the vaccine, and the history of the vaccine itself is filled with stories of trial and error, successes and paralytic reactions. Nonetheless, outbreaks of polio in the United States have not occurred since the widespread use of the vaccine, though all new cases of the disease in more than thirty years have been directly related to the use of OPV. The Centers for Disease Control and the American Academy of Pediatrics have recently recommended that OPV be used only in special circumstances and that the inactivated polio vaccine (IPV) be used instead. Polio is rare in the Western Hemisphere, though it still occurs worldwide.

Symptoms

As stated earlier, poliovirus infection is generally asymptomatic. When infection does occur, it is likely to manifest in one of the following three ways, after an incubation period of seven to fourteen days:

1. *Minor illness.* There are a few days of mild illness with symptoms of fever, malaise, drowsiness, headache, nausea, vomiting, constipation, sore throat, or some combination of these symptoms.

2. *Aseptic meningitis.* There are symptoms of fever, headache, malaise, nausea, and abdominal pain, followed a couple of days later by stiff neck and back, possibly with vomiting, which last two to ten days before disappearing completely. In a small number of cases there is temporary mild muscle weakness or paralysis.

3. *Paralytic poliomyelitis.* Either following the symptoms just described (especially in young children) or suddenly, paralysis, sometimes severe, with loss of muscle tone occurs. If there is brain involvement, there may also be painful spasms in nonparalyzed muscles.[51] Paralysis can last for months, with severe residual weakness lasting much longer. In severe cases, paralytic involvement of the respiratory muscles can lead to the need for aggressive intervention and may be fatal.

Wild polio generally affects varying age groups as follows:

- Children under five years of age generally develop paralysis or weakness in one leg.

- Those aged five to fifteen develop weakness of one arm, or a leg and arm.

- Adults are the most likely to develop paralysis of both legs and arms, with bladder paralysis and respiratory complications most frequent in this age group.[52]

Risks and Complications

Widespread polio outbreaks in the 1940s and 1950s left a mark of fear on our nation and others who experienced the devastating effects of this disease, though the complications associated with this disease "are surprisingly few."[53] The most poignant memory for many seems to be the iron lungs, assisted ventilation chambers for those who experienced respiratory paralysis. Those crippled by the disease, which can cause deformity due to atrophy of various muscle groups, as well as their friends, neighbors, and family members, were not spared from the impression that poliomyelitis can be a devastating illness. Even when paralysis does occur, 50 percent of cases recover completely, and another 25 percent have only mild residual paralysis.[54] Death is rare and occurs when there is respiratory involvement. When we consider that fewer than 1 percent of a population experienced symptomatic cases, this seems a small number, but it must be remembered that even 0.5 percent of several million is a statistically significant number of people. Nonetheless, as we will see in later chapters, the live vaccine itself has also contributed to the ongoing exposure of the American public to this disease. Although only small numbers of people have contracted the disease from the vaccine, these have been the only new cases of this disease in the United States in more than three decades—also a significant fact.

Postpolio syndrome has been shown to occur in individuals years after paralytic poliomyelitis. It is thought that aging exacerbates muscle weakness from the initial infection, with this problem affecting as many as 25 percent of the 300,000 people who had paralytic polio in the 1940s and 1950s.[55]

Conventional Treatment

Bed rest is recommended during the acute phase of the illness, and gentle massage and range-of-motion exercise can be done to relieve muscle pain and keep the body in proper alignment. Hot baths and hot packs can be given, as can analgesics or mild sedatives to keep anxiety at bay and promote calm. Emotional support is very important as well, as paralysis is difficult to cope with for most patients. Patients with polio must be observed closely for respiratory problems, and a clear airway must be maintained. Oxygen is provided as needed, and emergency measures for maintaining an airway should be on hand.

Food for Thought

It is interesting to note that there are several predisposing factors to poliomyelitis during outbreaks, including tonsillectomy and other surgeries to the nose and throat such as removal of the adenoids (with tonsillectomy, quite popular in the 1950s), routine vaccinations, excessive physical exertion, and fatigue, with pregnant women having a higher rate of susceptibility as well.[56]

Given that polio is no longer considered a threat in Western nations, and that the only incidences of the disease in the United States are currently vaccine related (with the OPV vaccine being discontinued only in the past year), the choice of whether to vaccinate for polio must be weighed against the odds of contracting the disease in individual circumstances. Clearly, the choice of using IPV is superior to OPV.

CHICKEN POX

While it has long been known that chicken pox, caused by a member of the varicella family of viruses, can lead to complications, it is considered a mild, albeit uncomfortable, reality of childhood that confers lifelong immunity. In recent years, however, since the introduction of the varicella vaccine, the disease has been treated with a more serious tone. There are even television commercials extolling the hazards of natural chicken pox infection, encouraging parents to be certain they vaccinate their children against this potentially dreadful illness.

According to the package insert for the Merck Varivax, Varicella Live Virus Vaccine, "Varicella is a highly communicable disease in children, adolescents, and adults caused by the varicella-zoster virus. . . . Approximately 3.5 million cases of varicella occurred annually from 1980–1994 in the United States with the peak incidence occurring in children five to nine years of age. The incidence rate of chickenpox is 8.3–9.1% per year in children 1–9 years of age. . . . Although it is *generally a benign, self-limiting disease* [emphasis mine], varicella may be associated with serious complications (e.g., bacterial superinfection, pneumonia, encephalitis, Reye's syndrome) and/or death."[57]

Approximately 75 percent of all children will contract varicella by age fifteen. Epidemics occur most frequently in winter and in spring. Chicken pox and herpes zoster (shingles) are two different disease manifestations of the same virus. Varicella is highly contagious and is spread by airborne droplets.

Symptoms

After an incubation period of two to three weeks, though on average thirteen to seventeen days, there appears an eruption of chicken pox on the back and chest, which then spreads to other areas. This stage is usually accompanied by a fever, which becomes further elevated as the rash progresses over the course of two to three days. The eruptions, small pimplelike bumps that can number from ten spots to hundreds, go through stages of being small, red, elevated areas that turn into blisters and then open and crust over. New eruptions continue to occur, each taking about thirty-six hours to crust over. The scabs last for a week or two and then fall off, leaving freshly healed skin. Rarely is scarring a problem.

The extremities are generally less affected than the trunk of the body. Younger children tend to have fewer lesions than older children and adults. The pocks can be extremely itchy, and the child may experience some malaise and likely a good bit of irritability, primarily from being so itchy. The illness usually lasts two to three weeks, and the child is considered contagious from five days before the skin eruption until all of the blisters have dried up and formed scabs. Chicken pox is so highly contagious that most who are susceptible who come in contact with it with contract it, and only 10 percent of those over fifteen have never had it.

Risks and Complications

Complications include the formation of infection at the site of the eruptions as a result of scratching, as well as complications resulting from the chicken pox affecting the eyes or the larynx, the latter causing swelling of the throat and subsequent breathing difficulties. Rarely, encephalitis may occur, as may arthritis, appendicitis, pneumonitis, orchitis, pericarditis, and glomerulonephritis, all unusual complications of the disease. Reye's syndrome was mentioned earlier as a possible complication of chicken pox, but this is the result of children having been given aspirin during the course of the illness. It is now more widely known that giving aspirin to children with viral infections is quite dangerous and can result in this complication and therefore should never be done.

Chicken pox in adults is often more severe and thus dangerous, with up to 14 percent of adults experiencing varicella pneumonia, and up to 20 percent of fatalities occurring in those over thirty.[58] Varicella also poses significant risks to the fetus whose mother contracts the illness during the eighth to fifteenth week of pregnancy, with the possibility of low birth weight, skin lesions, eye abnormalities, and evidence of brain damage and mental retardation.[59] When the mother contracts varicella just before or after the birth, the newborn may contract a severe or fatal form of the disease.

According to Barbara Loe Fisher of the National Vaccine Information Center (NVIC), "About 158,000 cases of chickenpox and 100 deaths from complications were reported in 1992. The Centers for Disease Control states that 'approximately 3.7 million cases of varicella occur annually in the United States; of these an estimated 4 to 5 percent are reported.' Although reported cases of chickenpox account for only a fraction of the total number of cases that occur every year, reports of deaths associated with chickenpox complications are estimated to be more accurate."[60]

Conventional Treatment

Standard treatment consists of restraining children from scratching the lesions, and using topical medications to relieve itching and irritation. Care should be taken to prevent the sores from becoming infected, and hygiene is an important part of this.

Susceptible adults who are exposed to the disease may be given an injection of varicella-zoster immune globulin (VZIG) within seventy-two hours of exposure to prevent infection or reduce its severity. This should also be given to immunocompromised children in whom chicken pox can be a life-threatening illness, to pregnant women who are susceptible and have been exposed, and to newborns whose mothers develop chicken pox within five days before birth or forty-eight hours after. However, giving VZIG to pregnant women will not prevent the fetus from becoming infected or harmed by the varicella virus.[61]

Food for Thought

The greatest risk from not vaccinating is that of not contracting the disease during childhood and later contracting it as an adolescent or adult. As more of the population is vaccinated, opportunities for exposure to the natural disease in the United States decrease, leaving the child susceptible. International travel or even natural cases in the United States then lead to the possibility of exposure later in life. We do not know whether varicella vaccine immunity will wane over time and lead to the types of shifting epidemiologies we have seen with measles and rubella, which are also viral infections, but this possibility certainly exists, with the possibility that boosters will be required in order to protect those who become susceptible later in life. This can be especially problematic for pregnant women, as contracting the disease in the first trimester or just after birth can cause severe and life-threatening consequences for the neonate.

HIB (*HAEMOPHILUS INFLUENZAE* TYPE B)

Originally thought to be the organism that causes flu (and thus its confusing name, influenza, though it does not cause flu), we now know that hemophilus influenza is a bacterium that can cause invasive diseases, most notably meningitis.

Hib resides in the respiratory tracts, nasal passages, and throats of up to 90 percent of all healthy individuals.[62] It is spread by respiratory droplets, as from coughing and sneezing, as well as by contact with contaminated respiratory secretions. For a number of years now, invasive Hib has been considered a significant public health problem primarily for young children, being the leading cause of bacterial meningitis in the United States.[63] In 1984 at least 20,000 cases of invasive disease occurred in the United States, with approximately 12,000 of these resulting in meningitis. These rates are the highest ever recorded. It is important to note that the disease has increased at least fourfold since 1946. This is primary attributed to the organism's having become antibiotic resistant.[64] Approximately 85 percent of all cases of invasive Hib occur in children under five years old, with invasive disease very unusual in infants under six months old, especially those that are breast-fed.[65] The greatest incidence of meningitis occurs in babies six to twelve months old and declines substantially after two years of age.[66] In the absence of prompt and effective medical treatment, the disease has a high mortality rate of up to 5 percent, as well as a high rate of seizures and other complications of the nervous system, up to 30 percent. Neurological complications include hearing loss, language delay or problems, learning disabilities, retardation, seizure disorders, and vision problems. Other complications include pneumonia, pericarditis, abscesses, septic arthritis, cellulitis, bacteremia, and epiglottitis. Similar strains of *Haemophilus* are associated with noninvasive diseases of the mucous membranes, including otitis media, sinusitis, conjunctivitis, bronchitis, and urinary tract infections.[67]

There are a number of factors that clearly increase the risk of exposure to, and contracting, Hib, including:

- Attending a day care center

- Crowded households

- Large households

- Low socioeconomic status

- Young age

- Ethnicity, with Native Americans, Inuits, blacks, and Hispanics being at greatest risk

- Lack of breast-feeding

- Household, hospital, or institutional exposure

- Immunocompromise, sickle-cell anemia, cancer[68]

By the age of five years old, it is thought that most children have achieved levels of normal colonization of Hib to confer resistance to disease, thus rates drop dramatically.

Symptoms

The incubation period of Hib-related disease is very hard to determine, as the organism is carried by most healthy members of society and so is often passed by asymptomatic carriers, for example, an older school-aged child bringing it home to a younger sibling. Symptoms of Hib infection include fever, chills, headache, cough, fatigue, lack of appetite, and vomiting. Headache may be severe. Meningitis will progress to stiff neck or back, which should be taken as a sign that your child needs emergency medical attention. Symptoms can progress to convulsions, confusion, shock, coma, and death, all of which can occur within just a few hours of the onset of symptoms. Aggressive medical treatment is required. Recovery from Hib infection may, or may not, confer permanent immunity.

Upper respiratory infections caused by Hib-related organisms do not generally take on invasive forms, but of course, all children with upper respiratory infections should be closely observed by parents.

Risks and Complications

As previously described, complications from Hib infection include a high mortality rate of up to 5 percent; seizures; neurological complications, including hearing loss, language delay or problems, learning disabilities, retardation, seizure disorders, and vision problems; as well as pneumonia, pericarditis, abscesses, septic arthritis, cellulitis, bacteremia, and epiglottitis.

Conventional Treatment

Treatment consists of aggressive antibiotic therapy as well as prophylactic treatment of other susceptible members of the household.

Food for Thought

Resistance to antibiotics is increasingly common among bacterial strains. What happens is that when one is sick with a bacterial infection and takes an antibiotic, the least resistant of the organisms are killed off, leaving those that are most resistant. Furthermore, bacteria can mutate to become increasingly resistant. It is therefore important to avoid unnecessary and excessive use of antibiotics for mild illnesses, reducing the likelihood of antibiotic-resistant organisms in the individual and in the environment. In addition, the frequent use of antibiotics can reduce immunity and increase susceptibility to pathogenic organisms. One might wonder if there is a connection between unnecessary treatment of childhood ear infections with increasingly strong antibiotics and the increases in Hib infection seen prior to the introduction of the vaccine.

HEPATITIS B

Hepatitis B virus is one of the several strains of hepatitis virus that lead to systemic infection and significant liver diseases. *Hepatitis* itself simply means "inflammation of the liver." The incidence of hepatitis B has increased by more than 37 percent in the last ten years, with more than 300,000 new infections and more than 5,000 deaths each year in the United States.[69] The CDC attempted to create programs to target high-risk populations, especially homosexuals, intravenous drug users, and health workers, but because these programs have had limited effectiveness, strategies were implemented in 1991 to accomplish universal vaccination of newborns.[70] The theory behind this is that not only will coverage protect those infants born to women with hepatitis B, but it will create a population of youngsters who will not be susceptible to the disease when they enter adulthood, when high-risk practices are more likely to occur and create opportunities for exposure. Furthermore, antibody responses are higher in younger recipients of the hepatitis B vaccine, and a smaller dose is required to vaccinate infants and children than adults. The latter issue is believed to make universal vaccination of infants cost-effective, but it should be remembered that most of the population would never contract hepatitis B and thus not require the vaccine, making cost-effectiveness a debatable argument.

Another reason for vaccinating infants is that those born to infected mothers can become chronic carriers, and the younger a person is at the time of infection, the greater the likelihood that the person will become a chronic carrier. It is estimated that of infected infants, 90 to 95 percent will become chronic carriers, as opposed to adolescent and adult exposures, where only 0.3 to 0.9 percent of people will become chronic carriers.[71] The CDC estimates that there are approximately 200 to 300 million chronic carriers internationally, but in developed nations fewer than 1 percent of the population are chronic carriers.[72] In western Europe and the United States it is estimated that only 2 to 7 percent of the population have ever been infected with hepatitis B and that fewer than 1 percent are chronically infected. Of course, 1 percent of millions of people is a significant number. Exposure occurs through contact with contaminated blood and other infected body fluids.

Most people will recover from hepatitis B infection after a few months, and only one case in 5 or 10 million will lead to mortality.[73] Even chronic carriers can eventually revert to noncarrier status, even if the virus has been carried for many years.[74] The most significant question to keep in mind is whether universal vaccination of newborns is justified given that most are not in high-risk groups.

Symptoms

Hepatitis B has an incubation period from 45 to 160 days. Initial symptoms may be very mild or entirely absent in young children. They can progress to nausea, vomiting, fatigue, anorexia, changes in taste and smell, skin rash, arthritis, headache, and cough. This is followed one to two weeks later by dark urine and pale, clay-colored bowel movements, after which jaundice appears. An enlarged liver can lead to tenderness in the upper-right abdomen.

Risks and Complications

Complications are rare but include severe inflammation of the brain, bleeding in the gastrointestinal tract, kidney and liver failure, and respiratory and cardiac collapse. Coma and death can result. Immunocompromised patients, the elderly, those in poor health, and those in compromised living conditions are most susceptible to these risks. Ninety percent of patients recover spontaneously, and most do not require hospitalization.[75]

Conventional Treatment

Treatment includes the following: limiting physical exertion, providing a nutritious diet, and observing for complications, which should be treated appropriately.

Food for Thought

Hepatitis B vaccine has come under recent scrutiny owing to its inclusion of thimerosal, a mercury derivative used as a preservative. Thimerosal, aside from causing reactions in those sensitive to the substance, may lead to excessively high mercury levels in the newborn, who is likely to have already absorbed considerable levels transplacentally from maternal environmental exposure. Because of this it was suspended from use in the newborn while further research was conducted. Within six months it was back on the market with the recommendation that thimerosal-free vaccine be used for the neonate. Unfortunately, thimerosal-free hepatitis B vaccine is costly; therefore, current recommendations are that newborns be vaccinated with thimerosal-containing vaccine if the other is unavailable. All children over six months can be given thimerosal-containing vaccine.

Concerns about hepatitis B vaccine safety, in combination with the low risk of infection in the general population, have led many parents to wonder whether the vaccine is justifiable. In fact, it is not only parents who have shown concern and doubt. Evaluation of family-practice physician acceptance of universal hepatitis B vaccine has shown conclusively that only between 17 and 32 percent of these practitioners agree with CDC recommendations calling for newborn vaccination.[76]

FIVE

What about the Risks?

Many people consider the benefits of vaccines to society unquestionable, but only recently has society begun to acknowledge that the risks of vaccines to the individual are less well studied.[1] Because this generation of parents doesn't have to wonder whether their child will contract polio or diphtheria from the kid next door, as these diseases barely exist in our society anymore, parents face a new concern: Do the small risks of an adverse vaccine reaction outweigh the small risks of contracting one of these now-rare diseases? Indeed, this is a concern that increasingly plagues parents who choose to vaccinate as well as those who choose no to do so.[2] Yet modern concern about vaccine safety is not new. As early as 1933 it was recognized that there is a possibility of encephalitis's being associated with the pertussis vaccine.[3] Concern during the past few decades has led to the creation of a number of vaccine-related consumer groups in the United States, including the National Vaccine Information Center, Concerned Health Professionals and Others, Parents Concerned about the Safety of Vaccines, and Determined Parents to Stop Hurting Our Tots.[4] In addition, numerous books have been published, and increasing numbers of articles appear in magazines and newspapers as diverse as *Atlantic Monthly*, *Money*, and the *Wall Street Journal*. National television programs have also aired specials on vaccination concerns.

Many think it impossible that vaccines, which are a ubiquitous and seemingly indispensable part of pediatric care and safety, could possibly be associated with harmful consequences. But there may be much about pediatric care that is less well evaluated than we might otherwise expect. For example, the Pharmaco-Epidemiology and Central Drug Monitoring and Medical Department of CIBA-GEIGY in Switzerland stated in 1991: "The surveillance of adverse drug reactions (ADR) in children represents a special challenge. . . .

There is a surprising scarcity of epidemiology projects on ADRs."[5] Many of the reports that do exist are directed to national authorities and appear in the literature but may never make it back to the manufacturers.[6] While surveillance for vaccines is likely more stringent than for other drugs, as the American public does not tolerate as well the idea of giving medications to healthy subjects, there may be room for questioning the adequacy of surveillance in this market as well.

The Power of a Small Group

Margaret Mead said that we should never doubt the power of a small group of people, as, indeed, she reminds us, this is where change comes from. The power of vaccine citizen action groups, publications, and television programs, particularly the 1982 showing of "DPT: Vaccine Roulette" and the 1985 publication of *DPT: A Shot in the Dark* by Harris Coulter and Barbara Loe Fisher, led the United States Congress to begin investigation of vaccine-related adverse reactions. Furthermore, the number of lawsuits levied by parents against vaccine manufacturers was growing, and litigation and claim costs led several manufacturers to cease vaccine research-and-development programs. Some even ceased production of already-licensed vaccines. These combined factors led to the passage of the National Childhood Vaccine Injury Act (NCVIA).[7] This program established a no-fault compensation program as a first recourse for those who felt that they or their child had been vaccine injured. This compensation program, the National Vaccine Injury Compensation Program, is administered by the federal government, but ironically, the program is financed by a tax placed on the sale of the vaccines included in the program.[8] In other words, the recipient is paying for vaccine injury insurance by paying higher prices for each mandatory vaccine received.[9]

The program also requires mandatory reporting of specific adverse events related to required vaccines, including measles, mumps, rubella, diphtheria, pertussis, and polio. The adverse-events reporting system as well as compensation will be discussed in greater depth later in this chapter. The significance here is that it was the initial step in the national government's recognition that vaccines can—and do—lead to severe consequences that are sometimes permanently debilitating or fatal.

Since 1986 new vaccines have been developed and vaccine practices changed to reflect concerns about adverse reactions. For example, it was only recently that the highly reactive whole-cell pertussis vaccine was replaced by acellular pertussis, and that the live polio vaccine was replaced by the inacti-vated (killed) virus. Indeed, ten years ago the reactiveness of the whole-cell pertussis was minimized by vaccine proponents. The rotavirus vaccine was on the market for a relatively short time (it was introduced in August 1998 and suspended by July 1999) before its use was halted by the CDC after reports of diarrhea, vomiting, and serious bowel obstruction (intussusception) in infants started coming in.

According to *Newsweek* magazine authors Claudia Kalb and Donna Foote, these changes might be fair reason for parents to pause and think twice about their vaccination decisions.[10] Public health officials, researchers, and physi-cians readily acknowledge that vaccinations are not without risk.[11] Dr. Robert Chen, chief of vaccine safety and development activity for the CDC in 1998, commented that while vaccines are responsible for "preventing death and dis-ability from disease," it is "also recognized that no vaccine is perfectly safe or effective. Some people will experience side effects from vaccines, and a few may not experience a complete immunological response to a vaccine, leaving the individual susceptible to diseases."[12] Furthermore, "denials of association despite accumulating evidence can also undermine public confidence" in vac-cination programs.[13]

This chapter will look at each of the adverse reactions associated with the vaccines commonly and routinely administered to children. In addition to cit-ing common mild reactions and rarer severe reactions, we will look at evi-dence that connects a number of chronic health problems with routine child-hood vaccines. Whether one chooses to vaccinate must be based on an in-formed decision. The choice not to vaccinate should be made with a clear understanding of the risks of childhood diseases; the choice to vaccinate must be accompanied by awareness of the attendant risks of the vaccines. Finally, this chapter will take a closer look at the realities behind vaccine reporting policies and the national vaccine compensation program.

A Range of Reactions

Vaccinations are associated with a wide range of reactions, from mild responses that can be expected with as many as 70 percent of all vaccinations given, to the severely devastating reactions that occur with great infrequency.[14] Between these extremes is a large gray area of chronic problems, especially those affect-ing the neurological and immune systems, which are becoming increasingly associated with vaccinations. Persistent allergies, multiple sclerosis, Crohn's disease, and asthma are among a few of the disorders for which a causal relationship with vaccinations has been established. Conjecture also exists linking such problems as cancer, autism, attention deficit hyperactivity disorder, and childhood violence with vaccines. It can be difficult to establish causal relationships between vaccines and chronic health problems, as many manifest years after the inoculations have been given.[15] Adverse-reaction reporting systems are also only minimally reliable, as many adverse reactions that are reported are not related to vaccines, and many adverse reactions that are related go unreported.[16] Furthermore, risk assessment must take into consideration; it is only theoretical that a child might be exposed to the disease. A one-in-a-million risk is small, but many parents who question vaccines bear two concerns in mind: that a child is definitely being exposed to risk, and that one in a million seems much larger when your child is that one.

Limitations in Vaccine Safety Research

While a great deal of research and development goes into vaccines, particularly isolating new vaccines and trying to limit the number of injections children receive by creating multiple combination vaccines, there are a number of problems that limit vaccine safety and efficacy testing.[17] For example, of seventy-six adverse events related to vaccines studied by a committee from the Institute of Medicine (IOM) in 1986, 66 percent of these had no research done to investigate them. The IOM acknowledged that the following limitations existed:

- Insufficient knowledge of the biological mechanisms involved in adverse events

- Insufficient or inconsistent information from case reports

- Inadequate size or length of studies relating to specific populations

- Inadequacies in surveillance systems

- Small number or experimental studies published compared with the number of epidemiological studies published[18]

Such limitations exist because of lack of funding as well as ethical and safety issues that prevent direct investigation.[19] According to Mortimer, "the climate for testing in humans is currently poor in the United States, and studies necessary to develop answers to some questions are often unacceptable to study subjects."[20] Nonetheless, in many ways, human experimentation is exactly what has persisted for the past several decades, if only because of the presumed obvious benefits of vaccines in reducing infectious disease rates. The diphtheria vaccine is but one example of a vaccine that was "not subjected originally to well-designed, prospective controlled field trials that would meet current standards."[21] The proof of benefit was considered self-evident and the proof of lack of harm equally apparent in the low adverse-reaction rates. Furthermore, even testing methods in humans can be less than reliable or useful. Evidence of antibody production in the blood (serologic testing) when blood levels are tested in a given time after a vaccine is administered should theoretically provide evidence of immunity. However, presence of antibody in the blood is not always an accurate predictor of immunity, and conversely, lack of antibody to the disease does not equate with susceptibility.[22]

Vaccines are also tested both before and after public use is sanctioned by government vaccine licensing agencies. Prelicensure testing of vaccines is based on extensive laboratory evaluation, then animal testing; finally, human clinical trials are conducted.[23] Remember, that means human testing is done before the vaccine is proven safe for humans. "Because rare reactions, delayed reactions, or reactions within sub-populations may not be detected before vaccines are licensed, post-licensure (also called post-marketing) evaluations of vaccine safety when millions of persons may be vaccinated" is also conducted. In other words, they are still getting the bugs out, if you will excuse the metaphor, after the vaccine is released to the general public for use in newborns and small children.[24]

Prelicensing decisions are not always based on the safety of the new vaccine but sometimes on other considerations. According to Dr. Stanley Plotkin, medical and scientific advisor to Aventis Pasteur Pharmaceutical Company, reflecting on the prelicensing debates that occurred regarding the ability of the oral polio vaccine to revert to its virulent state, "the kind of safety studies that would have had to be done (today) probably would have prevented or delayed licensure of the vaccine. But at the time we felt that prevention of polio was worth the risk, so the vaccine was licensed."[25] In retrospect, had a little more research been done, we might have stuck with the inactivated poliovirus now used almost exclusively because of the sometimes virulent nature of the oral poliovirus.

Postlicensure evaluation is done through passive reporting systems such as the Vaccine Adverse Event Reporting System (VAERS—see the following page), randomly exercised epidemiological studies, and computer databases. According to Chen, "Because vaccines are biologic rather than chemical in nature, variation in rates of adverse events (and immunogenicity) by manufacturer or even by lot might be expected." He proceeded to explain that postmarket surveillance can help detect potentially irregular lots in a "timely manner." Timely before what? one might wonder. And what has to happen in the market for an "irregular lot" to be detected? Irregular responses to childhood vaccinations?

The implication in Chen's remarks is that there could, indeed, be what are known in the vaccine community as "hot lots." Hot lots are batches of vaccine that, for various reasons, such as inadequate attenuation of the organism, may lead to an inordinate number of adverse reactions in children who are vaccinated from that particular batch. Interestingly, *Six Common Misconceptions about Vaccination and How to Respond to Them*, a booklet jointly published in 1996 by the U.S. Department of Health and Human Services and the Centers for Disease Control, clearly to dispel antivaccination "misinformation," tries to quell anxiety about "hot lots." The anonymous authors state that the FDA "reviews the week's VAERS reports for each lot, searching for unusual patterns. The FDA would recall a lot of vaccine at the first sign of problems. There is not benefit to either the FDA or the manufacturer in allowing unsafe vaccine to remain on the market. . . . The mere fact that a vaccine lot is still in distribution says that the FDA considers it safe."[26] I have full confidence that the FDA really wants what is best for American children. I just wonder whose child gets vaccine damaged enough for them to realize a "bad batch" was on the market. The booklet encourages parents not to consult VAERS reports, which list lot numbers associated with reactions, to try to determine which lots may be problematic because a report made to the VAERS doesn't mean that the reaction was truly caused by the vaccine in question. The booklet claims that no vaccine lot in the modern era (the VAERS has existed only in the *recent* modern era) has been found to be unsafe on the basis of a VAERS report. What they don't say is whether questionable lots associated with VAERS reports were recalled for other reasons, nor do they mention, as stated earlier in this chapter, that while there are many VAERS reports that may not be causally related to vaccines, there are also at least as many adverse vaccine reactions that go unreported to the VAERS.

Vaccine Injury Compensation and Vaccine Adverse Event Reporting System

The National Childhood Vaccine Injury Act of 1986 entitles a monetary award to those who have suffered a reaction to a mandatory childhood vaccine that has caused an excess of one thousand dollars in medical expenses or that has persisted longer than six months. By 1997 approximately one thousand vaccine injury victims had received remuneration totaling almost $750 million. The petition process can be extremely tedious, takes effort and persistence, and can be disappointing, as it is extremely difficult to prove that injuries are vaccine related rather than peripherally associated or coincidental. Furthermore, highly specific parameters that define exactly what constitutes a vaccine-related injury must be met. For example, it must be medically and scientifically established that a certain adverse reaction can be caused by a specific vaccine. Also, reactions must occur within narrowly defined and specific time frames after vaccination.

The Vaccine Adverse Event Reporting System was designed specifically for reporting events that are temporally related to the receipt of a vaccine. This means that the relationship between vaccine and reaction is speculative or unproved; therefore, having an event recorded in the VAERS does not mean that it was truly caused by a vaccination. The VAERS began functioning in November 1990, and by July 31, 1992, there were more than 17,000 reports registered. More than 11,000 of these reports concerned vaccines that are covered by the NVCIA. Slightly more than 2,500 of these reports concerned serious events, including death, prolonged life-threatening illness, or a reaction that led to a long-term hospitalization or permanent disability.[27] By 1994 more than 38,787 adverse events had been reported.[28] Most of the incidents occurred in the first three months of life, with a gradual decline after nine months, and most deaths are attributed to sudden infant death syndrome (SIDS), though the report on which these observations are based emphasizes that SIDS deaths are common during these months anyway, and that no causal association has been made between vaccines and SIDS. Nonetheless, it is interesting to note that of all adverse events, 92.5 percent occurred within two weeks of vaccination, with 45.5 percent of these occurring the day the vaccinations were administered, and an additional 20.4 percent by the second day after vaccination.[29]

Reports to the VAERS can be made by physicians, nurses, parents, relatives, or even neighbors of a patient. Forms are available at pharmacies, or one can make a report by phone, using the toll-free number (800-822-7967). Health care providers are obligated by law to report certain adverse reactions designated by the NCVIA, including those to diphtheria, pertussis, tetanus, polio, measles, mumps, and rubella vaccines.[30] (Other childhood vaccines are not covered under the compensation program.) In fact, federal law requires health care professionals who administer vaccines to follow these guidelines:

- All patients, or in the case of minors, their guardians, must be apprised of the risks of vaccines prior to administration of the vaccine.

- Adverse events must be reported within thirty days of vaccination. All adverse events must be reported regardless of whether it is the doctor's (or other care provider's) opinion that the event was related to the vaccine.

- Adverse events must be recorded in the patient's permanent medical record.

- A permanent record must be kept of the date, manufacturer's name, and lot number of all vaccines administered.[31]

Refusal to follow these guidelines constitutes breaking federal law, yet it is suspected that many doctors do not report vaccine reactions to health authorities, leading to a dramatic underreporting of vaccine reactions and deaths. Many doctors continue to claim that the vaccines had nothing to do with the reaction, whether for fear of litigation or from true belief that the events are unrelated. Fear of declining vaccination rates should parents become concerned about vaccines is another possible reason for downplaying reactions. Nonetheless, a number of parents have been awarded money from NCVIA for pertussis deaths that were originally classified as SIDS deaths.[32]

Liability-Free Manufacturers

While the vaccine compensation act was a milestone for many parents and a public acknowledgment of risks and damages associated with vaccines, in many ways the act safeguarded vaccine manufacturers from liability. "The law was enacted to help prevent vaccine manufacturers from being driven out of business by rising liability costs. . . . But in practice the reform effectively removed one of the drug industry's most compelling incentives to ensure that its products are as safe as possible."[33] According to *Money*, the program has cost taxpayers more than half a billion dollars, while profits to manufacturers have risen. Costs to vaccinate a child have escalated 243 percent since 1986. Revenues for some vaccines companies (including Connaught Laboratories and Wyeth-Lederle) have risen more than 300 percent since 1986, according to David Molowa, an international pharmaceutical analyst at Bear Stearns, a Wall Street investment firm.[34] Compulsory vaccines and no manufacturer liability create somewhat of a captive audience for the vaccine market.

Questions about profit over safety really arise when one learns that vaccine manufacturer Wyeth-Lederle, the only U.S. company producing the oral polio vaccine, mounted a strong lobbying effort to maintain its $230 million grip on the oral polio vaccine market when recommendations were shifting away from OPV to IPV. Fortunately, good sense won out and now OPV is used only in special circumstances. However, this change took some time. The initial CDC recommendation was that two doses of OPV be given after two of IPV. Now only IPV is given, for four doses. Incidentally, according to Robert Chen, "The CDC purchases and distributes more than half of the childhood vaccines administered in the United States."[35]

Who Profits?

In reality, nobody profits when a society's children are being damaged, and something is clearly going on in America when more than 10 percent of its children have been diagnosed with learning disabilities, school shootings are becoming commonplace, and more than 50 percent of the population has allergies. Yet vaccinations are largely ignored when causative factors for such phenomena are explored. Undoubtedly there is great and earnest belief that nothing as seemingly beneficial as vaccination could be a contributing factor, but even if vaccines were clearly causal, the belief might still persist that chronic behavioral problems and other consequences are still preferable to the rampant disease from infectious organisms that some postulate would occur in the absence of vaccine programs.

But could there also be a profit motive behind the fact that vaccines are so clearly overlooked as part of the increasingly poor immunity of children in our culture, or as part of the increase of chronic health problems? *Money* magazine investigator Andrea Rock, in a 1996 special report, revealed that the vaccine industry is booming, with "estimated revenues of more than $1 billion in the U.S. alone, up from $500 million in 1990."[36] Rock goes on to say, " *Money* found that health officials publicly downplay the lethal risks [of vaccines]. In addition, medical experts with financial ties to vaccine manufacturers heavily influence government decisions that have endangered the health of immunized kids while enhancing the bottom line of drug companies."[37] This, in spite of the fact that their research indicated that "DPT shots cause brain damage at the rate of one case for every 62,000 fully immunized kids . . . and that the shots kill at least two to four people a year, according to a federally funded Institute of Medicine Study."[38]

Some may be curious to learn that in the United Kingdom, physicians are given a financial incentive by the government to keep their vaccine rates high, with monetary bonuses given for vaccine rates higher than 70 to 90 percent among patients.[39]

Classifying Vaccine Reactions

Vaccine reactions are generally classified by frequency (whether they are common or rare), extent (whether local or systemic), severity (whether they lead to hospitalization, disability, or death), causality (whether the reaction can be definitively associated with the vaccine), and preventability (whether better handling of the vaccine, for example, might have prevented the reaction). Chen suggests the following classification of adverse vaccine reactions:

- Vaccine-induced reactions, where the reaction would not have occurred in the absence of the vaccine (for example, vaccine-associated paralytic poliomyelitis)

- Vaccine-potentiated, meaning the vaccine precipitated a reaction that would have occurred anyway, such as the first febrile seizure a child has

- Programmatic errors, meaning the reaction happened because of improper vaccine production, handling, or administration

- Coincidental reactions, where by chance a health problem arose concurrent with the administration of a vaccine, such as the presence of an underlying Hib infection, with Hib disease onset occurring just after Hib vaccine was given[40]

It is important to understand how vaccines are classified in order to understand how reactions and adverse-event reports are interpreted, especially since the reports are always interpreted retrospectively (after the event occurred) and with an underlying predisposition of most researchers to lean in favor of the vaccines. Thus, in the example of a child who is given a Hib vaccine and within five days develops Hib infection, the vaccine is not generally considered responsible; rather, it is said that the child had a latent Hib infection that just became symptomatic after vaccination. In the case of febrile seizures, how can one know that the child would have had febrile seizures without the vaccine? How can we ever know whether the DPT vaccine triggered an underlying tendency or caused the problem? Because of the speculative nature of such interpretations and the underlying biases inherent in this topic, one must

interpret reaction data with a critical mind. In some cases causality is established based solely on the length of time between the vaccine and the reaction.
Reactions that occur within a given time, under this classification system, qualify
the event as causal.[41] Unfortunately, this system can be unduly limited. For
example, if the criteria establish that a seizure occurring within twenty-four
hours of a DPT shot is considered causal and qualifies one for monetary compensation, and a child has a seizure twenty-five hours after the vaccine is administered, the case is no longer eligible for vaccine-damage compensation.
Frequently the criteria are narrower than vaccine critics think they ought to
be. Vaccine-reaction studies are also often based on similarly limited param-
eters. For example, in a survey of Los Angeles physicians asked to report all
adverse reactions to vaccinations in a forty-eight-hour period over two years,
several reactions, including deaths, were excluded from the study, as they occurred outside the allocated time parameter. One child became ill within hours
of the vaccine but died four days later—greater than the forty-eight-hour limit.[42]

Mild Vaccine Reactions

Reactions to vaccines can be expected in most cases and vary somewhat for
each vaccine, but in general they include fever, irritability, loss of appetite,
redness and/or soreness at the injection site, rash, swollen glands, headache,
tiredness (with increased sleeping in babies and young children), vomiting,
inconsolable crying, and even high-pitched screaming. Some of these reactions may occur in up to 50 percent of vaccine recipients, while others occur in
one out of fourteen to twenty vaccinations. Such reactions generally occur
within the first twenty-four to forty-eight hours of receipt of a vaccine.[43]

These reactions are considered by the medical profession to be mild and
inconsequential. The recommended prophylaxis is to give the child acetaminophen the morning of the vaccination appointment, which is thought to prevent fever and some of the other associated discomforts. Vaccine critics, however, suggest that these reactions may indeed be consequential and might represent mild levels of cerebral inflammation and irritation, which in turn may
be responsible for some of the postulated long-term effects of vaccines, such as
learning disabilities, autism, and even aggressive tendencies due to irritation of
the nervous system. It is now well known that many of the documented reactions to vaccinations involve the nervous system and that encephalopathy may
be a direct result of at least the DPT vaccine. Therefore it is quite plausible that
some of the so-called mild vaccine reactions are merely milder and seemingly
more benign versions of the overtly tragic and rare reactions.

Vaccinations may also be responsible for decreasing general immunity for some time after they are administered, thus possibly increasing susceptibility to other infectious organisms. For example, the *New England Journal of Medicine* published a report showing that tetanus booster vaccine has been associated with a temporary decline in T-lymphocyte blood counts to below normal levels; Hib infection is not uncommon within two weeks of receiving the Hib vaccine, and poliomyelitis is a more common occurrence in those who have been recently vaccinated, although in the latter instance, injections of other substances (for example, antibiotics) also increase poliomyelitis, particularly in the injected limb. Therefore, injection itself, rather than vaccine material, may be the culprit with poliomyelitis.[44]

Although it is not one of the mandatory childhood vaccines, I can't resist mentioning that the typical mild reactions to the flu vaccine are fever and aches—awfully similar to the disease, eh?

Severe and Immediate Vaccine Reactions

While severe or immediate vaccine reactions are considered rare, they can and do occur. This is important for parents to recognize so that such a reaction does not go undetected, untreated, or unreported. Such reactions can occur within minutes, hours, days, or weeks of a child's receiving a vaccine and include the following symptoms and conditions: high fever (in excess of 105 degrees Fahrenheit), inconsolable high-pitched screaming, listlessness, apnea (lack of breathing), cyanosis (turning blue), hives, severe allergic reaction, anaphylactic shock, change in consciousness, loss of consciousness, coma, death. With the DPT vaccine, nonstop crying, classified as prolonged for more than three hours, occurs in 100 of every 10,000 doses; fever of 105 degrees Fahrenheit or higher occurs in 30 of every 10,000 doses; seizures occur in 6 of every 10,000 doses, and limpness, pallor, and loss of alertness occur in 6 of every 10,000 doses.[45] (They are less common when acellular pertussis is used in the DTaP vaccine, but many doctors still use DPT, and reactions can still occur with DTaP.) As we will see shortly, each vaccine also has associated with it specific immediate as well as long-term severe reactions.

A Word about Multiple Vaccines

Because each child receiving the full complement of childhood vaccines would need an inordinate number of injections—as many as fifteen to nineteen injections by the age of six years old, with twelve of these by eighteen months—concerted efforts have been made to create singular multivalent injections. In other words, as many as seven vaccines are combined into one shot. This approach is considered by many vaccine researchers to be preferable, reducing discomfort for the child as well as stress for parents, nurses, and physicians who must watch the child suffer discomfort or inflict the discomfort on the child.[46]

While proponents of this approach are adamant that multivalent vaccines do not increase the risk of reactions, parents may want to be cautious about this approach for two reasons. The first is that there is no guarantee that the new multivalent vaccines confer adequate immunity, though a new seven-valent pneumococcal vaccine was licensed earlier this year.[47] Although the "U.S. Food and Drug Administration (FDA) requires that combination vaccines not be inferior in purity, potency, immunogenicity, or efficacy to each agent given separately," researchers are unsure of how to test for safety and effectiveness.[48] Traditional approaches to measuring these qualities may not be practical or possible, as large studies would need to be done and the components may yet be unlicensed.

Furthermore, though medical authorities continue to refute arguments that multiple vaccines may be overwhelming to young immune systems, there may still be cause for concern. Their counterargument is that because exposure to multiple foreign antigens is a common part of normal extrauterine life, exposure to multivalent vaccines is comparable to such exposure. For example, a single episode of an upper respiratory viral infection can lead to exposure to between four and ten foreign antigens, whereas "strep throat" can lead to exposure to somewhere between twenty-five and fifty foreign proteins. Exposure to foods, new bacteria in the intestinal tract, and bacteria that routinely enter the nose and throat occur uneventfully every day and lead to the development of antibodies as well. The Institute of Medicine concludes, "In the face of these normal events, it seems unlikely that the number of separate antigens contained in childhood vaccines, whether given orally or by vaccines, would represent an appreciable added burden on the immune system that would be immunosuppressive." They add, "Nevertheless, it is theoretically possible that some vaccine constituent might predispose an individual to infection through its action as an antigen or some other means."[49] What the IOM doesn't state is that though regular exposure to large numbers of ubiquitous microorganisms and foreign proteins is a normal part of extrauterine life (the womb is generally a germ-free environment), children are not regularly and directly inoculated with organisms and fragments of organisms that are known to be pathogenic to the point of being highly lethal. Common sense tells us that it is highly unlikely that in any one day a child would naturally be exposed to measles, mumps, and rubella, or diphtheria, pertussis, and tetanus, let alone seven infectious agents. In addition, children are exposed to infectious organisms most commonly through the respiratory passages, not through injection.

Furthermore, it is incongruent that vaccine recommendations for adult travelers prescribe getting vaccinations individually rather than in one visit, in order to reduce vaccine reactions, while recommendations for children eschew this concern. Still, a recent medical article evaluating reactions associated with multiple vaccines administered to travelers concludes, "Side-effects for vaccination of travelers are common. Increasing the number of vaccines is associated with increasing rates of local and systemic reactions."[50] While they emphasize that reactions are mild and vaccines should not be withheld when needed, the comment does provide some interesting food for thought.

To Each Its Own

While there are general reactions that might occur from any of the vaccines, each vaccine also has certain reactions with which it is associated with greater frequency or likelihood. The following discussion provides detailed and current information on each of the commonly used childhood vaccines and associated adverse reactions or problems. I have noted whether a causal relationship has been clearly established or whether the association is suspected but unproved. The order in which the vaccines are listed is identical to that for the corresponding diseases reviewed in the previous chapter, to facilitate the reader's ease of reference. Some of the medical terms below may be unfamiliar to the reader. Many of these are explained in the text, and most are described in the glossary found at the end of this book.

MEASLES, MUMPS, AND RUBELLA VACCINE

Because these vaccines are given in one trivalent vaccine (three vaccines in one shot), reactions to each individual vaccine may be hard to separate from the whole. The reactions most frequently associated with the MMR vaccine include "burning and stinging at the injection site, fatigue, sore throat, runny nose, headache, dizziness, fever, rash, nausea, vomiting or diarrhea, and sore lymph glands."[51] One vaccine manufacturer (Merck and Company) lists the following as some of the possible adverse effects of their MMR vaccine: panniculitis (inflammation of the fatty layer of connective tissue inside the abdomen), atypical measles, fever, syncope (loss of consciousness), headache, dizziness, malaise, irritability, vasculitis (inflammation of blood or lymph vessels), pancreatitis, diarrhea, vomiting, parotitis, nausea, diabetes mellitus, thrombocytopenia, lymphadenopathy, leukocytosis, anaphylaxis, arthritis, arthralgia, encephalitis, encephalopathy, subacute sclerosing panencephalitis (SSPE), Guillain-Barré syndrome (GBS), convulsions (both febrile and afebrile), ataxia (defective motor coordination), paresthesia (numbness or prickling sensations, hypersensitivity to sensations), sore throat, pneumonitis, rash, hives, cough, rhinitis, burning and stinging at injection site, otitis media, nerve deafness, orchitis, death.

Anaphylactic shock is a severe, acute, potentially lethal systemic allergic reaction. It generally occurs within a few minutes to a few hours of the exposure to the antigenic substance. Death can occur as a result of airway obstruction or spasm of the bronchial passages, or cardiovascular failure. It usually resolves without harmful consequences if treated immediately, usually with epinephrine. It is advised that epinephrine always be present when vaccines are administered. As MMR is grown on chicken embryo tissue, egg-related proteins can be found in this vaccine, predisposing those with egg-related allergies to anaphylaxis from this vaccine. However, vaccine-related anaphylaxis can be unpredictable and occur as easily in those with no previous history of sensitivity.[52] Furthermore, those with egg-related sensitivity do not always show sensitivity to the vaccine. Those with neomycin sensitivity may also be predisposed to a reaction to this vaccine, which contains trace amounts of the antibiotic. The IOM concludes that there is a causal relationship between MMR vaccine and anaphylactic reactions, and death from anaphylactic reactions, though these are considered rare.[53]

The following is a discussion of some of the risks associated with each component of the MMR vaccine.

Measles Vaccine

The live measles vaccine is currently in use, as it was discovered a few years after its introduction that the killed measles vaccine used between 1963 and 1967 provided only moderate immunity that eventually waned and led to the subsequent development of atypical measles in those previously vaccinated who later contracted wild-type measles. Atypical measles, as discussed earlier, was associated with severe reactions.[54] Between 1963 and 1993 in the United States, more than 230 million doses of measles vaccine were distributed.

Currently between 5 and 15 percent of all measles vaccine recipients develop a fever of 103 degrees Fahrenheit or higher, generally beginning five to twelve days after vaccination. Fever is sometimes accompanied by febrile seizures. Temporary rashes also develop in 5 percent of recipients.[55] The 1981 British National Childhood Encephalopathy Study determined that there was "a statistically significant association between measles vaccination and the onset of serious neurological disorder within 14 days of receiving measles vaccine. The risk for previously normal children was estimated to be 1 in 87,000 measles vaccinations."[56] In 1994 the IOM concluded that it is biologically plausible that measles vaccine can lead to encephalopathy. Vaccine advocates remind us that natural measles infection is also associated with the development of this disorder, hence the continued use of the vaccine.

Epidemiological evidence clearly connects encephalitis and other neurological disorders with the receipt of the measles vaccine. Encephalopathy refers to "acute or chronic acquired abnormality of, injury to, or impairment of the brain function."[57] Symptoms include changes in consciousness or behavior, convulsions, headache, and neurological damage. Encephalitis describes encephalopathy caused by brain inflammation and is typically accompanied by bacterial growth in the cerebrospinal fluid. Frequently, however, the terms are found interchangeably in the vaccine literature. The following are several examples of measles/MMR-related cases of encephalopathy:

- Twenty-three cases of neurological disease following measles vaccine were documented between 1965 and 1967 in the United States; 18 of the cases involved encephalitis, which is described as including sensory disturbances, seizures, major loss of motor function, and cerebral swelling.

- Eighty-four patients with neurological disorders within thirty days of the vaccine were reported to the CDC between 1963 and 1971; 26 recovered fully, 5 died, and 19 had permanent neurological damage.

- Between 1968 and 1974 in the United Kingdom 47 cases of what appeared to be encephalitis were reported in relationship to the vaccine.

- In the former East Germany, 7 cases of central nervous system (CNS) complications were reported out of 174,725 measles vaccines given, with 4 cases of encephalopathy, 2 cases of febfile seizures, and 1 case of encephalitis (1 left with residual paralysis) and 1 who later died of leukemia.

- Reports from Japan between 1928 and 1983 reveal 12 cases of encephalitis or encephalopathy for a rate of 3.7 cases per million.

- Two hundred twelve adverse events after MMR vaccine were reported to the Swedish government between 1982 and 1984 (based on 700,000 doses sold), with 17 cases of transient but serious neurological symptoms, 10 encephalitis cases, 5 with acute motor difficulties, 1 with fever and seizures, and 1 with hemiparesis (paralysis affecting one side of the body).[58] Please note that 700,000 sold doses does not clearly indicate how many children were actually vaccinated, and so does not give us information on the rate of reactions.

Thrombocytopenia, a disorder characterized by a decrease in blood platelet count (the cells responsible for proper blood clotting), has been associated with the measles vaccine, with an estimated incidence of 1 case per 30,000 to 40,000 vaccinated children.[59] In most instances it is a mild, transient problem, but severe cases can lead to thrombocytopenia purpura, spontaneous bleeding with bleeding into the skin, which can be fatal.[60] Thrombocytopenia can also be responsible for nosebleeds, a tendency to bruise easily, and prolonged bleeding from cuts. Most cases of thrombocytopenia occur after the first dose of measles vaccine, but it can occur after the second dose as well. One study found that measles vaccine can suppress bone marrow, with a significant drop in hemoglobin concentration both one and two weeks after the administration of live attenuated measles vaccine.[61] Natural measles vaccine is not generally associated with bleeding disorders; however, in impoverished countries where measles can be a devastating disease because of underlying malnutrition, "black measles" can occur, with bleeding in the skin.

Measles vaccine and natural measles can both be associated with residual seizure disorders (RSD). The literature and case reviews conducted by the IOM indicate that "there is evidence that acute seizures are possible sequelae of immunization with measles (and mumps) vaccines" and that it is "biologically plausible that there is a connection between immunization and RSD," though a causal relationship has not been established.[62] With residual seizure disorder, neurological problems persist beyond the initial acute episode of fever and seizures. Most initial seizures occur within thirty days of vaccination. Seizures may also initially occur in the absence of fever. When vaccine reports are assessed, it may be more common to dismiss seizures associated with vaccines as febrile seizures when fever is present, thereby obscuring the actual number of seizures as a result of measles vaccinations. In one Canadian study that evaluated the occurrence of seizures related to vaccine, cases were included only if the seizures had been diagnosed by a physician.[63] Obviously, not all such seizures occur in the doctor's presence, clearly limiting the numbers included in at least this research study, and presumably others as well.

Live virus vaccine, of which measles vaccine is one, have been implicated in demyelinating disorders. One such condition, optic neuritis, results in unilateral or bilateral vision impairment, which can be temporary or permanent. While the two have not been determined to have a proven association, the IOM concluded that "there is demonstrated biological plausibility of a causal relationship between optic neuritis and measles vaccine, in that measles is associated with demyelinating disorders."[64] Similarly, transverse myelitis, an acute-onset disease involving the sensory nerves of the spinal cord, may also be associated with measles vaccine. The incidence of this disorder in the general population is less than 1 per 100,000; the vaccine-related incidence appears to be low, but no studies large enough to determine this have yet been conducted.

Guillain-Barré syndrome, characterized by sudden onset of extreme muscle weakness, decrease in reflex response, and inflammatory demyelination of the peripheral nerves, is similarly and plausibly related to measles vaccines, but a causal association remains yet unproved. It is considered an immune-mediated disorder and has been associated with several viruses, including measles, mumps, and rubella, as well as varicella zoster, Coxsackie B, Epstein-Barr, and cytomegalovirus. In the 1970s large numbers of people were diagnosed after influenza vaccination, and it has been reported following a number of vaccines, including MMR.[65] In the case of a sixteen-month-old girl who developed severe generalized weakness of the arms and legs, inability to walk, and difficulty drinking and coughing, her doctors concluded that "immunization was the probable trigger for the development of Guillain-Barré Syndrome in this child."[66] The child required several months of treatment before regaining her ability to walk. Further case details regarding recovery were not provided.

Subacute sclerosing panencephalitis (SSPE) is recognized as a possible consequence of natural measles infection and is also associated with receipt of the vaccine. SSPE is a rare, subacute form of encephalitis that is accompanied by demyelination, meaning the removal of the myelin sheath (protective coating) surrounding the nerves. It generally begins as long as seven years after measles infection or vaccination and is a disease of slowly progressive deterioration. Eventually the victim, after a twelve- to twenty-four-month period, becomes vegetative and death ensues, though some periods of remission can occur. The first documented case in a vaccine recipient who had never had natural measles infection occurred in 1968. Though the risk of SSPE from the measles vaccine is clearly plausible, it has been well documented that the risk of SSPE from the vaccine is significantly less than that from natural measles infection.[67]

In a 1983 report, the Adverse Drug Reactions Advisory Committee (ADRAC) cites having received fifteen reports of adverse reactions occurring within thirty minutes of vaccination with live measles virus.[68] The most commonly reported symptom was the child turning moderately or severely blue, referred to as cyanosis, which can be a result of poor oxygen flow from breathing difficulty. All of the children apparently recovered from the episode. Reactions to measles vaccine are extremely common in India to the point where mild to moderate reactions are accepted by parents, though severe reactions and deaths are also not entirely infrequent. It is thought by health authorities and the World Health Organization that the frequency of reactions is due to contamination of the vaccine either in reconstitution or from the vials, leading to toxic shock syndrome from the use of contaminated products and unsterile needles.[69] Problems such as these have fueled research on the development of foods genetically engineered to contain vaccine viruses, and aerosol vaccines.[70] Another impetus for the development of foods genetically engineered to contain measles virus is to reduce measles infection in children under age one, commonly victims of this disease in the developing world.[71]

The use of genetically engineered foods containing viral and bacterial components opens up many ethical and safety concerns and issues beyond the scope of this book. However, it must be remembered that the "environmental cost of genetically altered foods presents a less obvious, but no less serious health risk. . . . This is because modified organisms, once introduced into the food chain, can never be recalled from the environment and will have unlimited and totally unpredictable effects on our health and ecosystems."[72] Research is under way to "medically engineer" bananas, rice, potatoes, and soy products, and research has been conducted using at least hepatitis B and measles virus.

In a 1995 letter to the editor in the *Lancet*, twenty-four notifications of temporary gait disturbances after MMR vaccinations in Denmark were reported in fifteen-month-old children (remember, MMR is not given until then), as well as two such reports in older patients—a thirteen-year-old boy and a twenty-two-year-old woman. The gait disturbances are reported in previously normal children, all of whom began to exhibit gait changes within three to twenty-five days of receiving the MMR vaccine (median time was six days).[73] These children began to demonstrate unsteadiness in walking and "tended to fall, walk into doors, and bump into tables." Most recovered, though one child had residual gait disturbances three months later. "In 16 out of 24 cases the symptoms were preceded by a febrile episode, and in 10 cases a rash was noticed. Symptoms such as irritability, high-pitched screaming, and difficulty with focusing the eyes were also seen in numerous of these cases. Cerebral involvement can indicate more severe disorders, and symptoms can last several months." It is unknown whether these children will develop long-term consequences. While it is considered rare for such disorders to occur, and they can also be associated with natural measles infection, it is clear that "any of the components of the M-M-RII vaccine or combinations of them might be responsible for the gait disturbances."[74]

Another report in the *Lancet* clearly connects sensorineural hearing loss (nerve deafness) with measles vaccine, citing it as a complication of both measles virus infection and measles vaccination. The authors state, "The incidence of neurological sequelae following measles vaccination was found to be 1 per 1.6 million doses of the vaccine," and report the case of a thirteen-month-old who developed fatal encephalitis after receipt of the vaccine, and in whom measles virus was clearly causal. However, they state that deafness after MMR is rare from the measles component, with only one case in the literature causally related to measles, and may be more likely to be a result of the mumps and rubella components of the vaccine.[75]

One of the most curious associations is that between the measles vaccine and inflammatory bowel disease (IBD), a quickly increasing problem in the U.S. population. Measles infection in early childhood has been linked to the development of IBD, especially Crohn's disease. It is now recognized that vaccination with the live attenuated measles vaccine may similarly "predispose to the later development of IBD, provoking concern about the safety of the vaccine."[76] Ulcerative colitis may be similarly linked to measles vaccine.[77] The authors of the 1995 *Lancet* report indicate that "the incidence of inflammatory bowel disease has increased over the past few decades, during which the use of live measles vaccine has become routine."[78] The etiology of this phenomenon, both with natural measles infection and measles vaccine, is persistence of viral infections. It is uncertain whether the vaccine strain is more likely to persist than that of wild-type measles virus.

Age at exposure may also be a factor, as exposure at birth to natural measles infection is implicated as a risk factor in later development of Crohn's disease (though not ulcerative colitis). The authors state that the mean incidence of measles vaccination is fifteen months, whereas the peak incidence in childhood of natural measles infection is four to five years of age. Measles virus infection can cause persistent disturbance of immune function, especially of helper-T response.[79] Measles vaccination with live virus may also lead to persistent immunosuppression to varying degrees. In countering this argument, Peter Patriarca and Judy Beeler of the Center for Biologics Evaluation and Research of the FDA state that in other geographic areas, the incidence of ulcerative colitis has been lower since the introduction of the vaccine, and they counter that the previously cited study overlooks familial tendencies toward these diseases. Nonetheless, they state that "a plausible hypothesis that would accord the results of the study is that immunological events leading to IBD must be initiated early in life, and may therefore have been more likely to occur in the cohort who had received measles vaccine (at age 10–24 months) than in the cohort who had wild virus infection (at variable times through age 11 years)."[80]

Of course, while not a direct "adverse reaction" to measles virus, the shifting epidemiology of measles to adolescence and adulthood discussed in previous chapters must certainly be considered an undesirable effect of mass vaccination programs for the prevention of this disease.

Mumps Vaccine

Aseptic meningitis is well documented to occur after administration of the MMR vaccine and is most likely associated with the mumps vaccine component. This is an inflammation of the meninges, the membranes of the spinal cord, associated with an increased number of white blood cells in the cerebrospinal fluid. In one study from 1991, of 630,157 recipients of the Urabe Am-9 strain, there were at least 311 cases of aseptic meningitis reported, with mumps virus related to the strain detected in the cerebrospinal fluid.[81]

Between February 1990 and January 1992 there were fifteen confirmed cases of vaccine-associated mumps meningitis cases reported, according to Norman Begg of the Communicable Disease Surveillance Center in London. He reports that rates of 10 per 100,000, a rate consistent with observations in other countries, is probably most accurate. However, according to Begg, "the low rate (1.5 per 100,000) derived from BPSU [British Pediatric Surveillance Unit] reports may be due to the fact that pediatricians did not link the illness (which was usually mild) to measles, mumps, rubella vaccination, which had been given up to 28 days previously."[82] The 1994 IOM report estimates reactions from the Urabe strain to have been as high as several per 1,000 doses. Few attempts have been made to assess the incidence of reactions from the Jeryl Lynn strain used in the United States, and even when aseptic meningitis has been reported, the strain of virus has not been isolated or identified.[83]

Regardless of whether aseptic meningitis turns out be a nonserious disease, children who are suspected of having meningitis will generally be subjected to aggressive assessment and treatment protocols, including spinal tap to assess for bacteria in the cerebrospinal fluid, antibiotics, and some length of hospitalization for observation. A 1989 paper in the *Lancet* states: "The most common neurological reaction to mumps-containing live vaccines is meningitis, which *carries the same favorable prognosis as that so often found in the course of natural mumps infection* [emphasis mine]."[84]

A Canadian report from 1989 discusses twenty-four cases of mumps vaccine–related meningoencephalitis, sixteen between 1973 and 1977, three between 1978 and 1985, and five between 1986 and 1988. Only four cases were related to the Urabe Am-9 strain, released in Canada in 1986 and associated internationally with high rates of aseptic meningitis.[85] Symptoms included fever, vomiting, meningismus (irritation of the brain and spinal cord without actual inflammation but with symptoms simulating meningitis), headache, parotitis, and seizures. Meningismus occurred in 70 percent of cases, while seizures, the least common of the symptoms, occurred in as many as 30 percent of all cases.

The Urabe Am-9 strain was withdrawn from the market in Great Britain in September 1992, leading to a subsequent withdrawal of the vaccine from the worldwide market. Though not all researchers considered the risk of problems from the vaccine significant enough to warrant this decision, it was deemed a practical decision, so that "bad press, a negative image, and liability suits" didn't inevitably follow.[86]

In spite of the incidence of neurological involvement in reactions to this vaccine, and the fact that 30 to 40 percent of natural mumps cases are so mild as to be asymptomatic, many researchers feel that the risks of the vaccine are entirely justified, as they consider the possible long-term consequences of natural mumps disease, such as permanent nerve deafness, to be of greater likelihood and consequence.[87] Nonetheless, I find the following statement regarding mumps vaccine meningitis untenable and wonder how many physicians support this attitude: "These observations should not be taken as an argument against mumps vaccination. I think because of the extreme rarity of this complication, parents need not be told about the risk before deciding on vaccination."[88]

The incidence of insulin-dependent (type I) diabetes mellitus (IDDM) has increased in children in the past decade. It is now questioned whether certain vaccines may play a role in the development of this disease in the pediatric population. Approximately 12 to 14 new cases per 100,000 children are reported in the United States annually, among children from infancy to sixteen years old. Researchers are uncertain of the etiology of this disorder, but among other factors, such as environment and genetics, are viruses, which may play a role in the destruction of the pancreatic beta cells or in the viral triggering of an autoimmune response.[89] Furthermore, viral toxins may lead to cumulative damage to these pancreatic cells.[90] While there are numerous reports in the literature suggesting a connection between mumps vaccines and IDDM, the IOM concludes that because IDDM is a disease with multifactorial causes, there is insufficient evidence to accept or reject the notion that the vaccine causes the disease. Genetic factors, previous pancreatic damage, and environmental factors may already be present, increasing susceptibility to any possible vaccine-related association with the disease.[91]

Allergic reactions to mumps vaccine are uncommon but do occasionally occur and are probably related to vaccine components, such as gelatin stabilizers or egg-related proteins from the culture medium on which the vaccine is grown. In general, most vaccine anaphylactic reactions "occur in individuals who have no known risk factors for reactions to these vaccines; thus, no special precautions can be taken."[92]

Regarding mumps vaccine, Edward Mortimer comments, "Immunization against mumps is carried out primarily because the disease is a nuisance. Mortality from mumps is essentially unheard of; aseptic meningitis is a frequent and unpleasant complication without permanent sequelae. Very rarely, sterility or permanent nerve deafness occurs. Reporting of mumps is haphazard, the disease so often misdiagnosed, and complications so rare that the effects of widespread mumps immunization are unmeasured."[93]

Rubella Vaccine

Rubella vaccine, as discussed earlier, has led to a significant reduction in congenital rubella syndrome, an important contribution to the prevention of deafness, mental retardation, and fetal death associated with this disease when contracted by the fetus during pregnancy. In addition, however, it has been associated with a shift in epidemiology away from being a benign disease of childhood to one that adolescents and adults may be susceptible to owing to waning vaccine protection. In addition, it has been associated with other short- and long-term health consequences. While we, of course, should not simply abandon the vaccine and return to the days of high rates of congenital rubella syndrome, we must also acknowledge some of the adverse effects with which this vaccine is associated, most notably arthritis complaints and persistent rubella infection that may lead to insulin-dependent diabetes mellitus or autism.

An article in the *New England Journal of Medicine* links persistent measles virus infection from the vaccine with chronic arthritis in children.[94] It is stated in the report that it is possible to isolate rubella virus from arthritic joints in children even months after vaccination. It is thought that this problem can recur for years. In an article in *Science* in 1970 the Department of Health, Education, and Welfare (HEW) reported that "as much as 26 percent of children receiving rubella vaccination in national testing programs developed arthralgia and arthritis."[95] It is well established that arthritis, which can be caused by rubella infection, is the most significant side effect of this vaccine.[96] Several different rubella vaccines that have been on the market have been capable of causing such reactions, both in adults and in children.[97] While many different joints can be affected, knees and fingers are the most common, whereas the hips are rarely effected.

The mechanism of joint inflammation is through the direct infection of synovial tissue with the rubella virus. Arthritis resulting from the vaccine, however, is considered less frequent than that resulting from rubella infection, the latter group experiencing this side effect 30 percent of the time and the former experiencing arthritic symptoms in 5 percent of cases.[98] Nonetheless, the association between the vaccine and side effects may be significant enough to cause medical workers to refuse vaccination, including obstetricians who are regularly in contact with pregnant women, the very group the vaccine was designed to protect from exposure to disease. In one study of medical doctors who were offered the vaccine as a booster up to 90 percent of obstetricians and more than 75 percent of pediatricians refused the vaccine.[99] Physicians cited fear of unforeseen vaccine reactions as their reason for refusal.[100]

The idea that viral infections can persist in our bodies months or years after vaccination is quite disturbing and may shed light on another adverse effect associated with rubella immunization: chronic fatigue immunodeficiency syndrome (CFIDS). According to Allen D. Allen in an article in *Medical Hypotheses*, "Adult women are over-represented in the population of patients with chronic fatigue, and are especially susceptible to developing such symptoms following vaccine exposure to attenuated rubella virus."[101]

The author goes on to discuss the fact that within three years of the introduction of a new and more potent strain of live rubella vaccine onto the market in 1979, reports of CFIDS began appearing in the medical literature. He concludes that multiple rubella viral antibodies found in patients with CFIDS and the ability of the virus to produce characteristic CFIDS symptoms suggest that persistent rubella infection from the vaccine may indeed play a role in the etiology of this syndrome. He furthermore suggests that adults may be susceptible to the respiratory secretions from children who have been recently vaccinated with this vaccine, which creates persistent exposure for the adults. This also indicates that rubella virus from the vaccine can linger in children's systems and be passed to adults through casual contact.[102]

Furthermore, persistent infections with viruses have clearly been linked to IDDM. Based on studies of patients with congenital rubella syndrome, it is apparent that patients with a genetic predisposition to diabetes may develop IDDM after MMR vaccination.[103]

Other side effects resulting from development of mild rubella infection associated with rubella vaccine include rash, swollen lymph nodes, fever, sore throat, and headache, with reactions the least prevalent in infants and greatest in women (up to 50 percent of women who receive the vaccine). Other more serious reactions include polyneuropathy, with nerve disorders of the arms and knees most common, as well as carpal tunnel syndrome, and Horner's syndrome (which involves facial nerves and muscles). The symptoms usually begin approximately forty days after vaccination.[104] Optic neuritis, transverse myelitis, Guillain-Barré syndrome, and the ability to temporarily suppress nonspecific cellular immunity have also been reported.[105]

MMR and Autism

Possible links between autism and MMR vaccine have received considerable press coverage recently, as congressional hearings have been conducted to review evidence of a link between the two. Autism is a complex, lifelong developmental disability manifesting as difficulty with language, social interactions, communication, and behavior. The degree of autism can vary dramatically, and children with this disorder can score variably on IQ tests from ranges suggesting profound mental retardation to above-average abilities. About 30 percent of children with autism may also have epilepsy, and boys are three to four times more likely to be affected by autism than are girls. Early in the history of autism it was thought that the disorder might affect higher socioeconomic brackets with greater frequency than other populations, but autism now occurs in all racial and ethnic groups and social strata. The incidence of autism has increased dramatically in the past decade, now with as many as 1 in 300 children being affected, compared with 1 in 10,000 cases suspected in 1978.[106] Currently there is no known cause or cure, though many causal pathways have been suggested, including genetic predisposition, metabolic disorders, infectious disease, and environmental factors, and a number of interventions and treatments may reduce the expression of the symptoms.[107] While many vaccine proponents have adamantly denied a connection between the MMR vaccine and the subsequent development of autism, the evidence linking the two is compelling. Senator Dan Burton initiated the congressional hearings after his own previously healthy grandchild developed autism after receiving his routine childhood vaccinations.[108]

The most striking features of the association between MMR and autism are that the prevalence of the disorder has increased significantly coincident with the introduction of the trivalent vaccine in the 1980s (previously, measles, mumps, and rubella vaccines were given separately) and the fact that the children who developed autism were entirely healthy and developmentally normal prior to receipt of the vaccine. Parents have literally watched as their active, communicative, and intelligent children reverted to preverbal states, became withdrawn and behaviorally difficult, and sometimes resorted to self-inflicting damage, such as repeated head banging. Several mechanisms have been established by researchers suggesting a causal effect. One mechanism is the already established persistent viral infection leading to autoimmunity, particularly against myelin-basic protein of the myelin sheath, resulting in destruction of the protective coating of the nerve fibers that are essential for higher brain activities. It has already been clearly established that vaccines can lead to demyelinating disorders.[109] In one research study it was found that up to 80 percent of autistic children demonstrated evidence of autoantibodies specific to brain structures, while 0 to 0.5 percent of nonautistic children have such antibodies.[110] However, recent studies cited in the *Wall Street Journal* dismiss any connection between MMR vaccine and autism.

Vaccine-related autism has also been found concurrent with chronic bowel inflammation known as reactive ileal-lymphoid-nodular hyperplasia, not a surprising finding, as many live viral infections may persist in bowel tissue. Of twelve children studied with this bowel disorder, eight had onset of related behavioral symptoms after MMR vaccination.[111] Behavioral symptoms may occur as early as days or as long as several months after MMR vaccination, but in the eight children in the study, the average interval from exposure to onset of behavioral symptoms was 6.3 days.[112] Gluten and wheat sensitivities, prevalent in autistic children, may also be related to this phenomenon, and the connection between behavioral disorders and celiac disease was first described by Hans Asperger as early as 1961. It is thought that inflamed or dysfunctional intestine plays a part in behavioral changes, perhaps in part owing to incomplete breakdown and excessive absorption of components found in certain foods, including barley, rye, and oats, and casein from milk and dairy products.[113] These "opioid" substances, as they are called, may have direct deleterious central nervous system effects.[114]

Another mechanism that might come into play involves depletion of the existing supply of vitamin A by live measles vaccine, which may alter metabolic pathways necessary for appropriate neurotransmitter functioning. Decreased immunity and increase of autoimmunity may also be related to vitamin A depletion, gut disturbance, and related behavioral problems as previously described.[115] It has been shown that enhanced nutritional supplementation has improved symptoms of autism, reducing behavioral problems and increasing communication and sociability.[116]

While the connection between autism and MMR vaccine is hotly disputed by many medical professionals, the evidence linking the two, at least in the eyes of the parents of thousands of autistic children, seems apparent. In his Committee on Government Reform presentation, Bernard Rimland, Ph.D., states that though it is claimed that vaccines are safe, "physicians are indoctrinated to disbelieve claims of harm and are not trained to recognize . . . adverse reactions. From 90% to 99% of the adverse reactions reported to doctors are never reported by those doctors to . . .VAERS." Andrew Wakefield suggests that one solution to the problem of multivalent MMR's leading to the development of autism is to widely space the administration of the doses of these vaccines, giving them separately, not as a trivalent. It appears that it is the combination of the three that is especially problematic, with each possibly interfering with the actions of the other and creating unpredictable effects on the immune system.[117]

Another relationship between autism and vaccination exists when susceptible women are given rubella vaccine postnatally and then proceed to breastfeed. A significant correlation has been found between the vaccine and adverse reactions in the women, as well as significant adverse effects to the child, notably the development of autism, when the child receives routine rubella vaccination (MMR) at approximately fifteen months.[118]

DIPHTHERIA, PERTUSSIS, AND TETANUS VACCINES

Of all the childhood vaccines, none has come under such great scrutiny as the DPT vaccine, owing to a high rate of complications associated with it, particularly the pertussis component. While the United States has recently switched to using the acellular pertussis vaccine (DTaP) rather than whole-cell pertussis vaccine, because of evidence that it may be less reactogenic, it is important to look at the whole-cell pertussis vaccine for several reasons: Some doctors still administer it; it has been in continual use for decades in the United States despite evidence of its reactogenicity; it has been the focus of tremendous vaccine controversy and has left its mark on many families who have experienced adverse reactions as a result of its use; although it is now considered reactogenic, concerns regarding its use were to a great extent previously dismissed. Even now, controversy lingers regarding the effects it wrought, particularly in relation to SIDS deaths. Furthermore, it is not certain the new acellular pertussis vaccine is not reactogenic; it may just be less reactogenic than its predecessor.

Manufacturer-listed adverse reactions to DPT (also abbreviated as DTP), which are considered frequent, include the following: local redness, warmth, induration with or without tenderness, hives, rash, fever, drowsiness, fretfulness, and appetite loss. High fever, inconsolable crying, a palpable nodule at the injection site lasting several weeks, sterile abscesses at the injection site, anaphylaxis, and death have also been reported. Neurological illnesses temporally associated with the vaccine include cochlear lesion (damage to the inner ear), brachial plexus nerve damage, EEG disturbances, encephalopathy, and Guillain-Barré syndrome. There may be seizures and hypotonic-hyporesponsive collapse, onset of infantile spasms, intracranial pressure with distension of the anterior fontanel in infants, and other neurological consequences. SIDS has been associated with DPT, though a causal link has not been made. This is addressed below in the discussion of pertussis vaccine.

Diphtheria Vaccine

According to an article in *Vaccine*, "Adverse side-effects to tetanus and diphtheria toxoids have been known for many years and there have been ways to minimize these reactions. These procedures did not get widespread acceptance because the current . . . vaccines meet the regulatory requirements and the manufacturers are reluctant to change the established procedures of production due to the amount of work involved in the regulatory issues under the current Good Manufacturing Practices (GMP)."[119]

The diphtheria vaccine currently in use is an aluminum-adsorbed preparation, meaning it is combined with aluminum to increase the availability of the diphtheria toxoid in the body. Indeed, the question of metal toxicity and adverse effects requires further investigation. Metal toxicity, particularly from aluminum and mercury, may turn out to be implicated in many of the adverse neurological consequences associated with vaccines, such as the link between MMR and autism.[120] In her report to the Committee on Government Reform hearings on autism, one mother of an autistic child inquires: "Could someone please explain to me why it is acceptable to have products on the market that exposed my child to 37.5 micrograms of mercury in one day when at that time he should not have been exposed to more than .59 micrograms given his body weight? Even a body as big as mine shouldn't be exposed to more than 5 micrograms of mercury in one day. That is completely unacceptable. One size does not fit all when it comes to vaccines."[121]

Earlier vaccines were associated with higher rates of reaction than the more highly purified one used now, though the authors of the *Vaccine* article quoted above suggest that the current one could be more highly purified and a less reactogenic adjuvant could be used.[122] There is an association between the diphtheria vaccine and the subsequent development of encephalopathy. In the early 1980s the Italian Ministry of Health investigated forty-five reports of reactions associated with the DT vaccine, including encephalopathy, coma (cause unknown), Reye's syndrome, respiratory distress from coma, and death.[123] Encephalopathy in these cases is believed to be a result of the tetanus portion of the vaccine rather than the diphtheria component. There may be a link between diphtheria and tetanus toxoid administration and arthritis, but evidence pointing to this association is limited.[124] It is plausible that diphtheria toxoid can lead to the development of erythema multiforme (EM), an inflammatory eruption characterized by red lesions of varying appearance affecting the skin and mucous membranes.[125] The lesions typically have a bull's eye or target appearance. Allergic reactions (sometimes severe) can occur as a result of hypersensitivity to the aluminum component of the vaccine.

Pertussis Vaccine

The whole-cell pertussis vaccine, in use in the United States until just recently, has been at the center of the vaccine safety controversy, owing to its relatively higher rate of reactogenicity than other childhood vaccines. Indeed, it has served as a catalyst in bringing the vaccine-safety debate to public attention. "The controversy involves not only the interface among epidemiology, politics, and policy, but also legal and economic issues, ethical concerns, emotional overlays, and the role of the media."[126] For at least thirty years, numerous cases of pertussis vaccine–related adverse events resulting in neurological damage have been reported in the literature, and more significantly, reported to doctors by parents but often denied. Any acknowledged reactions have generally been dismissed as an unfortunate but acceptable risk of the vaccine, seen as so critical to preventing pertussis outbreaks.[127] Often cited is the fact that when the United Kingdom suspended the use of the whole-cell pertussis vaccine in the early 1970s, because of frequency of severe reactions, major pertussis epidemics were experienced there (between 1977 and 1982). Similar trends were seen in Japan, where the vaccine was suspended for the same reason. Vaccine proponents estimate that without the pertussis vaccine there would be outrageous rates of infection with severe outcomes.

Unfortunately, much of the evidence regarding just how much disease incidence there would be without the vaccine is speculative and has at times been based on data from eras when the disease incidence was greatest. Gordon Stewart from the University of Glasgow Hospital remarks that it is "assumed that if there were no vaccination program, the incidence, complications, and death rate would now be what they were in . . . 1940 to 1950. This is surely untrue of any infectious disease. Secondly, they assume that the vaccine gives 70 percent protection. This figure overlooks recent reports from North America and from Australia and the United Kingdom that 30 to 50 percent of cases occur in vaccinated children. Thirdly . . . recent reports from the United States indicate much higher frequencies of toxicity."[128] Alan Hinman comments: "Much of the evidence for the benefits of pertussis vaccination arises from epidemiologic studies regarding the incidence of the disease and the effectiveness of the vaccine in preventing it. The very nature of epidemiologic data has contributed to the controversy, since there is virtually no epidemiologic study with absolutely incontrovertible results that allow only one interpretation."[129] For example, it is well known that pertussis is widely underdiagnosed and underreported in the United States, making it hard to determine the exact efficacy of the vaccine.[130] Prior to the late-1970s epidemic of pertussis, only 10 percent of people diagnosed with the disease were hospitalized. Strikingly, during this epidemic, only 4 percent were hospitalized.[131] We cannot minimize the potentially devastating effects of this disease, particularly in those who are malnourished or immunocompromised, which in 1982 in the United Kingdom led to an epidemic involving 65,000 people and caused 14 deaths.

Pertussis continues to persist, both in unvaccinated and vaccinated populations. For example, in one study among a population in Nova Scotia, 91.2 percent of those who developed pertussis were fully vaccinated, a 45 percent vaccine efficacy rate.[132] The authors of this study stated that older children, adolescents, and adults are susceptible because vaccine efficacy wanes with increasing intervals after a booster dose. Nonetheless, peak incidence in this community was in the one- to five-year-olds, the group that should have been optimally protected.[133]

Records from 1974 to 1975 in the United Kingdom indicate 8,092 cases of pertussis. The rates of hospitalization varied, as did deaths, but for both, negative outcomes were higher in the youngest age range. In those below six months, 7 deaths were reported in 545 cases (1.3 percent); in ages six months to five years, 3 deaths were reported in 7,464 cases (0.04 percent). Two cases of encephalitis were recorded (0.025 percent).[134]

Whole-cell pertussis vaccine is associated with a very high frequency of reactions. Barkin and Pichichero conducted a study of vaccine reactions occurring within forty-eight hours of receipt of DPT among 1,232 respondents to a questionnaire and determined the following: "Only 7% reported no reaction, while 336 (27.3%) reported mild, 722 (58.6%) moderate, and 88 (7.1%) severe reactions. Over 50% experienced temperatures of at least 100°F, and 80% noted behavioral changes."[135] Acknowledged mild reactions include sore arm or leg, fever, fussiness, appetite loss, tiredness, and vomiting. Acknowledged moderate to serious reactions include persistent crying (categorized as three hours or more, occurring in 100 of every 10,000 doses), fever of 105 degrees Fahrenheit or higher (occurring in 30 of every 10,000 doses), seizures (occurring in 6 of every 10,000 doses), and hypotonic-hyporesponsive episodes (child becomes limp, pale, experiences loss of or altered consciousness; occurs in 6 of every 10,000 doses). Acknowledged severe reactions include anaphylactic shock from allergic reaction and severe neurological consequences (long seizure, coma, persistent loss of consciousness).[136] One paper in *Pediatrics* describes the DPT vaccine as having "high reactogenicity in a pediatric population receiving the product in accordance with current recommendations."[137]

A 1979 article in the *New England Journal of Medicine* states that data from Sweden estimate severe reactions to occur at a rate of 1 in 3,100 vaccinations, consisting of convulsions, shock, pallor, and cyanosis lasting up to thirty minutes; meningeal involvement; and persistent crying lasting more than twelve hours or requiring hospitalization. The authors estimate severe reactions, consisting of repeated convulsions, to be 1 in 34,000 vaccinations, and encephalitis to be 1 in 170,000 vaccine recipients.[138] Unpublished data from the Netherlands estimated the risks to be even higher for major reactions, with encephalitis occurring in 4 of 190,000 vaccine recipients, a rate similar to that determined for Scotland.[139] The authors of this study conclude that maintaining vaccine programs is still desirable; they assert that encephalitis occurs twice as often with a vaccine program as without but that deaths are almost four times more likely in the absence of a vaccine program. Hinman and Koplan corroborate this statement: "Deaths from pertussis decline from 457 to 44 with a program.

However, there is also an increase in the total number of children with re-sidual defects from encephalitis with the vaccination program (54 vs. 29 with-out a program)."[140] Barkin and Pichichero comment that "the acceptance of significant risks associated with pertussis vaccine is further complicated by evi-dence that immunity is not sustained. Susceptibility to pertussis 12 years after immunization may be as high as 95%, as noted in an epidemic among hospital personnel in Cincinnati."[141]

Contrary to this opinion, Dr. Gordon Stewart of the University of Glasgow in the United Kingdom states that "the claim by official bodies that the risks of whooping cough exceed those of vaccination is questionable, at least in the U.K."[142] He emphasizes that surveillance systems are inadequate, both nation-ally and internationally, and that when valid comparisons are made between vaccinated and unvaccinated children, attack rates may be lower and fewer in vaccinated children, but confounding variables such as overcrowding and so-cioeconomic differences are not considered. The issue of confounding vari-ables is again raised in the July 1992 issue of the *American Journal of Epidemi-ology*, where the authors state, "Studies that fail to control adequately for such confounding factors are likely to underestimate the risks of adverse events attributable to vaccination."[143]

While the relationships between the pertussis component of the vaccine and short-term neurological consequences, persistent neurological problems, and SIDS have been downplayed by many U.S. scientists and public health officials, there has been a groundswell of parents, physicians, and others who have seen the devastating effects of this vaccine with their own eyes and have no question that the pertussis vaccine can cause such problems. According to Barkin and Pichichero, the actual incidence of reactions such as encephalitis, seizures, and other severe neurological complications is unclear because of the absence of data.[144] They explain that estimates vary from as many as 1 in 3,600 children to 1 in 500,000 children. The British National Childhood Encepha-lopathy Study estimated the increased risk of acute encephalopathy from per-tussis vaccine to be 1 case for every 110,000 doses of DPT, and for encephal-opathy with residual damage one year later to be 1 per 310,000 doses.[145] Keep in mind that as children receive four doses of this vaccine by the time they are fifteen months old, 110,000 doses may represent only 35,000 children.

In spite of such clear findings of a relatively frequent association between pertussis vaccine and adverse neurological consequences, one report attempts to dismiss the intensified reports of anaphylaxis, collapse, convulsions, and neurological complications in the northwest Thames region of England over a seven-year period as possibly just a response to negative publicity accorded the pertussis vaccine during that time.[146] In contrast to this, nationwide coverage of the television program that minimized the risks of pertussis while emphasizing risks and alleged risks of the vaccine did not have a significant impact on pertussis use in the U.S. population at the time.[147] Another report from as recently as 1990, published in the *Journal of Pediatrics*, states that although pertussis vaccine encephalopathy was first reported fifty-six years ago, "analysis of the recent literature . . . does not support the existence of such a syndrome and suggests that neurological events after immunization are chance temporal associations of neurologic conditions that occur in the target age group, even in the absence of immunization."[148] In other words, neurological damage occurring after a DPT vaccine is purely coincidental.[149]

According to *Morbidity and Mortality Weekly Report*, "Update: Vaccine Side Effects, Adverse Reactions, Contraindications, and Precautions":

- the National Childhood Encephalopathy Study and other controlled epidemiological studies have provided evidence that DTP can cause acute encephalopathy,

- children with chronic nervous system dysfunction were more likely than children in a control group to have received DTP within seven days of onset of serious acute neurological illness,

- children who had an acute neurological illness after DTP administration were significantly more likely than the control group to have nervous system dysfunction ten years later, and

- DTP vaccine may cause chronic nervous system dysfunction or it may trigger a predisposition to nervous system dysfunction in children who have chronic underlying brain or metabolic disorders.[150]

The ACIP committee that prepared the report calculated that hypotonic-hyporesponsive episodes occur in 1 per 1,750 doses and convulsions occur at this same rate.[151] Children with a history of convulsions, or a family history of convulsive disorders, may be especially susceptible to such a reaction to the vaccine. An article in the *Journal of Pediatrics* indicates a risk of a neurological event after a DPT vaccine to be 7.2 percent higher for those with prior risk.[152] The authors recommend that children with such histories not receive DPT vaccine until it is known whether they have any evidence of neurological disorder, and if they do, they should receive DT only.[153] Nonetheless, in 1988 the *Report of the Task Force on Pertussis and Pertussis Immunization* claimed that the majority of cases of vaccine-related encephalopathy in the United States "in reality represent the onset of epilepsy."[154]

While several studies conclude that the long-term effects of vaccine-related seizures and hypotonic-hyporesponsive events are nonexistent or negligible, we must keep in mind that there are studies in the medical literature from as recently as the early 1990s that deny a causal relationship between the vaccine and these events, despite clear evidence to the contrary.[155] What is perhaps most significant and at the same time most greatly disregarded about serious adverse reactions to vaccines is that they repeatedly occur in children who parents assert were previously entirely normal, healthy children. These children, after receiving their routine vaccinations, begin to exhibit behaviors they have never before displayed. Furthermore, when there is a familial tendency to vaccine reaction, the parents may see this pattern each time one of their children gets vaccinated. This is frequently the case when there is no preexisting individual or family history of vaccine-reaction–like behaviors.

In addition to children with a direct or familial history of convulsions, it has long been recognized that children allergic to substances such as eggs and gelatin might be more prone to adverse reactions as a result of allergic response to vaccine components such as the gelatin base stabilizer, or protein fragments from mediums upon which vaccine cultures are grown, such as chicken embryo. Recent articles appearing in the literature, however, suggest that even children who have had a history of serious reactions may continue their vaccine program. The authors of one study conclude: "We successfully vaccinated children with histories of serious reactions to vaccination including HHEs, convulsions, apnea, high temperatures and persistent screaming, as well as those with egg allergy."[156] This is in spite of the fact that numerous medical authorities on vaccination, including the CDC Advisory Committee on Immunization Practices, contraindicate giving the DPT vaccine to children with such a history of serious adverse reaction to prior DPT vaccination.[157] Adverse reactions may also be caused by ingredients in the vaccines other than the pertussis organism or components, particularly aluminum compounds such as aluminum phosphate and aluminum hydroxide. Furthermore, it is unclear what effect such metals, found in both the DPT and the DTaP vaccines, might have on long-term health.[158] It is clear that parents must use their common sense and evaluate each child and each vaccine individually.

In addition to the reactions already described, the DPT vaccine, and particularly the pertussis vaccine, are associated with increased development of allergy-related respiratory problems and asthma.[159] According to a recent article in the *Journal of Manipulative Physiologic Therapy*, "DTP or tetanus vaccination appears to increase the risk of allergies and related respiratory symptoms in children and adolescents."[160] According to Dr. Michel Odent, "Among the 243 immunized children, 26 were diagnosed as having asthma, compared with four of the 203 children who had not been immunized."[161] The pertussis vaccine seemed to create the greatest statistical significance in the likelihood of developing asthma.

Diphtheria–tetanus–acellular-pertussis vaccine was licensed in the United States in 1991. Even as recently as 1994, the DTaP vaccine was recommended for use as the fourth and fifth booster shots only, as clinical efficacy and safety in young children had not been established.[162] Only more recently has DTaP primarily replaced the DPT vaccine. While most medical researchers seem optimistic that DTaP will result in significantly fewer adverse side effects than DPT, the safety of this vaccine is inconclusive.[163] According to James Cherry, an outspoken vaccine researcher and advocate, "Compared with the whole cell pertussis component DTP vaccine, the DTaP vaccines were found in reactogenicity and immunogenicity studies to be associated with less severe and less frequent adverse reactions" (implying that there are still somewhat frequent and somewhat severe reactions, or few reactions?). However, he says that the definition of pertussis established by the World Health Organization for vaccine efficacy trials excludes some laboratory-confirmed cases: "Vaccine efficacy appears better than it truly is, whereas less effective vaccines seem comparable with their more effective counterparts."[164] The incidence of adverse reactions increased after booster shots, and a previous severe reaction was a risk factor for a severe reaction after a booster dose.[165] A recent report from the Italian Institute of Health regarding the effects of acellular pertussis given to fifteen thousand children revealed that "the frequency of heavy adverse reactions was exactly identical for the two vaccines, acellular and cellular."[166] While the use of acellular pertussis is clearly associated with reduced rates of reactions in Japan, it should be noted that children there are not vaccinated with pertussis until they are two years old, a factor that itself may be responsible for reduced reactions.

Pertussis Vaccine and Sudden Infant Death Syndrome (SIDS)

The association between SIDS and pertussis vaccination has been repeatedly dismissed by the majority of medical authorities as an erroneous relationship, with no causal evidence to indicate that the DPT vaccine can cause SIDS. In fact, nearly every article encountered in the literature denies a causal effect between the two. Most reports state that any association between SIDS and

DPT is purely coincidental, highlighted by the fact that as SIDS generally occurs in the age range that DPT also happens to be given, it is inevitable that there would appear to be a relationship when there is none. An overly simplistic (and perhaps insulting), yet nonetheless typical, explanation to parents can be found in the CDC brochure *Common Misconceptions about Vaccination:*

DTP Vaccine and SIDS

One myth that won't seem to go away is that DTP vaccine causes sudden infant death syndrome (SIDS). This belief came about because a moderate proportion of children who die of SIDS have recently been vaccinated with DTP; and on the surface, this seems to point toward a causal connection. But this logic is faulty; you might as well say that eating bread causes car crashes, since most drivers who crash their cars could probably be shown to have eaten bread within the past 24 hours.

There are, however, many parents who insist that their previously healthy baby died in close proximity to receipt of this vaccine, with no doubt that the vaccine caused death, and a growing number of doctors who recognize that such adverse reactions may indeed be related to vaccinations. Furthermore, there clearly are SIDS deaths that occur within the time frame in which DPT vaccines are administered, and there are no clear mechanisms of differential diagnosis to determine whether an infant death occurred owing to vaccination or to SIDS, the causes of which remain unknown.[167] Indeed, many infant deaths are classified as SIDS when the cause is uncertain but appears natural and spontaneous. "Rarely will a coroner or doctor admit that a vaccine played any role in an infant's death."[168] Barbara Loe Fisher and Harris Coulter, in their book *DPT: A Shot in the Dark,* say with much common sense and logic: "The cause of SIDS is unknown. If the cause is unknown, then how can doctors rule out the possibility that vaccination was either the direct cause or at least a contributing cause in cases where the only common denominator was death? And yet Alan Hinman was quoted in the *Journal of the American Medical Association* as stating: 'We have received reports of 44 deaths occurring within 4 weeks of DPT immunization. Thirty-two of the deaths were SIDS. Of the other twelve, in only one was there autopsy or clinical information that would indicate that this was a neurologic or encephalopathic response to DPT.'"[169] Also, most of the studies conducted to determine if there is a relationship between SIDS and DPT only look at deaths within forty-eight or seventy-two hours of the vaccine as possibly related. It is well known that other vaccine reactions, such as symptoms of illness after a measles vaccine, can occur later after vaccination than this; why not SIDS death?

In one well-documented case in Tennessee in 1979, four SIDS deaths were clearly and specifically attributed to DPT vaccination by researchers, though even this association is frequently rebutted in medical journal articles. "On March 9, 1979, the Tennessee Department of Health reported to the Centers for Disease Control that four sudden and unexplained deaths had occurred since November, 1978, in infants who had been vaccinated during the 24-hour period prior to death. All four deaths were classified as sudden infant death syndrome, and all had received a first vaccination of diphtheria–tetanus toxoids–pertussis vaccine and oral polio vaccine."[170] An ensuing study looking at larger groups of infants indicated that "this evidence seems adequate to indicate an unusual temporal association between DTP vaccination with lot A [the particular lot used in the control group and associated with the deaths in Tennessee] and SIDS."[171] Of course, "fevers, seizures, and sudden unexplained death (SIDS) all occur during the first year of life in the unvaccinated as well as the vaccinated. Since 95 percent of children in the United States are vaccinated, it is difficult . . . to find a placebo control group."[172]

Tetanus Vaccine

Tetanus vaccination is associated with the lowest rate of adverse reactions of all of the vaccines currently in use. Nonetheless, a number of reactions are associated with the vaccine, including quite common minor local reactions such as pain, swelling, and redness at the injection site. Severe reactions are infrequent and are often accompanied by a sore, swollen arm, along with fever, malaise, and possibly other systemic responses. Severe reactions are usually associated with increasing doses of the vaccine and are rarely associated with the primary vaccination. Therefore, frequent booster shots increase the risk of a reaction.[173] Other reactions associated with tetanus vaccine include arthritis, temporary decreased immunity, and anaphylaxis. The latter of these risks is clearly documented and has occurred with enough frequency that a clear causal relationship between tetanus toxoid and anaphylaxis has been established, though again, in relationship to the number of doses given in the United States, the incidence is rare.[174] It was initially suspected that allergic reactions to tetanus vaccine were caused by proteins contaminating the vaccine, but nine cases have been reported since the removal of these proteins, using a more purified form of the vaccine.[175] Several additional cases have been reported to the VAERS but were dismissed on the grounds that they did not meet the criteria for anaphylactic shock.[176] In a review of all the cases of reactions to diphtheria and tetanus toxoids between 1952 and 1970, of 2.5 million doses of monovalent tetanus given to adults and 1.1 million doses of DT given to children in Denmark, 2 cases of what appear to be anaphylaxis occurred, both just after children received their first dose of the vaccine. In another retrospective study comparing reactions to DPT and DT among a total of 10,028 children, 13 developed pallor and cyanosis within five minutes to twenty-four hours of vaccination. These events were not classified as anaphylaxis, however, and both cases of anaphylaxis resolved automatically. The 1983 study of the northwest Thames region in Great Britain revealed 2 cases of what was called "acute collapse" among 135,000 children receiving their initial series of three doses of DT (meaning 1 in 45,000 children), with 6 additional episodes after DT booster among 221,000 children. The symptoms exhibited were coldness, clamminess, and lack of pulse, slight facial swelling, pallor, and vasovagal attacks (hyperventilation, pallor, sweating, accelerated heartbeat). Again, the IOM dismissed these symptoms as not indicative of anaphylaxis based on the definition determined for the IOM study. All of the children recovered from their reactions.

Guillain-Barré syndrome has also been recognized as an accepted, though uncommon, result of tetanus vaccination. Because both GBS and anaphylaxis can be fatal, a causal relationship between tetanus and death from these causes has been established, though it is considered "extraordinarily low."[177]

The actual risk of contracting tetanus is also quite low, with the greatest number of cases ever reported in one year in the United States since this has been a reportable disease purportedly being in the range of about 620. Most cases do appear to occur in those who have never received tetanus vaccination, or in those whose immunity has waned, particularly women over fifty years old. However, because the risk of a reaction increases with repeated exposure to the vaccine, care must be taken in giving booster doses to those with evidence of preexisting immunity from vaccination or to those who have received repeated boosters throughout their lives. Reactions are more common among groups likely to receive regular boosters, such as the military or veterinarians.

POLIO VACCINE

The 1990s brought us dramatic changes in poliovirus vaccine policy, with the initial recommendations of changing from four doses of live oral polio vaccine to two initial doses of killed polio vaccine followed by two live doses, to the current recommendation issued in 1999: to use only the killed poliovirus vaccine for all four of the doses. An official ban on OPV was expected to begin in the year 2000, as the American Academy of Pediatrics initially requested a partial ban only. Exceptions allowing the use of OPV should be made only if children will be traveling within four weeks of vaccination to an area where active polio infection occurs.

Despite the fact that Jonas Salk, a discoverer of the inactivated polio vaccine, has been commenting on the danger of live poliovirus vaccine for several decades, it took the CDC and other health authorities this long to acknowledge publicly that the only cases of polio infection in the United States occur as a result of direct exposure to the live vaccine or to someone who has received the live vaccine within several weeks. The latter is a risk because the vaccine recipient sheds live virus in saliva (for up to a week after vaccination) and bowel movements (up to eight weeks after vaccination). Yet many doctors have failed to make this policy change in their practices, according to Paul Offit of Children's Hospital in Philadelphia in a presentation at the Federal Advisory Committee on Immunization Practices meeting in Atlanta, Georgia, in 1999. He commented that 10 percent of pediatricians are still offering OPV, "ignoring the ban."[178] Prior to the ban the vaccine was responsible for at least eight cases of paralysis annually. According to the report by the Institute of Medicine, it has been known since the 1930s that OPV can cause polio: "The concept that live attenuated polio vaccine causes a small number of poliomyelitis cases thus has a history of six decades."[179] Between 1962 and 1964 alone there were 123 cases of paralytic polio that occurred within thirty days of vaccination, and it was determined that 57 of these met the criteria for vaccine-induced illness. Family members, unvaccinated playmates, and siblings were also at risk of contracting the disease, and numerous case reports of this occurring can be found as well.[180]

Product manufacturer (Lederle) inserts for OPV list paralytic polio and fatal paralytic polio in immunocompromised persons as possible adverse reactions to the vaccine. Adverse reactions listed (by Pasteur Merrieux Connaught) for IPV include the following: transient local redness at the injection site, irritability, sleepiness, fussiness, and crying. Loss of appetite and vomiting may occur. They note that Guillain-Barré syndrome has been temporally related to the administration of another manufacturer's brand of inactivated poliovirus vaccine. This connection was made after a 1976 report that indicated that there were ten cases of GBS in patients who had received IPV.[181] In one case involving a ten-month-old girl who developed GBS after receiving her vaccinations, throat cultures revealed that the GBS was actually caused by the measles vaccine.[182] Nonetheless, the risks of IPV appear to be significantly lower than for OPV.

It is interesting to note that the IOM specifically comments that "the possible causal relationship between polio vaccines and SIDS has rarely been studied," therefore "evidence is inadequate to accept or reject a causal relation between polio vaccine and SIDS." Why has this been inadequately studied when, like other vaccines, it is administered during those months when the risk of SIDS occurrence is greatest?

Another troubling aspect of the OPV vaccine is its association with Simian virus 40 (SV40), a virus of monkey origin, known for its ability to initiate insidious, aggressive cancerous tumors.[183] The story goes like this: In the early 1950s, Jonas Salk discovered that monkey kidneys could be used to culture poliovirus in quantities significant enough to meet the demands for mass-producing the polio vaccine. However, in 1960 SV40 was discovered, and shortly after that it was found in the polio vaccine. In 1961 it was discovered that the virus could cause tumors in laboratory rodents.[184] All recipients of injected polio vaccine between 1954 and 1963, and all those who received OPV between 1959 and 1961, may have received vaccine contaminated with SV40.[185] SV40 virus was also found in vaccines given to army personal to protect them against respiratory infections, as well as in an adenovirus vaccine given to more than 100,000 men in army camps during that time period.[186]

It was originally assumed that the virus could not infect humans, as interspecies transfer of viral infections was not suspected to occur.[187] Indeed, there seemed to be little concern regarding the presence of extraneous live viruses in the polio vaccine, which was considered so safe that it was also used for the treatment of herpes lesions.[188] However, a paper from 1964 published in the journal *Acta Biologica* revealed the presence on SV40 in the feces of numerous infants following the experimental vaccination of infants with poliovirus to test for serologic response from individual vaccines.[189] Clearly, interspecies transfer was possible and had occurred. However, the ramifications of this were yet unknown.

The position of the Centers for Disease Control and Prevention is that SV40 has not caused any harm, illness, or cancer in those who received vaccines contaminated with the virus.[190] However, they do admit that researchers have identified SV40 virus in human tumors and DNA samples from normal tissue and cancerous tissue. They state that they are unsure of the implications of such findings.[191] But a number of researchers have come to a very different conclusion. And indeed, the whole topic has an air of covert mystery surrounding it.

According to authors Debbie Bookchin and Jim Schumacher, when federal officials in 1961 discovered the presence of SV40 in vaccines, they ordered vaccine manufacturers to screen for and eliminate the virus from the vaccine. However, they kept the controversy quiet and did not recall existing stocks, resulting in an additional 2 million people receiving this vaccine for an additional two years.[192]

Although it was "determined" that SV40 did not harm humans, it has been used widely in cancer research because it causes a variety of tumors easily in animal experiments. Only recently has significant research gone into its effects as a cancer-causing agent in humans. But recently various international teams of researchers have found definitive evidence of the presence of this virus in human cancers, particularly mesothelioma, a lung cancer linked to exposure to asbestos. Michael Carbone, an Italian medical school graduate with a Ph.D. in human pathology and a leading researcher of SV40, states, "There is no doubt that SV40 is a human carcinogen" and is "definitely something you don't want in your body."[193] Since Carbone's first studies linking SV40 with human mesothelioma, scientists from seventeen other labs internationally have confirmed his findings, possibly clarifying why at least 20 percent of those with this type of cancer have no prior asbestos exposure. SV40 is also linked to brain tumors, bone tumors, Wilms' tumors, adenosarcomas, and rare uterine cancers. It has been isolated in many cancers that affect children who had not directly received the contaminated vaccine; researchers now recognize that the virus is transmittable from parents to children through DNA.[194] While the extent of this issue is beyond the scope of this book, it is fascinating and I encourage readers to access information on this topic, particularly the articles that appeared in *Atlantic Monthly* magazine and on the CDC vaccine information Web site. When I first encountered the issue I was concerned that perhaps this was a hoax or paranoid fantasy, but the research and evidence are easily available, and the presence of SV40 is a clearly demonstrable scientific fact supported by the FDA and the CDC.[195]

What is the significance of the SV40 issue for youngsters receiving vaccines today? Perhaps just the realization that we don't know exactly what is in our vaccines or how this might affect us in several decades. Just as there were extraneous viruses that went undetected in vaccines forty years ago, there may be other substances in our vaccines now that we don't even know to look for. And we don't know enough about immunology, virology, genetics, and interspecies transfer to assume that injecting our children with material derived from other animals isn't going to create long-term immunological problems.

VARICELLA VACCINE

Varicella vaccine is not yet mandated by most states, though the federal government does recommend it for all children over a year old who have not yet had the chicken pox.[196] Adverse reactions to varicella live virus vaccine include pain and redness at the injection site, upper respiratory illness, cough, irritability, nervousness, fatigue, disturbed sleep, diarrhea, appetite loss, vomiting, earache and/or infection, diaper rash, generalized rash, headache, malaise, abdominal pain, nausea, eye complaints, chills, swollen lymph nodes, muscle aches, lower respiratory illness, allergic reactions including hives or a rash, stiff neck, arthralgia, eczema, dry skin, itching, and constipation. Pneumonitis has been reported in a small number of children, as have febrile seizures.[197] Chicken pox lesions have been reported on the body within one to four weeks of vaccination.[198] More serious side effects cited by Merck include anaphylaxis, thrombocytopenia, encephalitis, nonfebrile seizures, Guillain-Barré syndrome, transverse myelitis, Bell's palsy, pharyngitis, and secondary skin infections, including shingles, impetigo, and cellulitis.[199]

The two most significant concerns regarding long-term effects of varicella vaccine are those of shifting disease epidemiology and the possibility for the virus to lie dormant in the body and reemerge later as zoster infection (shingles).

Varicella vaccine decreases in efficacy by 3 percent annually after vaccination, and the duration of protection from chicken pox is unknown.[200] This means that while children are protected from chicken pox during the age range of least vulnerability to severe consequences from the disease, adults who were vaccinated as children and therefore never contracted chicken pox naturally are susceptible to the illness. Chicken pox in adults carries significantly more risk. Furthermore, the likelihood of contracting the disease naturally is diminished as more children are vaccinated, though it is thought that vaccinated children can shed the virus, passing it on to susceptible others (pregnant women, infants, susceptible adults, and those who are immunocompromised). The risk of shifting the epidemiology of chicken pox to more vulnerable populations must be carefully considered against the generally benign nature of the naturally occurring illness.

The question of the development of shingles later in life owing to dormant varicella-zoster virus from the vaccine has not yet been answered. The suspected rate, based on available epidemiologic evidence to date, suggests a case rate of 18.5 cases of herpes zoster per 100,000 vaccine recipients.[201] According to Michiaki Takahashi, writing on this subject in *Vaccines*, "A long-term follow-up of vaccinated, healthy children will be required to answer this question."[202] In other words, nobody knows. And we are engaging in a live human experiment—with our children—to find out.

HIB VACCINE

Conjugated Hib vaccine was approved in 1988 for use in children eighteen months or older, after the unconjugated Hib vaccine failed to provide adequate protection for children under two, the population in which 75 percent of Hib cases occur. By 1991 Hib vaccine had been approved for use in those as young as two months. It is currently mandated in at least forty-four states. Hib meningitis is a particularly serious infection, especially prevalent among children in day-care settings. Adverse effects of Hib vaccine observed during clinical trials included seizures, hives, renal failure, and Guillain-Barré syndrome. SIDS deaths did occur in both the control group and the study groups and were not considered to be adverse reactions to the vaccine.[203] Local pain and tenderness at the injection site are common, and anywhere from 1 to 20 percent of vaccine recipients develop low-grade fever in the first twenty to seventy-two hours after vaccination.[204] Ten to 25 percent of conjugate recipients exhibit irritability after vaccination.

One of the most interesting "side effects" of Hib vaccine is the susceptibility of recipients to Hib infection shortly after vaccination, generally within seven days.[205] While some might assert that the children who develop Hib just after vaccination were actually already infected prior to vaccination and were in the prodromal stage of illness, significant evidence exists demonstrating that the vaccine itself may lower immunity, leading to increased postvaccination susceptibility.[206] Observations that vaccination can lead to decreased immunity were made as early as 1893, and again in 1896. Studies of those vaccinated against typhoid fever show increased susceptibility to the infection.[207]

Fisher reminds us that Hib "has not been evaluated for its carcinogenic, mutagenic potential, or impairment of fertility, and it is not known whether [the vaccine] can cause fetal harm when administered to a pregnant woman or can affect reproductive capacity."[208] Finally, as this vaccine is conjugated with tetanus toxoid, side effects of tetanus vaccine are applicable to Hib vaccine, as are side effects from sensitivity to additives and stabilizers.

HEPATITIS B VACCINE

Hepatitis B vaccination was recommended for pediatric use beginning in the immediate neonatal period as part of a broader attempt to stem the spread of this highly infectious virus, even though most neonates are at low risk for contracting the infection. Thus the Hep B requirement for newborns came under serious scrutiny when it was revealed in July 1999 that one of the components of the vaccine, thimerosal, a mercury derivative, could place the newborn at serious risk of mercury toxicity and, in fact, exceeded EPA limits for mercury in the first six months of life.[209] The vaccine was abruptly banned for all babies other than those born to mothers with infectious hepatitis B, and for those babies it was recommended that thimerosal-free vaccine be used. However, the vaccine was reinstated by 2000, with the suggestion that when thimerosal-free vaccine is available, it should be used in otherwise healthy newborns, but when it is not available, the thimerosal-containing vaccine should be used. High levels of systemic mercury can lead to learning disabilities and attention and language deficits, aside from serious poisoning.[210] According to Dr. Neal Halsey, director of the Johns Hopkins Institute for Vaccine Safety and former chairperson of the American Academy of Pediatrics Committee on Infectious Diseases, "For infants born to women with high mercury consumption [for example, from environmental exposure or consumption of large amounts of fish], no one knows what dose of mercury, if any, from vaccines is safe. . . . We can say there is no evidence of harm, but the truth is no one has looked."[211]

But the thimerosal issue is only one drawback to the hepatitis B vaccine, which is associated with a number of side effects. One of the immediate problems with postnatal injection with this vaccine is that it can cause unexplained elevated fever in the newborn.[212] This elevated temperature will frequently result in the neonate's being subjected to unnecessary procedures and treatment to diagnose the unexplained fever.[213]

Furthermore, hepatitis B vaccine is associated with significant rates of temporary and long-term arthritic complaints.[214] According to an IOM report, "An association between hepatitis B vaccine and acute arthralgia, arthritis, or both has been suggested since the initial use of plasma-derived hepatitis B vaccines."[215] The incidence is greater in adults than in children, and women seem especially susceptible to this complaint, with as many as 50 percent of greater women vaccine recipients reporting this side effect.

Central nervous system demyelination is also attributed to hepatitis B vaccination, with a possible link between the vaccine and multiple sclerosis, as well as Guillain-Barré syndrome.[216] A French medical journal article evaluated this relationship and concluded that "findings did not permit [the researchers] to exclude confidently an association between HB (hepatitis B) vaccine and the occurrence of a first CNS demyelinating episode."[217]

In addition to this, HB vaccine has been implicated in at least twenty-two cases of systemic lupus erythematosus (SLE, an autoimmune disorder) that were previously undiagnosed. The authors of one study conclude that "in SLE patients, hepatitis B vaccination may be followed by disease exacerbation."[218] While the authors admit that the connection may be coincidental and that they are positively in favor of hepatitis B vaccination, they raise questions about the vaccine for those with SLE. Keep in mind, however, that they describe cases in which SLE had previously been undiagnosed. Dr. Daniel Battafarano, another medical researcher, comments: "Individual vaccines and a combination of vaccines have been reported to be associated with the onset of SLE within 1–3 weeks of vaccination and typically after secondary or booster immunization. Hepatitis B vaccine is only one of many vaccines that have been temporally related to the development of SLE."[219] He, too, remarks that in spite of this, hepatitis B vaccine is extremely safe and well tolerated, even by SLE patients. It is hard to overlook the fact that both SLE and rheumatoid arthritis are autoimmune conditions, and that HB vaccine may have a not yet understood impact on the immune system that warrants cautious use.

In 1988 in New Zealand a massive vaccination campaign was begun, initially targeting children five years old or under, and extending over a few years to those up to sixteen years old. Prior to vaccination, the incidence of diabetes in the study groups was 11.2 cases per 100,000 per year, while after immunization the incidence rose to 18.2 per 100,000. Further longitudinal studies have not been done to see if the incidence has further increased.[220] While those vaccinated at birth demonstrated decreased incidence of diabetes mellitus, those vaccinated after six weeks of age showed evidence of increase of insulin-dependent diabetes mellitus. A letter to the *New Zealand Journal of Medicine* states: "The hepatitis B vaccines have been noted in the package inserts and Physicians Desk Reference to cause several autoimmune diseases, and the FDA has gone on record that the hepatitis B vaccines cause the autoimmune disease alopecia (U.S. FDA internet home page). The hepatitis B vaccine, as well as other vaccines, can potentially induce insulin dependent diabetes mellitus."[221]

Perhaps it is these problems, and concern about other adverse effects yet unknown, that have led many physicians to question the necessity and wisdom of universal hepatitis B vaccination for infants. One study undertook a random-sample survey of three hundred family physicians in North Carolina. Of the 78 percent who responded, only 17 percent agreed that it was warranted to vaccinate all the newborns in their practice for hepatitis B.[222] The same research team surveyed pediatricians and found a striking similarity: only 32 percent believed it was warranted in their practices.[223]

The Long-Term Picture

In examining some of the adverse effects of vaccinations, we have seen that they can have immediate short-term consequences that are both mild and serious. However, we also saw that vaccines are implicated in a number of chronic health problems, such as allergies, asthma, diabetes, and rheumatoid arthritis. When we consider the consequences of such insidious and pernicious problems as mercury toxicity and learning disabilities, the possibility of shingles in later life from dormant chicken pox virus, or the potential for other problems, including immune malfunctions such as Crohn's disease, to occur because of persistent viral infections, we must really think twice about whether avoiding certain diseases is a trade-off courting others. Our children deserve long and healthy lives. Vaccines offer benefits, but they are also a bit of a gamble. Perhaps vaccinations are only one small part of disease prevention and more emphasis needs to be placed on enhancing immunity through other (and safer) means.

SIX

Personal Choices and Public Policies

Contrary to the thinking behind mass vaccine programs, no single approach to vaccinations is best for all children. Medicine is not a one-size-fits-all garment. This chapter will

- discuss vaccination and responsibility issues

- explain informed consent

- explore the vaccine decision-making process, including whether to vaccinate, how and when to vaccinate, and how to do so selectively

- discuss reducing vaccine reactions

- evaluate the choices you will have to make regarding school, disease exposure, and medical care

- discuss issues regarding raising unvaccinated children

- explain contraindications to vaccinations

- explain vaccine exemptions

- explain adverse event reporting

- discuss vaccine laws in the United States

As you read this chapter, keep in mind that the question of whether to vaccinate is not an all-or-nothing issue. Many parents choose a middle ground of partial vaccination, delayed vaccination, or other strategies that feel safe and sensible for them. Furthermore, you do not have to make a decision right this minute. You can think about it, discuss it with friends and family, speak with your doctor or other doctors, and do some further research. Being a parent is a tremendous responsibility, and the decision about whether to vaccinate is formidable to parents who know both sides of the story. Either way you must feel confident in your choice and be willing to take responsibility for the ramifications of your decision. Therefore, think carefully and make a decision that is influenced by nothing but the best interest of your child.

Vaccinations and Personal Responsibility

From the moment most Americans are conceived, they are initiated into a sea of health care interventions. By the age of six months, most have been exposed to repeated ultrasounds, hospital delivery that is rife with medical interventions (sometimes of a surgical nature), medications (including pain medication used during the birth, antibiotics for earaches or colds, and so on), and a host of vaccinations. Few people ever question this when they come of age, simply going through life as a recipient of such medical treatments without question, either as a matter of routine care or when health conditions arise. That is, until they have been wrongfully treated and experience an iatrogenic (doctor-caused) problem, or until they realize that such methods are not fostering their wellness (or that of their children).

At this point, many people either engage in medical malpractice lawsuits or turn their backs on medical care. Iatrogenesis in medicine made the front pages of newspapers this year when it was acknowledged by the medical profession that as many as eighty thousand deaths occur annually as a result of medical mistakes, including botched surgeries, improper diagnosis of conditions, and, most significant to our discussion, the improper use of medications (wrong dose, wrong medication, wrong prescription to wrong person). That Americans are turning their backs on conventional medicine is evident in the growth of the alternative-medicine and natural-products markets to a $12 billion annual industry and in the prevalence of advertisements of natural products in magazines and television commercials and their presence in pharmacies and supermarkets.

However, there is no need either to be a victim of wrongfully practiced medicine or to turn one's back on medicine. Furthermore, unquestioning acceptance of alternative medicine is no more intelligent than unquestioning acceptance of conventional medicine. The key lies in taking responsibility for one's health care decisions and making sensible decisions based on accurate information and assessment of one's own circumstances. In regard to vaccines, this means making a well-educated choice and then accepting responsibility for that choice.

Being informed is the result of actively seeking information through research, questioning, and reflection. It requires being honest with oneself and feeling empowered to get what one needs. This may entail a decision to vaccinate your child fully or only partially or to decline vaccinations entirely. The outcomes of your decisions are your responsibility; thus it is essential to have a clear strategy for making a decision and clear plans for a response to circumstances that might arise as a result of your choices. Taking responsibility also means that you take a proactive approach to building your child's immunity. Merely hoping your child won't get sick isn't enough.

Informed Consent

Intrinsic to sensible decision making is informed consent. The meaning of informed consent may appear self-evident, but it is worth dissecting it a bit. Generally, in the medical arena, informed consent is a matter of formality—a physician or nurse superficially informs you of the risks and benefits of a procedure and you sign a paper consenting to have the procedure done. With minors, the guardian signs on behalf of the child. Informed consent rarely informs the patient of risks in any depth, almost never discusses alternatives, and primarily serves as a mechanism for protecting the medical practitioner from any future malpractice liability should the patient experience adverse effects as a result of the procedure. Indeed, the informed is frequently underinformed and occasionally misinformed, and the entire "informing" interaction entails only a few minutes. There may be little room for questions, with an indifferent or bothered response from the "informer," and the informing may be done with some level of emotional coercion on the part of the practitioner, should the practitioner be biased in favor of the procedure. For example, at a well-baby visit, at which vaccines are routinely administered, few doctors—or nurses, who are frequently the ones to give the vaccinations—spend more than fifteen minutes with the patient. This is barely enough time to ascertain how the child is feeling, what the child's eating and sleeping habits are, and how home life and school are going, before shots are administered.

Rarely do these care providers discuss the potential for severe adverse reactions beyond mentioning that these are extremely rare. Parents may simply be given CDC vaccine information sheets to review, which sorely deemphasize the potential for adverse reactions. Parents are told to give acetaminophen to reduce discomfort that might arise. Physicians are required by federal law to inform their patients of the risks of adverse vaccine reactions. Unfortunately, the minimal information provided by physicians may be interpreted as meeting the requirements of the law. Many care providers may overlook this step entirely, and most parents, assuming that vaccines are entirely safe and effective, never ask questions. This means that to be truly informed one must be self-motivated and proactive and not rely on medical practitioners, who may be too busy to keep up with the literature and share their findings with patients.

Consent is the second operative word in the informed-consent process. Consent implies that one has choices and has willfully chosen a particular course of action. Consent implies freedom to decline. Consent implies that parents have the following choices:

- To vaccinate their child(ren) fully

- To vaccinate their child(ren) selectively

- To decline all vaccinations

Parents have the legal right to make any of these choices. Unfortunately, as society supports only the first choice, that of vaccinating entirely, there is a price to pay for the other choices; thus this is not true freedom, and the notion of consent is not entirely accurate. Furthermore, if I pressure you into making a certain decision by emphasizing certain aspects of the issue and deemphasizing others, then one could argue that you were not entirely informed. Such is the case with vaccinations.

The prices to pay are apparent to many parents who choose not to vaccinate and need to interface with public institutions. For example, school attendance can be difficult without a vaccine waiver from a doctor. These can be difficult to obtain, as few doctors are willing to support parents who don't vaccinate their children. Attendance at day care can be similarly difficult without vaccine records. Parents who have chosen not to vaccinate their children often find it difficult to find a physician willing to have their children as patients in their practice, as many will only see children who receive vaccines routinely. Furthermore, many parents of unvaccinated children, and the children themselves, have received extremely demeaning and aggressive treatment from emergency room physicians or other hospital personnel when it is learned that the child is unvaccinated, even if the emergency for which care is sought is entirely unrelated to vaccine-preventable diseases.

Making an informed choice means being prepared for all the ramifications of that choice. For parents who choose to vaccinate, this means accepting the possibility of short-term mild and severe adverse reactions and knowing how to respond quickly and appropriately should the reaction be severe. It also means accepting the risks of long-term reactions that are known and those that may as yet be unknown and that might not manifest for years after receipt of the vaccine. Finally, those who choose to vaccinate should assume responsibility for reporting adverse reactions to the Vaccine Adverse Events Reporting System so that the CDC and federal government can track them. This is one of the few avenues parents have for knowing what reactions are occurring and how often, and it can provide a basis for demanding safer vaccines or changes in vaccine policies.

Parents who choose to vaccinate selectively or decline vaccines entirely must accept not only the medical consequences of their choice, including the possibility of their child contracting an illness that vaccines are designed to prevent, but also social consequences such as potential conflicts and confrontations with school personnel, medical personnel, and even friends and family who disagree with the choice. Vaccine disputes have arisen in divorce cases, involving custody battles over unvaccinated children. The vaccination issue may become a pivotal point in determining who is awarded custody, with the parent willing to vaccinate being awarded custody or the custodial parent being forced to vaccinate in order to maintain custody. Furthermore, there is an emotional burden that parents who choose not to vaccinate often face, bearing the weight of anxiety that comes with making a choice that they may be told (repeatedly) is endangering their child. Parents who choose not to vaccinate must go to extra effort to enroll their children in school, summer camp, day care, and college and must be aware of the possibility of their child's being exposed to children who may be contagious as a result of vaccination with communicable diseases, as was the case until the recent discontinuation of the routine use of the oral polio vaccine. Finally, parents who choose not to vaccinate may be faced with unique considerations should they choose to travel to areas where certain diseases are still active, or should an epidemic arise in this country. However, any child can be susceptible to such diseases, as no vaccines provide complete protection in every recipient.

Making Vaccine-Related Decisions

The most effective decision-making methods involve asking yourself questions and weighing the answers to arrive at the best choice(s). This can be done by making a "pros and cons" list for the choice to vaccinate and the choice not to vaccinate. These can then be compared and a decision can be made accordingly. It is important to include your values, beliefs, and feelings in your decision-making process, but a measure of objectivity may yield the most sensible decision. It may be necessary to repeat this process for each individual vaccination.

Parents ask themselves each of the following questions for each of their children, if an informed decision is to be made about vaccinating:

- How dangerous is the disease against which I am vaccinating? (This must be answered for each disease for which vaccines are given.)

- What is the likelihood of my child's contracting this disease if I don't vaccinate? If I do vaccinate? (Remember, vaccines are not 100 percent effective.)

- What are the risks of the vaccine and how likely are these to occur?

- Is my child at high risk for an adverse reaction to the vaccines?

- Can I minimize my child's risks of disease?

- Can I minimize my child's risks of a vaccine reaction?

- What legal concerns does my decision involve?

- Can I live comfortably with my decision if I choose not to vaccinate?

The information you have read in the previous chapters of this book has provided a foundation on which to answer many of these questions, particularly regarding the risks associated with the diseases and the vaccines. Furthermore, you have learned a great deal about each disease and conventional medical treatment. In subsequent chapters, you will learn about how you can minimize your child's risk of contracting illnesses and how to treat some childhood conditions safely at home. We will also look at minimizing the risks of adverse reactions to vaccinations, contradictions to vaccines, and legal considerations surrounding vaccination.

One question, however, that no academic information can answer for you is that of your ability to live with your decisions. The choice to not vaccinate your children can not only expose you to tremendous social criticism but also can create internal pressures. For example, some parents choose not to vaccinate because they are afraid of the harm the vaccine might cause. However, they also feel a certain amount of disease paranoia, worrying about tetanus every time their children run barefoot and wondering about disease every time they are around other ill or recently vaccinated children. This is a terrible burden to live with, as well as a tremendous amount of anxiety to project onto a child. Parents who choose not to vaccinate may occasionally question their decision; this is healthy and shows intelligence and reflection. But if you constantly feel worried about your decision and your child, it may be better for you to consider vaccinating your child, either fully or partially.

Finally, remember that your vaccination decision is your business. You are not obligated to discuss your vaccination decisions or your child's vaccination status with anyone, other than in relationship to disclosure for school or on a legal basis. Protecting yourself and your child from undue concern or even outright hostility is your right.

Strategies for Vaccinating

While some parents may choose to forgo vaccinations altogether, you may not feel comfortable with that decision for your own children. There are a number of ways to vaccinate selectively, so that your concerns for safety are addressed. Some parents may want their children protected from certain diseases by vaccines and want natural immunity to others (for example, chicken pox). Others may have concerns about the safety of certain vaccines but not others. Therefore you may choose to vaccinate selectively, by giving your child some vaccines and forgoing the ones you don't feel comfortable about or don't feel are necessary. Many parents who selectively vaccinate, for example, avoid the cellular pertussis vaccine and choose acellular instead, they allow only the inactivated polio vaccine, and they decline the chicken pox vaccine. Given the changes in American Academy of Pediatrics and Centers for Disease Control recommendations these past few years, such choices, which were formerly considered "radical," are now considered preferable. Other parents vaccinate with only tetanus and inactivated polio, feeling confident that their child is unlikely to be exposed to or adversely affected by other of the diseases for which we vaccinate.

Yet another set of strategies parents use for vaccinating is delayed vaccination, in which the child is not vaccinated until after the sixth month or first year of life. Many feel that this allows the child's immune system time to develop, enabling the child to tolerate vaccines better. This approach is often combined with selective vaccination. Parents may also choose to have the pediatrician administer vaccinations separately rather than several in one visit.

138

Regardless of whether you choose to vaccinate fully, partially, or not at all, remember: Make your own decision. Do not allow yourself to feel bullied into extreme positions, or any position at all. You and your child alone will have to live with the repercussions of your decisions. Make choices that you feel good about and to the best of your ability.

Reducing Vaccine Reaction

Parents who choose to vaccinate can exercise a variety of strategies for reducing adverse vaccine reactions. Some of these are scientifically documented, others are common sense.

Give acetaminophen prior to vaccination: An article that appeared in the *Pediatric Infectious Disease Journal* documents "significantly fewer local and systemic reactions . . . in acetaminophen-treated infants at 2 to 6 months of age."[1] This treatment, however, did not confer any benefits to those eighteen months or over, who had higher rates of systemic and local reactions than younger babies.

From the perspective of natural medicine, acetaminophen merely suppresses symptoms that the body is trying to express in response to a perceived threat—the vaccine. Furthermore, the vaccination itself creates a state of chronic viral or bacterial latency, also a form of suppression of illness. While the overt symptoms of illness that produce the greatest discomfort in the child are not manifest, leading to an appearance of a reduced reaction and increased comfort, this is not necessarily optimal for the child's immune wellness in the long run.

Two other medical journal articles suggest that adverse reactions may be reduced by choosing specific needle lengths for injection and specific injection sites. One study, which appeared in the May 1989 issue of *Pediatrics*, demonstrated that severe pain was reduced by giving DPT-polio injection in the arm rather than the thigh, whereas redness and swelling were observed more often after injection in the arm. The study concludes that parents reported more reactions as moderate to severe with injections in the thigh than in the arm. The study was conducted with children at eighteen months of age, and found that arm injection eliminated the limping for twenty-four to forty-eight hours after injection associated with vaccination in the thigh. There was more redness and swelling with a sixteen-millimeter needle compared with a twenty-five–millimeter needle.[2] According to L. J. Baraff and colleagues, some decreased reactivity was seen in injections in the buttocks rather than the thigh, but "no injection site was consistently associated with lower reaction rates."[3]

Note: Your doctor should have epinephrine on hand when vaccinations are administered, in case of an anaphylactic reaction. This is consistently emphasized in vaccine manufacturer package inserts.

Parents have found that perhaps the best strategy for reducing reactions is to avoid multiple vaccines, staggering vaccinations over an increased number of pediatric office visits. This is perfectly within the legal rights of parents to do.

Furthermore, ensuring that children are well when they receive their vaccines is of utmost importance. Defer vaccines if your child has a fever, a cold, an earache, or other visible signs of illness. Make sure the child is well rested prior to the pediatric visit, and schedule the visit for morning when you have a full day to observe your child for reactions.

The administration of vaccine may use up a high amount of vitamin C, and additionally, vitamin C may reduce adverse reactions; therefore, you may want to increase your child's intake of vitamin C with a children's vitamin C supplement with bioflavinoids. For children under two give 100 milligrams four times daily for three to five days prior to vaccinating. Older children may be given 250 milligrams of vitamin C four times daily for three to five days prior to vaccination.

Adequate vitamin A may also prevent severe reactions. However, some forms of vitamin A can be toxic to children. Give only beta-carotene or carotene, up to 1,000 international units once daily for children under two and up to 5,000 international units once daily for older children, for several days prior to vaccination.

Homeopathic physicians recommend the following to reduce the likelihood of an adverse vaccine reaction:

- Give ledum 30C, three doses daily for one day before and three days after vaccination *or* three doses thirty minutes apart after vaccination *and* give hypericum 30C, three doses daily as for ledum (above), along with the ledum at this same dosage.

  or

- Give nosode (homeopathic version of the organisms, for example, MMR nosode) in 200C dosage, one dose two days before vaccination and once immediately after vaccination.

  or

- Give thuja 30C, three doses twelve hours apart, after vaccination.

For polio vaccine give:

- Ledum and hypericum as described above *and* thuja 4C, one dose daily for two weeks before and two weeks after vaccination.[4]

Homeopathic medicine is based on the concept of "like cures like," meaning that a substance that can cause symptoms similar to a disease, when given in minute and specially potentized (done by vigorously shaking the dilution) forms, can treat such an illness. Because homeopathic preparations are so highly diluted as to contain virtually none of the physical substance from which they are derived, they are not able to be evaluated by conventional laboratory methods and are highly controversial. Many report excellent cures with homeopathic treatment; others report no benefit. Certainly there is no harm in adding the above remedies to a reaction-prevention scheme; however, should a serious adverse reaction arise, they should not be relied upon for primary medical treatment. Furthermore, it is unlikely that homeopathic remedies are adequate protection against serious diseases, and they do not substitute for conventional vaccination.

Remember, a child who has just been vaccinated has had one or more very serious infectious diseases injected into his or her body. This is why they often get "sick" after vaccination. Treat your child as if he is ill; that is, go home, rest your child, provide nourishing but simple foods, keep visitors at bay, and cozy in to your house for the day—or several, if your child has previously had a vaccine reaction or appears to be having a mild reaction. Acetaminophen may be advisable for children with a history of seizures, giving it every four hours for twenty-four hours. Other children may be given vitamin C, herbs such as echinacea to enhance immunity, or herbs to calm and ease the child, such as chamomile, lemon balm, and lavender (see chapter 8 for details on using herbs with children). Common sense and comfort measures may help to reduce discomfort and reactions.

Note: Should a serious vaccine reaction arise, consult with your doctor or take your child to a hospital emergency room immediately.

When Not to Vaccinate

Even the conventional medical establishment recognizes that vaccinations are contraindicated for certain children and under certain circumstances. The following information is based on the recommendations of the Advisory

Committee on Immunization Practices (ACIP) and those of the Committee on Infectious Diseases (Red Book Committee) of the American Academy of Pediatrics. These recommendations may vary for different manufacturers. The recommendations are current as of March 2000, were accessed by the author on August 22, 2000, and may be accessed by the reader at the CDC National Immunization Program Web site, www.cdc.gov/nip/recs/contraindications.htm. These recommendations are considered by the National Vaccine Information Center to be a very minimized and excessively restricted list of contraindications.[5] A broader discussion of contraindications will follow these. Items marked with an asterisk indicate areas of controversy. These are discussed in the subsequent section, "Playing It Safe."

ACCEPTED CONTRAINDICATIONS AND PRECAUTIONS FOR VACCINE ADMINISTRATION

Vaccine	True Contraindications and Precautions	Not True (Vaccines May Be Given)
General for all vaccines (DTP, DTaP, OPV, IPV, MMR, Hib, hepatitis B, varicella)	Anaphylactic reaction to a vaccine contra-indicates further doses of that vaccine	Mild to moderate local reactions following a dose of injectable antigen*
	Anaphylactic reaction to a vaccine contra-indicates the use of other vaccines containing that substance	Low-grade or moderate fever following a prior dose of vaccine*
		Mild or acute illness with or without a low-grade fever*
	Moderate or severe illness with or without a fever	Current antimicrobial therapy*
		Convalescent phase of an illness*
		Prematurity (same dosage and indications as for normal, full-term infants)*
		Recent exposure to infectious disease*
		Allergies or familial tendency to allergies*

142

ACCEPTED CONTRAINDICATIONS AND PRECAUTIONS
FOR VACCINE ADMINISTRATION*(cont'd)*

Vaccine	True Contraindications and Precautions	Not True (Vaccines May Be Given)
		Pregnancy of mother or household contact*
		Unvaccinated household member*
DTP/DTaP	Encephalopathy within 7 days of administration of previous dose of DTP/DTaP	Temperature of less than 105°F following a previous dose*
	Precautions: Fever of 105°F within 48 hours after a prior DTP/DTaP not attributable to other causes	Family history of convulsions*
		Family history of SIDS*
		Family history of an adverse event following DTP/DTaP vaccine*
	Collapse or shocklike state within 48 hours of prior DTP/DTaP	
	Seizures within 3 days of receipt of a prior DTP/DTaP	
	Persistent, inconsolable crying lasting 3 hours within 48 hours of a prior DTP/DTaP	
	Guillain-Barré syndrome within 6 weeks after a dose	
OPV	Infection with HIV or household contact with HIV	Breast-feeding*
		Current antimicrobial therapy
	Known immuno-deficiency; immuno-deficient household contact	Mild diarrhea
	Precaution: Pregnancy	

ACCEPTED CONTRAINDICATIONS AND PRECAUTIONS
FOR VACCINE ADMINISTRATION *(cont'd)*

Vaccine	True Contraindications and Precautions	Not True (Vaccines May Be Given)
IPV	Anaphylactic reaction to neomycin, strepto-mycin, or polymyxin B	
MMR	Anaphylactic reaction to neomycin or gelatin	Tuberculosis
		Simultaneous TB skin testing
	Pregnancy	
	Known immuno-deficiency	Breast-feeding
		Pregnancy of mother or household contact
	Precaution: Recent administration of a blood product or immune globulin preparation	HIV infection without evidence of severe immunosuppression
		Allergic reaction to eggs
	Thrombocytopenia	Nonanaphylactic reactions to neomycin
	History of thrombo-cytopenia purpura	
Hib	None	
Hepatitis B (HBV)	Anaphylactic reaction to baker's yeast	Pregnancy
Varicella	Anaphylactic reaction to neomycin or gelatin	Immunodeficiency of a household contact
	Pregnancy	HIV infection in a house-hold contact
	Known immuno-deficiency	Pregnancy in the mother or household contact
	Precaution: Receipt of immune globulin preparation within 5 months	

PLAYING IT SAFE

While the Centers for Disease Control, the Advisory Committee on Immuniza-tion Practices, and the American Academy of Pediatrics might play it conserva-tive, parents who are concerned about adverse reactions to vaccines may want to play it safe. In fact, based on medical literature, VAERS data, and the National Vaccine Information Center, many of the factors alleged by the CDC to be misconceptions should be cause for considerable concern. Let's briefly review those that should cause serious reflection before a vaccine is administered.

- *Mild to moderate local reactions following a dose of injectable antigen:* While previous mild reactions to a vaccine do not necessarily indicate that the child will have further reactions, a moderate reaction might be cause for concern, as some reactions get worse with increased numbers of doses.

- *Low-grade or moderate fever following a prior dose of vaccine:* Again, fever following vaccination is common and not necessarily indicative of a future adverse reaction but should be cause for utmost caution.

- *Mild or acute illness with or without a low-grade fever:* Common sense dictates that if a child is already mildly ill, one should not vaccinate until the child is well. Illness affects immunity; vaccination might reduce immunity. Why not just wait? Children who become ill after a vaccine should be watched closely after further vaccinations. Many parents whose children eventually have severe adverse reactions report that their child had mild reactions after previous vaccinations were administered.

- *Current antimicrobial therapy:* If the child is receiving antibiotic therapy because he or she is otherwise ill or has been fighting an infec-tion recently, this indicates temporarily decreased immunity. Again, vaccinations may also reduce immunity, so it may be prudent to wait until the child has had a chance to recover fully before administering vaccinations.

- *Convalescent phase of an illness:* See preceding paragraph.

- *Prematurity (same dosage and indications as for normal, full-term infants):* Premature infants have decreased liver function below that of normally immature liver function in healthy neonates. Immediate postnatal immunization of premie babies with hepatitis B vaccine may increase the likelihood of interventions owing to fever caused by the vaccine, may predispose to reactions, and may increase the likelihood of neonatal jaundice, also leading to additional interventions. Delaying vaccinations in hepatitis B–negative newborns does not increase the risk of contracting hepatitis B.

- *Recent exposure to infectious disease:* The same precaution as with mild illness at the time of vaccination. Why further compromise immunity in a child who may be in the early stages of fighting an infection?

- *Allergies or familial tendency toward allergies:* If the allergies have predisposed other family members to vaccine reactions, this is significant cause for caution, at least.

- *Pregnancy of mother or household contact:* It is unknown how many of the childhood vaccines would affect pregnant women, and some may predispose the pregnant woman to exposure to live viruses, such as with the rubella vaccine and varicella vaccine; therefore concern and caution are warranted.

- *Unvaccinated household member:* The only incidences of poliomyelitis in the United States in several decades have been a result of direct or indirect contact with live polio vaccine (OPV). This seems enough reason to avoid OPV if there are unvaccinated members of the household. This is clearly emphasized in the literature.

- *Temperature of 105 degrees Fahrenheit following a previous dose:* I don't know about other parents, but I'd be really concerned if my child developed a 105-degree temperature after anything, and would certainly exercise extreme caution before using that substance again.

- *Family history of convulsions:* A CDC study conducted in 1987 showed that children with a personal history of convulsions are nine times more likely to have a seizure following a DPT vaccination and children with a family history of convulsions are three times more likely to have a seizure following a DPT shot than those who do not have this history.[6]

- *Family history of SIDS:* If there is even a remote chance that certain vaccines contribute to SIDS, then it seems sensible to avoid those vaccines at least in those children with a family history of SIDS. Since there is no clear understanding of what causes SIDS, and SIDS deaths occur "coincidentally" with vaccinations, particularly DPT vaccines, then logically one cannot entirely rule out the association.

- *Family history of an adverse event following DTP/DTaP vaccine:*
  Again, common sense dictates extreme caution in this respect. Many
  families appear to exhibit a tendency toward reactions, and indeed, there
  are numerous testimonials from parents who have several children who
  have had adverse reactions after receiving vaccinations.

- *Breast-feeding:* This is likely to be a concern only for a polio-susceptible
  mother whose breast-feeding baby received OPV, exposing her to live
  poliovirus. This is also the case for non–breast-feeding susceptible
  mothers. Breast-feeding mothers who have not been vaccinated for polio
  should give their babies only IPV (inactivated). Doctors do not routinely
  ask about family vaccine history (though they are supposed to), so you
  must bring this up to your child's doctor.

Adverse-Event Reporting

To report an adverse event, complete the VAERS form (available at pharmacies) and submit it, or report the event by calling 800-822-7967. You may also
report adverse reactions to the National Vaccine Information Center (NVIC),
a clearinghouse of vaccine information that maintains a registry of adverse
vaccine reactions. Call NVIC at 703-983-DPT3.

Vaccine Laws and Exemptions

Each state has different vaccine requirements, and requirements also vary for
each vaccine. As of 1995, the CDC provided the following information on
vaccine requirements: Diphtheria, rubella, measles, and polio vaccines are required by all fifty states. The pertussis vaccine is required by all states except
the following: Idaho, Maine, Missouri, New York, Oregon, Pennsylvania, Texas,
and Washington. Mumps vaccine is required by all states but Alaska, Arkansas,
Iowa, Maryland, Missouri, New Mexico, Vermont, and West Virginia. Tetanus is required by all states except Missouri and New York. Hib vaccine is
required by most states for attendance at day care, Head Start programs, and
the like. Hepatitis B is required in about 50 percent of states and is recommended in most.[7]

Julius Landwirth, M.D., J.D., elucidates the legal status of vaccination in
the United States in his article in *Pediatric Clinics of North America:*

The state's authority to supercede otherwise constitutionally protected rights of parents to make health care decisions for their children rests in its "police power," a loosely defined doctrine under which government has the authority to enact coercive legislation in the interest of protecting the public's health and safety. The United States Supreme Court affirmed this doctrine in 1905 when it denied the claim by a Cambridge, Massachusetts, citizen that a municipal law requiring smallpox vaccination for all adults violated his personal liberty. The Court ruled that compulsory vaccination statutes, applied with discretion, are among the "manifold restraints to which every person is necessarily subject for the common good."[8]

Courts have since upheld that preventing admission to and denying access to education are not inconsistent with state vaccination requirements, and even the constitutionally guaranteed right to freedom of religion can be superceded by vaccine regulations.[9]

MEDICAL EXEMPTIONS

In the United States, each state, with the exception of Alaska, where vaccine laws are vague and vaccinations may not be mandatory, allows some form of exemption from vaccinations. In Mississippi and West Virginia, the only exemptions that appear to exist are medical exemptions, for which a medical doctor must verify that, for some reason, your child is medically unable to receive vaccinations.[10]

Medical exemptions can be very difficult to obtain, and as seen previously, the window for what qualifies as a true medical exemption by CDC, ACIP, and AAP standards is extremely narrow and limited. Finding a supportive pediatrician or family physician early on in your parenting career can serve as a terrific investment for you as your child grows and you face issues such as requiring a vaccine waiver for school.

RELIGIOUS EXEMPTION

All states offer religious exemptions, with the exceptions of Mississippi and West Virginia. However, for religious exemption to be granted, some states require proof of affiliation with a religious organization whose beliefs oppose vaccination. The states requiring proof include Arkansas, Hawaii, Iowa, Kansas, Nebraska, Oregon, South Carolina, South Dakota, and Texas.[11] According to medical ethicist Catherine Diodati, there have been several recent federal court rulings that have allowed parents to claim religious exemption without formal church membership.[12] Other states offer a broad definition of religious beliefs to include personal religious beliefs.

PHILOSOPHICAL EXEMPTION

Philosophical exemption allows parents to object to vaccinations on the basis of a personal philosophical belief. A family physician friend of mine recently informed me that her philosophical exemption for her own child was rescinded after she gave her son a tetanus vaccine. She was informed by the relevant state agency that she could no longer possibly have a philosophical conviction that prevented her from vaccinating, as she had clearly done so. She told me that several of her patients were being told that they must either give their children all of the vaccines or, to be awarded a philosophical exemption, give none. Furthermore, there have been national thrusts to enforce strict vaccine tracking systems, and a movement to eliminate philosophical exemptions. Fisher recommends that parents choosing a philosophical exemption keep a close watch on state legislation.[13] As of 1997, the following states allowed for philosophical exemption: Arizona, California, Colorado, Idaho, Louisiana, Maine, Michigan, Minnesota, New Mexico, North Dakota, Ohio, Oklahoma, Rhode Island, Utah, Vermont, Washington, and Wisconsin.[14]

SCHOOL AND THE UNVACCINATED CHILD

Public schools, private schools, day care centers, colleges, and any programs that receive public funding have the right to require that your child be vaccinated to be admitted to the program. Private and religious schools have the right to refuse exemptions, but publicly funded programs allow the state-permitted exemptions. State laws allow schools to deny your unvaccinated child admittance to the school in the event of an outbreak of a vaccine-preventable disease. You may be asked to sign a waiver from the school acknowledging that you understand this and that you assume full responsibility for consequences to your child's welfare in light of choosing not to vaccinate.

PROOF OF IMMUNITY

Some states and schools may accept proof of immunity as a satisfactory substitute for vaccination. You will need, at your expense, to take your child to a physician or private lab willing to run blood tests for you. The results must be within the range that demonstrates immunity. Proof of immunity can be admitted in the event of an outbreak so that your child can stay in school.[15]

EXEMPTION FORMS

Each state has its own requirements and, frequently, its own exemption forms. It is actually disadvantageous to use other forms, and therefore no sample forms are provided in this book. If you plan to apply for a state vaccination exemption, speak with your child's physician or contact the state health department to obtain the appropriate forms.

PUBLIC ASSISTANCE

Proof of vaccination is now being used as leverage against families requiring public assistance to ensure that their children are current on vaccinations. Financial assistance may be denied or reduced for mothers on welfare or women receiving assistance from the Special Supplemental Nutrition Program for Women, Infants, and Children (WIC). Reduced assistance usually occurs at a certain rate per unvaccinated child, such as reducing the number of WIC vouchers allocated.[16] This severely penalizes women who have a personal conviction not to vaccinate and is considered by public health servants to be one of the most effective means of assuring compliance with vaccine requirements.

EXEMPTION DENIED

The state does have the right to reject your request for exemption. As mentioned earlier, philosophical exemption has been denied on the basis of partial vaccination. Should this happen to you, request the reason for denial and resubmit your request, revising it as appropriate if necessary. If it is again denied, keep careful records of all conversations and contacts, and appeal to a higher authority in the administrative chain of command or to a higher official bureau. Continue to keep detailed records of all interactions, and consult an attorney if you are unable to get satisfaction independently. The National Vaccine Information Center can provide a referral (see Resources).

RECOMMENDATIONS, REQUIREMENTS, AND LEGAL PROBLEMS

Barbara Loe Fisher, in her eminently useful book *The Consumer's Guide to Childhood Vaccinations*, reminds us that recommendations and laws are not synonymous, and while your state may require certain vaccines, others may only be recommended. Therefore, it is important to inquire into the laws for your state. The National Vaccine Information Center (NVIC) will send summaries of state laws upon request (see Resources). If you become involved in a legal problem surrounding vaccination, there are attorneys who specialize in this area and are available for legal assistance. Contact NVIC for references.

I highly recommend that parents read Catherine Diodati's excellent book *Immunizations: History, Ethics, Law, and Health* for an intelligent discussion of the many ways that vaccine laws infringe on personal rights and how the very need to maintain exemptions is in itself an infringement of freedom. She crafts a cogent argument for individual freedom while recognizing the goal of the state to protect the larger community from the potential and alleged consequences of individual freedom.

I have made an effort to substantiate the information in this book by relying heavily on medical literature and not vaccine-critical books or popular health books so that you have a fairly objective view of vaccination issues. However, the information in vaccine-critical books is exactly what you do want if you are trying to weave your way through the educational system as a nonvaccinating parent. For this purpose, and to expand your research, I encourage you to read books and articles by Neil Miller, Randall Neustaedter, Walene James, and others. Books by Barbara Loe Fisher are consistently well researched and balanced in approach, while raising highly critical concerns about vaccines and vaccine politics. Furthermore, national vaccine education and resource groups can be helpful in providing detailed legal information.

Books

Unvaccinated Children and Exposure to Infectious Diseases

Parents who choose not to vaccinate have varying attitudes about their child and disease. Some complacently assume that if the child is apparently healthy, he or she will not become sick, but do not proactively build immunity. Others do proactively build immunity. Some plan to get medical treatment should an infectious disease arise or plan to vaccinate in the event of a disease epidemic. Others try to expose their child to the milder infectious diseases whenever possible, to give their children immunity to these diseases while still young. Toward this end, I have even heard of T-shirt swaps occurring among friends in different states. When one child gets the chicken pox, for example, his T-shirt is sent by overnight mail to a friend whose child has not had it; the shirt goes on that child, and hopefully a full-blown case of varicella results.

In general, proactively building immunity, natural exposure to appropriate infectious diseases (not necessarily via United States mail!), and a reasonable attitude toward vaccination should an epidemic of a serious disease such as diphtheria occur seem prudent. The assumption that healthy children don't get sick is erroneous and some illness is desirable because the immune system is stimulated and builds immunity on the basis of contracting infectious diseases. And healthy children do get sick. They have times of increased stress (teething, schoolwork, stress from home life, stress from school, puberty) resulting in decreased resistance. Some microorganisms are highly specialized and evolved to defeat even some of the most ingenious of our innate physical defenses. While the power of positive thinking cannot be underestimated for its potential for improving health, I think it goes a bit far to assume it can prevent all disease.

Nonetheless, generally healthy children with strong immune systems can mount a formidable resistance against disease, and indeed, this is the best defense we have both in preventing disease and in preventing adverse reactions to vaccinations. Healthy children also tend to have milder infections than their less-healthy counterparts. The extreme of this is seen in malnourished children from developing nations, or in immunocompromised children, who may be severely damaged even by generally mild childhood diseases such as chicken pox.

Health is built on excellent nutrition, moderate exercise, minimizing stress, and maximizing emotional wellness. This requires time and commitment on the part of parents and should involve the community at large. For example, school lunches should be healthy, not packaged and processed as they generally are; schools should offer recreational time outdoors each day and an inviting physical education program. Few do. And home life and school life have become increasingly stressful as divorce rates remain high and school crime rates soar. All of this can and does have an impact on children's immunity and thus their susceptibility to illness. The next chapter is devoted exclusively to natural approaches to children's health and immunity.

Traveling with Unvaccinated Children

Traveling with unvaccinated children can present unique challenges, particularly when traveling to areas with known endemic or epidemic infectious diseases. While we in the United States are privileged to live in a relatively infectious-disease–free region, many countries still face regular outbreaks of diphtheria, polio, measles, and tropical infectious diseases. Therefore, you will want to contact the Centers for Disease Control travel advisory services before traveling. They maintain up-to-date information on exactly what diseases are prevalent in different countries, whether there are currently outbreaks, when outbreaks typically occur (for example, malaria occurs most during the rainy season in central Africa), and what vaccines or medications are used to prevent infection. You might consider vaccinating for certain diseases prior to such travel. If you choose not to, you must have a clear emergency plan should your child contract an illness, especially if you plan an extended trip. Not only is your child more likely to be exposed to certain diseases in certain countries but it is also more likely that you will have difficulty finding adequate medical care that meets your standard.

Even if you travel to a developed European nation where adequate medical care is accessible, your chances of exposure to infectious disease are greater than in the United States, as people there travel more broadly and have exposure to immigrants from nations where diphtheria, for example, still surfaces somewhat regularly. Also, fewer people are vaccinated against pertussis, and outbreaks have occurred numerous times in recent decades. While you might not be concerned about pertussis for your healthy child, diphtheria can be serious. Keep in mind that travel itself predisposes one to illness, as it often necessitates changes in diet and sleep habits and exposure to large numbers of people and climatic changes. Traveling with an unvaccinated child, you must consider all of these factors.

If you choose to vaccinate because of travel plans, prepare to do so several months before your trip in order to give the number of shots required for adequate protection. Planning ahead also allows enough time for the vaccine to become effective and leaves enough time for using IPV rather than OPV, for example, minimizing the likelihood of an adverse reaction.

Medical Emergencies in Unvaccinated Children

Unvaccinated children break arms, need stitches, and so on, just as frequently as vaccinated kids. Unfortunately, it is all too common that parents of unvaccinated children are accosted by medical personnel when it is discovered that the child is unvaccinated. One friend of mine was harassed by doctors and nurses when she took her son to the hospital to get a tetanus immune globulin shot after a mild but swollen puncture wound. Not only was she verbally assaulted in front of her child for being an "irresponsible parent," but her son was treated unnecessarily aggressively.

The best way to protect yourself from this treatment is to seek out a supportive pediatrician who has hospital privileges; should a problem ever arise, you then have someone to call upon who knows your child's medical history.

If you don't have a supportive physician, then it may be best, depending upon the nature of the emergency, not to disclose your vaccine choices. However, *if the emergency is in any way possibly related to an illness for which children are typically vaccinated, it is essential that you disclose your child's vaccine history.* This information may be essential to your child's proper treatment. If anyone begins to hassle or berate you, tell them in a very calm manner that you would be happy to discuss you vaccine choices with them, but after your child has been attended to and when you feel calmer. Chances are they'll leave you alone after that. Remember, physicians are specifically trained to see every visit with a child as an opportunity to vaccinate. They consider themselves just to be doing their job. Confrontation in a medical setting is rarely helpful and tends to arouse hostility on the part of the medical staff. This is definitely not the time to go on an antivaccine crusade. Hold your ground, but keep a low profile and stay away from arguing. Your goal at that moment is to assure that your child is receiving appropriate medical care. If you continue to be hassled by the medical staff, ask to speak to the hospital social worker as a mediator, and explain your circumstances as calmly as possible.

Changing Your Mind about Vaccination

It is not uncommon for parents to have begun vaccinating their child, only to decide they don't want to continue vaccination or that they will vaccinate only selectively for the remainder of the vaccines. Conversely, parents may choose not to vaccinate but later decide they'd feel more secure if their child received vaccines. Or other circumstances such as travel or summer camp may necessitate certain vaccines. Changing your mind is part of your prerogative. Parents grow along with their children, and what you once thought may be different from what you think today.

If you choose not to continue vaccinating, you must simply comply with the exemptions if your child is enrolled in school or other programs requiring vaccination. If you choose to vaccinate a previously unvaccinated child, be certain to check on the appropriate vaccine schedules for different ages. For example, pertussis vaccine should never be given to children over seven years old; instead, DT should be given. Hib vaccine is probably not necessary for children over two years old, and hepatitis B may trigger untoward reactions in adolescent girls. Similarly, rubella vaccine can cause some arthralgia and arthritis in women and may better be given to girls in their early years of puberty rather than in their twenties or older, though it can be given safely then as well. Check with the CDC for recommendations and vaccine schedules, as these change periodically, new vaccines may be introduced, and old ones are occasionally discontinued.

Health Consequences of Legal Exemptions

Most of the critique of vaccine exemptions focuses on the fear that increasing exemptions equals decreasing vaccinations equals increased disease rates. However, this may be an extremely limited equation, lacking critical variables, namely, potential benefits derived from decreased administration of vaccines. In response to an article in the *Journal of the American Medical Association* in 1999 entitled "Health Consequences of Religious and Philosophical Exemptions from Immunization Laws: Individual and Societal Risks of Measles," physician Richard Fried of the Kimberton Clinic in Kimberton, Pennsylvania, states:

> Several studies have indicated an inverse correlation between measles disease and development of atopic illnesses. A recent report [published in *Lancet* 353 (1999): 1485–88] demonstrates that among children with an "anthropological lifestyle," there was a significant reduction in atopy. Notable among these children is a low immunization rate and a high incidence of natural measles infection.
>
> Western medicine has been criticized for focusing too much on narrow parameters and losing sight of the human being. Although these issues may be difficult to analyze scientifically, we need to have the courage to examine all possibilities of the short- and long-term advantages and possible disadvantages of a widespread immunization policy and not just fall back on the judgment that anyone who questions the benefit of immunizations is either a quack or a religious fanatic.[17]

SEVEN

Natural Approaches to Health and Immunity

Exposure to infectious organisms stimulates the development of immunity, thus some measure of mild illness may even be desirable for healthy growth and development. However, parents understandably want to protect their children from serious, debilitating, and life-threatening diseases, so vaccines have a natural appeal. But there is more to health and disease prevention than can be accomplished by inoculating the body with thousands of microorganisms and parts of microorganisms. Furthermore, that approach, while certainly reducing some degree of infectious disease, as we have seen, may predispose to vulnerability to chronic disease, including autoimmune disorders. In this chapter we will look at true immunity, how it can be fostered through nutrition, breastfeeding, emotional wellness, and healthy lifestyle. In chapter 8 we will explore the role of natural medicine in preventing and treating infectious disease, as well as the appropriate role of conventional medicine.

Healthy Living

Lifestyle habits can also contribute to or detract from immunity. Regular sleep patterns, for example, with enough hours of rest each night, allow the body to rejuvenate and give the body time to replenish, heal, and grow. It is important for children to get to bed at an age-appropriate hour each night. For teenagers it may be beneficial to immunity to sleep late in the morning, as their bodies once again require extra rest. While this may not be possible on weekdays, letting teens sleep in on weekends and encouraging them to get to bed at a reasonable hour on both weekdays and weekends are advisable. Supporting emotional expression and communication, taking time for recreation and re-laxation, and making sure to laugh and have some fun on a regular basis are positive contributors to healthy immunity that cannot be overemphasized. Furthermore, it is the parents' responsibility to shield younger children from undue stress and to help adolescents navigate stress gracefully and efficiently. Reduced stress means improved health. Enjoying time outdoors in natural spaces can do wonders for mental and physical wellness, improving sleep and health.

Hold on to Those Tonsils

Children who have had their tonsils removed are at significantly greater risk of contracting infections, especially through the upper respiratory passages. If your child has chronically swollen tonsils, think twice and try natural alterna-tives before resorting to surgery. The tonsils are major glands, placed at the portal of our upper respiratory tracts for protection. Chronically swollen ton-sils indicate an already compromised immune system. Work with diet, nutri-tional supplements, and topical and internal herbal treatments to improve immunity and avoid tonsillectomy.

Hygiene

Recall that two of the most important contributors to disease reduction in this century have been improved living conditions and hygiene. While exposure to people and germs is critical for the healthy development of immunity, com-mon sense dictates observing basic hygiene rules.

Wash hands before meals. Many microorganisms are passed hand to mouth. Use disposable tissues rather than handkerchiefs during colds, and teach your child to wash hands after blowing his or her nose. Cover your mouth when coughing and wash hands. Don't touch the hands of a baby—they go right to the baby's mouth. Ask strangers or even friends or relatives who seem sick not to touch baby's hands and to keep a distance if noticeably contagious. Don't share a drinking glass or a water, soda, or juice bottle with a friend who has drunk out of the container, even among members of communal households. Teach children to wash hands after bathroom use, and you should do the same after changing a baby's diaper. Public swimming pools and water parks are breeding grounds for infectious microorganisms. Pools that smell heavily of chlorine may have high levels of contamination, as the ammonia in urine reacts strongly with chlorine, causing the chlorine to give off an increased odor. Teach your kids not to drink pool water, and rinse them off in the shower after public bathing.

Common sense? Many people don't observe such basic rules.

Nutrition and Immunity

As discussed previously, the immune system is a marvelous and cohesive network of interactions and sensitivities that allows us to maintain individual integrity while living in and being inhabited by a sea of microorganisms. Indeed, some of these microorganisms have become a part of us, living in a symbiotic community relationship. However, we are also regularly exposed to organisms that would prefer not to live symbiotically, their programming rather tending toward parasitism, or worse, host destruction, the latter scenario being least desirable for the parasitic microorganism, whose existence becomes dependent on that of its host. In the case of bacteria, no host, no food. For viruses, no host, no functioning or replication. The human body has evolved masterful mechanisms for responding to such challenging microorganisms. Immunity involves a complicated interplay of actions and reactions that deter would-be "intruders." Most of these mechanisms are bypassed by vaccinations, particularly those that are given by injection. At least with the oral route, there is closer approximation to the way most vaccine-preventable microorganisms (with the exception of tetanus) enter the body—via respiratory and gastric routes. Unfortunately, we have seen that live oral polio has consequences of its own, perhaps because nature never intended us to swallow an orange-flavored concentrate of live poliovirus.

Nonetheless, humans are at a tremendous biological crossroads, as we have been at no other time in our history. We have evolved over millions of years to be capable of contracting, for example, measles virus, with relatively few people succumbing to it. This is an enormous feat, as in populations exposed to the virus for the first time, most people will become extremely sick and a significant portion will die. Theoretically, then, and most likely so if we look at evolution, we are only generations away from the natural exposure to measles being a consistently mild childhood disease, as it actually has become during the past century. Seen from this perspective, the antigen is but "a small perturbation in a rich ongoing network."[1]

Richard Moskowitz, medical doctor, homeopath, and outspoken vaccine critic, addressing the Society of Homeopaths in the United Kingdom, eloquently contrasts natural and artificial immunity, also using measles as an example:

> In its natural state, the measles virus enters the body of a susceptible person through the nose and mouth and incubates silently for about 14 days in the lymphoid tissues of the naso-pharynx, the regional lymph nodes, and finally in the liver, spleen, bone marrow, and the lymphocytes and macrophages of the peripheral blood. The illness known as the measles is the process by which the virus is expelled from the blood through the same orifices that it came in, and involves a concerted and massive effort of the entire immune system. Once specific antibodies have succeeded in targeting the virus, the ability to synthe-size them on short notice remains as a code "memory" of the whole experience, a virtual guarantee that people who have recovered from the measles will never get it again, no matter how many times they are re-exposed.
>
> In addition to conferring this specific immunity, the process of recovering from the natural disease also "primes" the organism non-specifically to respond promptly and efficiently to other microorganisms in the future. A crucial step in the maturation of a healthy immune system, the ability to mount a vigorous, acute response to infection unquestionably represents a major ingredient of optimum health and well-being in general.
>
> Finally, measles is about 20% fatal in populations exposed to it for the first time. It has taken us many centuries of adaptation and "herd immunity" to convert it into an ordinary childhood disease. . . . In that historical sense, the permanent immunity acquired by recovery from the natural disease represents an absolute net gain for the total health of the race as well. However, the vac-cines act inside the human body, true natural immunity or any other qualitative benefit cannot be ascribed to them: their effectiveness is a mere statistic, and the resulting "immunity" a narrowly defined technicality.
>
> Thus, in contrast with the natural disease, the vaccine produces no local sensitization at the portal of entry, no incubation, no massive outpouring, and no acute disease of any kind. It can elicit long-term antibody production solely by surviving in latent form in the lymphocytes and macrophages of the blood. But then the vaccinated individual would have no way to get rid of it, and the technical feat of antibody synthesis could at most represent the memory of this chronic infection.[2]

We have seen clear evidence that viruses are retained in the body, some-times for decades, later manifesting as Crohn's disease, multiple sclerosis, and other related autoimmune and nervous system conditions.[3] That the body har-bors these microorganisms, keeping us in a state of chronic infection, should be no surprise to readers. Chronic infection debilitates immunity and renders us more vulnerable to other microorganisms and conditions.

Remember, it is also the responsibility of the immune system to prevent tumor growth and cancer.[4] How can our bodies work efficiently and effectively if preoccupied by chronic illness? Perhaps the saddest part of this is our self-destruction in the face of chronic infection. Autoimmunity is a result of our chronically harboring foreign material in our own cells. Our bodies, in their beautiful effort to protect us by eliminating foreign matter, mistakenly destroy their own cells, which they read as foreign owing to the antigenic material they contain.

In spite of our wonderful natural evolutionary potential, we have chosen to bypass natural immunity and supplant it with artificially raised measles virus, grown on media that are also introduced into our bodies, carrying their own fragments of genetic information and potential. In a sense, we are undermining our own integrity. As a society we have chosen to take the road of technology and control over nature. Perhaps there is a road that runs alongside this one that would allow us to access that road as needed but that honors the body and its inherent wisdom and propensity for life.

The Road Less Traveled

Walene James states that one of the cornerstones upon which vaccinations rest is the belief that "vaccinations are the only practical and dependable way to prevent both epidemics and potentially dangerous diseases."[5] Clearly, vaccines are not the only way to prevent disease; it has been estimated that "the frequency of unnoticed infections outnumbered clinical illnesses by at least one hundred fold," with "evidence of this substantiated by the high proportion of adults who have virus-neutralizing substances in their blood serum and the number who, during an epidemic, excrete virus without being ill."[6] Furthermore, many substances, including nutrients and herbs, have been shown repeatedly in clinical trials, as well as in in vitro and in vivo studies, to reduce, prevent, and eliminate infection.

There is a growing consortium of scientists who have begun to corroborate the belief long held by traditional healers that the body is a self-healing entity and that healthy organisms are more likely to resist infection. There is also a growing recognition that suppressing symptoms such as fever and inflammation may not be entirely recommendable and may have contributed to the increases in chronic pediatric problems that we have seen in the past couple of decades.

Furthermore, there is increasing awareness of the power of nutrition, natural products such as herbs, and the mind-body connection in creating health and resisting disease. We are also seeing new terminology arising, such as "cooperation with nature" and "supporting the body's natural defenses" in our society, as individuals become disenchanted with the medico-military model of "destroying foreign invaders," which seems so often just to create stronger "foreign invaders," as with the overprescription of antibiotics. People are also seeking a less blame-oriented approach to disease and a more integrative approach to healing. Disease is seen less an a punishment for wrongdoing, or something by which we are victimized, and recognized as a necessary adaptive process for life on this planet.

People are seeking a model that emphasizes improving health and creating a stable, responsive, internal environment. Such a model can lead us away from the direction of immunocompromise that we have stumbled headlong into and toward a direction of immunocompetence, which our bodies were designed to create. This is a model that can be reinforced whether or not parents choose to vaccinate their children. Until recently such views were counterculture, radical, or alternative, but now they are becoming accepted enough that raising your child on an organic diet and using herbal supplements would not meet with laughter or derision but with interest and support.

Breast-feeding

Breast-feeding no longer confers passive immunity to the common childhood diseases it once protected against, since most mothers no longer possess natural antibodies as a result of having had the natural infection. However, breast-feeding is still one of the most important contributors to childhood immunity, a fact that the medical literature readily substantiates.

One of the primary ways in which breast-feeding promotes immunity in the baby is through the provision of large amounts of IgA (immunoglobulin A) through the breast milk.[7] This enhances immune activity at the mucosal level, which, we have learned, is a main avenue for the entry of infectious organisms into the body and a first line of protection for us. In addition to IgA, breast milk is rich in a great variety of other immunologic factors, including the nonspecific humoral factors lactoferrin and lysozyme, and various types of immunoglobulin, including IgG and IgM.[8]

The specific activity of IgA has been shown against a number of organisms that cause infections of the respiratory and digestive tracts.[9] Cellular immunity is also enhanced through the activity of breast milk macrophages on the infant's intestine.[10] Indeed, the mechanisms of conferring immunity from mother to offspring are so effective that they may be more than just passive immunity and be a model of active immunization.[11] The complement system is also stronger in breast-fed infants than those not breast-fed, with the neu-trophils showing increased activity and the serum of breast-fed infants dem-onstrating greater chemoattractant capability.[12] According to an article in the international medical journal *Acta Pediatrica*, "Convincing studies demonstrate significant protection during breast-feeding against diarrhea, respiratory tract infections, otitis media, bacteremia, bacterial meningitis, botulism, urinary tract infections, and necrotizing enterocolitis."[13] This protection may last for years after breast-feeding and may also protect against Hib infection and wheezing bronchitis.[14] Breast-feeding actually stimulates the maturity of the immune system of infants.[15] An interesting finding, discussed in the *European Journal of Pediatrics*, is the considerably larger thymus gland of breast-fed infants at four months compared with the non–breast-fed. The thymic gland, once consid-ered useless, is now recognized to be a significant contributor to immune func-tion and is the site where T-lymphocytes mature. This difference in size was still present at ten months, size being directly correlated to the number of times the infant breast-fed daily. Immune-enhancing factors in breast milk are considered responsible for enhanced thymic size.[16]

Other benefits to the infant appear to be increased IQ and academic per-formance, decreased risk of certain malignancies (cancer), inflammatory bowel disease, autoimmune disease, allergy, and juvenile diabetes, all of which con-tinue much beyond the end of the breast-feeding relationship.[17] The IgA anti-bodies in breast milk have been shown to be effective against cholera, campylobacter, shigella, and giardia, among other organisms, appearing to decrease the ability of certain microorganisms to adhere to the mucosal mem-branes. This also protects against *Haemophilus influenzae* and pneumococci, possibly explaining why breast-fed babies have fewer ear infections than non–breast-fed infants.[18] In fact, breast-feeding is now encouraged as a prophylac-tic measure against the staggering number of upper respiratory infections in the pediatric population, particularly those children who attend day care and nursery school.[19] It is clear that breast-feeding protects the newborn from in-testinal and systemic infections.[20] This protection is especially critical for the premature infant, who is susceptible to a greater number of infections as well as damage caused by inflammatory processes.[21] In fact, internationally, infant morbidity and mortality have been directly affected by a decline in breast-feeding.[22]

The role of breast-feeding in the prevention of cancer later in childhood is still being studied. It is thought that infants who were never breast-fed, and those who were breast-fed short-term only, have a higher risk of developing cancer than those who were breast-fed for six months or longer.[23] The reason for this may be that the antimicrobial activity of breast milk, which seems to stimulate early development of the infant immune system, may also enable the baby to "better negotiate future carcinogenic insults . . . directly developing the long-term development of the immune system."[24] Of course, the fact that breast milk is an excellent source of nutrients for infants, and excellent nutrition prevents infections, should not be underestimated in its immunoprotective roles.[25]

What is particularly interesting about immunity conferred by breast-feeding is that it appears to last for some years after breast-feeding has been discontinued.[26] Weaning itself may be associated with a peak in intestinal immune activation, which coincides with the development of tolerance to food.[27] Toward the goal of immunocompetence, it is clear that breast-feeding is a significant step: "Besides providing optimal nutrition for the normal newborn, breast milk has several distinctive non-nutritive advantages that make it a superior choice over formula. Among those are the fact that it contains phagocytic and *immunocompetent* [emphasis mine] cells and promotes intestinal mucosal maturation."[28] The composition of breast milk makes it the "gold standard" choice for feeding to infants.[29]

Breast-feeding is also known to protect babies from SIDS, probably through its actions on gastrointestinal immunity. Not only are formula-fed infants at greater risk of dying from SIDS, but many have gastrointestinal infections prior to death.[30]

It is interesting to note that breast-feeding is not only protective against many infections and medical problems but also is specifically protective against some of those associated with vaccinations, for example, irritable bowel syndrome, allergies, increased rates of upper respiratory infections, and even SIDS. Logic has it, then, that parents who are choosing not to vaccinate must consider breast-feeding an important part of their proactive plan for enhancing immune functioning. In addition, parents who breast-feed and also plan to vaccinate may find that their children have extra protection against long-term adverse reactions that children who are vaccinated but not breast-fed do not have.

A final word about breast-feeding. Much research has been done on the positive effects of breast milk on short- and long-term immunity; indeed, much research has been presented to you in this chapter. True to the tendency of reductionism in scientific research, it is the breast milk that is studied and not the significance of the breast-feeding relationship. While breast milk has clearly evidenced effectiveness against pathogenic organisms, how many of the positive effects of the substances found in breast milk are enhanced by the loving, nurturing relationship engendered by the activity itself? It was well known by the early 1900s that infants in orphanages who received little touch died of wasting diseases, in fact, in epidemic proportions. It is well worth considering that while breast milk is an independently effective agent against infectious diseases, it is likely that the full effects of a positive breast-feeding relationship cannot be overvalued and could never be recreated in a formula designed to match the biochemical factors in breast milk. Immeasurable aspects of human life may eventually be discovered to be the axis around which all biochemical activities revolve.

The Importance of Nutrition in Immunocompetence

Breast-fed babies definitely have an advantage, but even if you did not breast-feed your children, immunologic health can be fostered through excellent nutrition. Perhaps more than any other factor, nutrition is implicated in the continuing health of the immune system. To see the impact of poor nutrition on immunity, one need only look at the correlation between severe malnutrition and high disease rates for less privileged nations and compare them with countries such as the United States or western European nations. In countries where malnourishment is rampant (in addition to overcrowding, frequently indecent working conditions, and other hallmarks of poverty), diseases that might otherwise be common childhood illnesses are akin to plagues. Measles takes its most virulent and destructive form in such places, not infrequently manifesting as a severe hemorrhagic disease. In such places vaccines may indeed be essential, life-preserving tools. However, we must remember that even vaccines are only a Band-Aid on a wound of greater social injustices that allow such malnutrition and poverty to exist in a world of plenty.

Still, even in privileged nations, nutrient deficiencies can occur, as a result of both insufficient dietary intake of nutrients and of dietary excesses that are associated with their own nutritional deficiencies. According to leading researchers on nutrition and immunity R. K. and S. Chandra, "The immune system plays a key role in the body's ability to fight infection and reduce the risk of developing tumors, autoimmune, and degenerative disease. Nutritional deficiencies and excesses influence various components of the immune system."[31] Despite the seeming affluence of our nation, there are many who live at or below the poverty line, who suffer from malnutrition and have higher rates of infectious diseases than the rest of the population. Such social disparities explain why many Native Americans and African Americans have a greater susceptibility to vaccine-preventable infectious diseases than the general population.

While the relationship between health and diet has long been recognized by the alternative medicine community, its significance has been largely ignored by conventional medicine. Only recently has science begun to acknowledge the dramatic role of nutrition in disease prevention. Yet "the complex interactions between nutrition, infection, and immunity are still poorly understood and the precise role of each factor is difficult to ascertain."[32] Infection itself causes profound metabolic changes, altering nutritional needs. It is clear, however, that "nutrition is a critical determinant of immune responses and malnutrition is the most common cause of immunodeficiency world-wide.[33] For about thirty years now, systematic studies have proven that nutrient deficiency reduces immune system function, increasing susceptibility to and severity of infections, particularly in children.[34] Not only are opportunistic infections reduced by good nutrition, but so is tumor development.[35] Nutrition plays such a dramatic role that it is a wonder that more emphasis isn't placed on nutrition education at prenatal visits for pregnant women, routine well-baby visits, and pediatric visits and in schools. The role of nutrition in immunity is of significant public health importance yet is largely overlooked.[36]

PRENATAL NUTRITION AND LOW-BIRTH-WEIGHT BABIES

Parents have the opportunity to begin to foster a healthy immune system for their baby even before birth. By ensuring an excellent diet for the pregnant mother, the chances of giving birth to a premature or low-birth-weight baby are reduced. Smoking, alcohol consumption, and drug use may also lead to prematurity, low birth weight, and other damage as well, so it is best to avoid these during pregnancy (and preferably for six months prior to conception and while breast-feeding). Any factors that hinder fetal growth and development interfere with immunologic maturation.[37] Early immunocompromise can be significant and can persist for months, or even years, after birth.[38] Discuss optimal prenatal nutrition with your midwife or doctor, and do your own research to get your baby off to a healthy start.

Specific Nutrients and Immunity

While research into nutrition and immunity is still in its infancy, a number of interesting associations have been made generally, as well as for specific nutrients and their influence on specific immunologic functions. It is clear that

165

"there is a strict and cyclical relationship between infection, immune function, and nutritional status, with changes in one influencing the other two. Impermanence of immune function can occur even in healthy subjects in apparently good nutritional status as a consequence of some nutrient deficiencies."[39] Recognizing this, it is important as a first line of proactive measures for parents to take stock of their children's nutritional status. But before we get into dietary improvement, let's take a look at what research literature indicates about specific nutrients and immunity.

ANTIOXIDANTS

The immune system is highly dependent on cell-to-cell communication for optimal functioning. Damages to this signaling system will reduce immune response. Free-radical damage is particularly problematic. Antioxidant vitamins A, C, and E have demonstrated, in many epidemiological studies, the ability to reduce oxidative damage and improve immune function, as well as reduce cancer risk. There is evidence that adequate intake of antioxidant nutrients from an early age can improve cellular immunity and prevent degenerative diseases.[40] Polyunsaturated fats are implicated in adverse effects on immune function. The antioxidant nutrients, particularly vitamins A, C, and E, can work together synergistically to mitigate the adverse effects of polyunsaturated fatty acids on immune functions.[41] Furthermore, antioxidants have exhibited the ability to increase the phagocytic activity of the macrophage, allowing the body to more effectively and efficiently eliminate pathogenic microorganisms.[42]

Vitamin A

Vitamin A and related vitamin A compounds (retinoic acids and carotenes) have been studied extensively, as their impact on the immune system is significant. They are considered to have an important immunomodulatory effect in both adults and children. The mechanisms for this include an immune modulating effect on the gut immune system, which we have seen is a primary site of contact with pathogenic microorganisms.[43] Vitamin A has been shown to play a major role in the expression of various immune components (cytokines, mucins, and keratins), the production of lymphocytes, regulation of apoptosis (cell death), the production of antibodies, and the function of neutrophils, natural killer cells, macrophages, and T- and B-lymphocytes.[44]

Recent research conducted at Johns Hopkins University School of Medicine demonstrated the effectiveness of vitamin A supplementation in reducing morbidity and mortality from a variety of infectious diseases, including measles, diarrheal disease, measles-related pneumonia, HIV infection, and malaria.[45] It not only enhances resistance to infection, but reduces autoimmunity.[46] A study from the International Center for Diarrheal Research (diarrhea is one of the biggest killers of children in the world) in Bangladesh concluded that cell-mediated immunity was consistently better in well-nourished infants, irrespective of supplementation, but that vitamin A supplementation in already generally adequately nourished infants did improve immune activity.[47]

Vitamin A induces the increase of cellular immunity, including phagocytic activity and tumor-destructive responses. Low plasma levels of vitamin A impair immune responsiveness and also have a damaging effect on the health and functioning of the mucous membranes.[48] Vitamin A not only reduces the tendency to infection and enhances immunity, it also enhances the body's response to vaccination, increasing the antibody response to such vaccines as DPT and measles.[49] Thus, optimal nutrition benefits all children, regardless of their parents' vaccine choices.

Vitamin E

Vitamin E, a major fat-soluble antioxidant vitamin, is present in all cellular membranes and is essential for maximum immune function. Animal studies have indicated that supplementation of the diet with vitamin E enhances immunity and may also partially compensate for selenium deficiency, which leads to immunosuppression.[50] Vitamin E increases complement activity and protects against autoimmune disease.[51] Excessive intake of vitamin E is immunosuppressive, so careful supplementation, with an emphasis on dietary sources, is important.[52]

Vitamin C

Vitamin C, a water-soluble antioxidant nutrient, has long been associated with reduction in infection. High levels of vitamin C can also preserve levels of vitamin E in the body, contributing to its immune-enhancing qualities as well.[53] Furthermore, vitamin C demonstrates all of the benefits associated with antioxidants in protecting immune function and cellular communication. However, at least in one study, lower levels of ascorbate were associated with reduction in iron in the plasma, which led to an increase in the activity of macrophages.[54] Overall, however, the benefits of adequate vitamin C far outweigh any concerns.

ADDITIONAL NUTRIENTS

A number of other nutrients appear to have the ability to specifically enhance immunocompetence. Zinc appears to have the ability to enhance immune function and improve gut integrity.[55] It was shown to be critical for the development of both T- and B-cell function and the maintenance of vigorous cellular immunity.[56] Vitamin B_6, copper, iron, folate, and selenium have also been well studied and are shown to have a significant impact on immune function.[57] Selenium deficiency has been linked to viral infection, and supplementation has resulted in enhanced T-cell function and increases in natural killer-cell activity, while copper has been shown to reduce infection in some animal species.[58]

PROTEIN

Protein deficiency is strongly linked to immune system underfunctioning, depressing a variety of immune functions.[59]

Excessive Supplementation

While optimal nutrition is important, excessive supplementation can also be detrimental, as the interaction between nutrients can limit their functions or actually inhibit certain immune functions. For example, mildly excessive iron intake can reduce immunity, and excessive calcium inhibits leukocyte function.[60] It is therefore important to derive as much nutrition from healthy food sources as possible, and to do research or consult a qualified nutrition advisor before using individual nutrient supplements in large quantities. It is also preferable to supplement groups of nutrients rather than to isolate and supplement individual nutrients. For example, multivitamin-multimineral supplements designed for children may be better than giving your child separate nutrients.

Weight and Immunity

Interestingly, while malnutrition is a significant contributor to decreased immunity, so is obesity. Childhood obesity and diabetes have risen dramatically in the past decade. Many studies have correlated a positive relationship between lower caloric intake in the presence of adequate nutrient intake and optimum immune function, with a reduction not only in infections but also tumor formation.[61] A reduction in caloric intake and fat intake, as well as supplementation with fish oil, enhances immunologic functioning and increases life span.[62]

Teaching your child good eating habits early on, including what foods to eat and to eat only when hungry, not when bored or emotionally stressed, and ensuring adequate physical activity can prevent these problems and all of the complications that go along with them, while enhancing your child's immune system.

Optimal Nutrition for Children

Ensuring that your child receives optimal (better than adequate) nutrition takes some time and planning but will quickly become a way of life for you if you are committed to doing so. It is much easier to introduce healthy eating habits if you begin when your children are young. Since most parents in the stages of deciding whether to vaccinate have young children, you are in luck.

Healthy eating habits include eating a wide variety of healthful foods, eating regularly, eating proper amounts, and ideally, eating in pleasant surroundings with a minimum of stress.

This chapter focuses on healthy foods for optimum immunity. For further information on childhood nutrition I encourage you to read *SuperImmunity for Kids* by Leo Galland, a book I have referred to over and over again since my oldest children were young.

Book

Natural and Organic

There is almost no end to the list of pesticides, herbicides, preservatives, colorings, and flavorings in foods. In addition, an increasing number of foods are irradiated or genetically engineered. Nobody knows how this is going to affect health, in either the short or long term. Speculation is that we might be in for some trouble. The only way to prevent individual harm from these substances and processes (and reduce the harmful impact on our lovely green-and-blue planet) is to eat foods that are naturally raised and organically grown. This is especially important for dairy and meat products. While the prices of organic foods may be higher than conventional fare, the latter have their own price, too. Increased illness means medical expenses, missed work, and stress.

Large natural food store chains now enable you to eat most of your familiar foods in natural varieties, so you don't have to give your family "weird stuff" like tofu and seaweed. But the growth in the natural foods market even offers creative ways to serve these foods, and plenty of cookbooks for recipes and ideas. Again, children who begin to eat this way from birth won't flinch at a bowl of miso soup with tofu and sea veggies, but if you have older kids who are new to this haute cuisine, you can still serve a hamburger (organic beef) on a bun (whole wheat) with the trimmings. Naturally, there is a lot more to healthful eating than substituting organic varieties for the common stuff—ice cream is ice cream is ice cream on some level—but it's a start. Eventually you can introduce whole grains, beans, and a variety of vegetables. My kids do eat their greens, love beans and brown rice, and will enjoy a carrot for a snack. This is what they know. Sure they have preferences; a couple of them detest tofu, they all HATE cooked spinach, and none loves raw mushrooms. They all LOVE ice cream. It's all about firmness, with a healthy dose of flexibility and fun.

Wide Variety

One of the best ways to ensure optimal nutrition is to eat a wide variety of foods from a wide variety of food groups. Too often kids' diets are redundant and limited—pizza, macaroni and cheese, cereal and milk, peanut butter and jelly, tuna sandwiches, burgers and fries, and too many fast foods. This does not provide a variety of nutrients and, furthermore, tends to create food sensitivities to wheat, peanuts, and dairy.

The food pyramid provides a good foundation for understanding the basic food groups and which choices are needed daily in what quantities.

FOOD PYRAMID

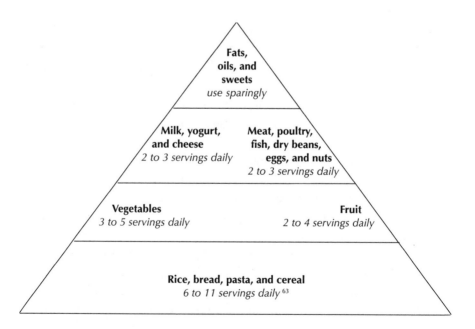

Fats, oils, and sweets
use sparingly

Milk, yogurt, and cheese
2 to 3 servings daily

Meat, poultry, fish, dry beans, eggs, and nuts
2 to 3 servings daily

Vegetables
3 to 5 servings daily

Fruit
2 to 4 servings daily

Rice, bread, pasta, and cereal
6 to 11 servings daily [63]

What to Feed Your Kids: Nutrients for Optimal Health

The following discussion supplies a list of the common nutrients kids need for optimal growth and development and indicates which foods provide these. Combined with the information from the food pyramid, you'll have a good idea of what kinds of foods provide which nutrients and how much your child needs and how often. As each child's needs will be slightly different, you will need to adjust the pyramid servings and foods slightly for each child. For example, an athletic child may need a full ten servings of rice, bread, pasta, or cereal daily, whereas a more sedentary child may need only six servings. A child who is sensitive to dairy may need foods other than dairy to supply calcium, and this may also require additional servings to assure that needs are met. The following information is geared toward school-age children. For infants and adolescents, refer to *SuperImmunity for Kids* by Leo Galland, M.D., or *Smart Medicine for a Healthier Child* by my friend and colleague Janet Zand, O.M.D., with Rachel Waltron, R.N., and Bob Rountree, M.D. Dosage is based on a range for children four to fifteen years old.

WATER

The body is two-thirds water and needs plenty of it to function. Dehydration can lead to increased susceptibility to infection and is dangerous during fevers. Insufficient water can also cause mental dullness, depression, irritability, and constipation. Water is necessary for the utilization of water-soluble vitamins. This is the healthiest beverage for children. Sodas, juice, and milk are not substitutes on a daily basis. Noncaffeinated herbal teas made with herbs safe for use with children and soups or broth may be substituted occasionally. Filtered water is preferable to tap water, which is full of chemicals used to purify what would otherwise be unthinkable to consume.

Amount: 6 to 8 glasses daily

COMPLEX CARBOHYDRATES

Complex carbohydrates are slow-burning fuels, complex sugars that provide the body with lasting energy. They are also needed for digestion and elimination and to provide dietary fiber.

Best sources: whole grains such as rice, whole wheat, millet, oats, barley, and cornmeal, as well as dried beans

Amount: 6 to 11 servings daily

PROTEIN

Protein is essential for the growth, development, and repair of all tissue, as well as for heat, energy, and hormone production. While small amounts of meat in the diet are fine, it is preferable to eat a variety of beans and whole grains and keep red meat consumption to a minimum, particularly for children under five years old. Children who are extremely fair and tend to catch colds and sickness can benefit from the regular addition of red meat to the diet—a small amount (a piece the size of the child's palm) a few times weekly.

Best sources: red meat, fish, poultry, cheese, milk, yogurt, nuts and seeds, grains and beans when eaten together, tofu

Amount: 2 to 3 servings daily

FATS

Healthy fats are essential for regulating body temperature, building cell walls, and the healthy development of hair, skin, and nails. They are also essential in optimal immune function, mental function, and hormone regulation.

Best sources: cold-pressed oils, including olive, walnut, safflower, sunflower, flax, and canola

Amount: sparingly each day

Note: Butter can be used in moderation, but margarine should *never* be used, nor should other partially hydrogenated or hydrogenated oils, or saturated fats such as coconut or palm kernel oils. The formation of molecules that occurs in margarine is not found in nature and is entirely foreign to our bodies. Dairy and meat products should be kept to a minimum, as they too are high in saturated fats. Saturated fats and hydrogenated oils increase the need for essential fatty acids (see below), reduce immunity, and damage cell walls.

ESSENTIAL FATTY ACIDS

Herbalist and naturopathic doctor Mary Bove states, "Modern research and clinical observation suggest that essential fatty acids (EFAs) are a key to optimal health and healthy development of the immune system throughout life."[64] They are converted in the body to a substance known as prostaglandin, which reduces inflammation, enhances immunity, and reduces allergic responses. Unfortunately, the body does not make its own EFAs, so they must be derived through the diet or nutritional supplementation. EFAs are most abundant in raw nuts and seeds, dried beans, cold-water fish, and the oil from certain plants, including evening primrose, flax, black currant, and borage.

There are two distinct types of EFAs: omega-6 oils and omega-3 oils. The former are found in safflower, sunflower, corn, and evening primrose oils. This is usually not deficient in children whose diets include some of these sources and who are otherwise well nourished so that they have the minerals necessary for using these oils. The omega-3 oils, however, are commonly lacking in the typical diet and are most abundant in fresh cold-water fish such as salmon, tuna, mackerel, and cod, as well as flaxseed oil and flaxseeds. Beans and fresh nuts and seeds eaten regularly, according to Bove, provide an excellent source of both omega-3 and -6 oils.

If your child has a tendency to get sick often or has chronic allergy problems or chronic inflammatory problems (for example, eczema), consider supplementing the diet using either food sources or a high-quality supplement. If you choose to supplement with flaxseed oil, choose a high-quality brand and only purchase a product that is kept in the refrigerator section of the health food store, as it goes rancid easily at room temperature. Store it in the refrigerator at home. Add it to salad dressing or to food after cooking. If your child can't tolerate the flavor and is old enough to swallow pills, use evening primrose oil in soft gel capsules.

Amount: supplement with 500 to 1,000 milligrams of evening primrose oil daily, or 2 teaspoons of flaxseed oil daily

WATER-SOLUBLE VITAMINS

B_1 (Thiamine)

Thiamine is important for the heart, nervous system, and muscles, as well as for carbohydrate metabolism.

Best sources: acorn squash, black beans, brown and white rice, corn, lentils, navy beans, peas, pinto beans, pine nuts, pork, quinoa, salmon, sunflower seeds, tempeh, trout, tuna, wheat germ

Amount: 0.9 to 1.3 milligrams daily

B_2 (Riboflavin)

Riboflavin assists fat and carbohydrate metabolism, builds healthy hair, skin, and nails, is important for vision, and is needed for cell growth.

Best sources: almonds, asparagus, avocados, bananas, broccoli, brussels sprouts, cheddar cheese, cottage cheese, dandelion greens, eggs, feta cheese, green leafy vegetables, ham, lentils, mango, mushrooms, peas, raspberries, ricotta cheese, salmon, soybeans, Swiss cheese, tempeh, tuna, wheat germ, yogurt

Amount: 1.1 to 1.5 milligrams daily

B₃ (Niacin)

Niacin is necessary for breaking down carbohydrates, fats, and protein; helps form red blood cells and hormones; and is necessary for healthy skin, the digestive tract, and the nervous system.

Best sources: avocados, barley, beef, brown and white rice, chicken, corn, eggs, milk, mushrooms, nectarines, peas, peanuts, raspberries, salmon, tempeh, tuna, turkey, whole grains

Amount: 12 to 15 milligrams daily

B₅ (Pantothenic Acid)

Pantothenic acid supports the adrenal glands, builds a healthy nervous system and skin, assists carbohydrate and fat metabolism, is important for healthy sinuses, and is needed for production of essential fatty acids and neurotransmitters.

Best sources: avocados, beans, brown and white rice, cheese, chicken, eggs, lentils, lobster, mushrooms, salmon, sunflower seeds, wheat germ, whole grains, yogurt

Amount: 3 to 7 milligrams daily

B₆ (Pyridoxine)

Pyridoxine helps to metabolize proteins and amino acids into hormones, builds red blood cells and antibodies, and is essential for central nervous system function.

Best sources: avocados, bananas, cauliflower, chicken, chickpeas, Chinese cabbage, green and red peppers, legumes, lentils, oatmeal, potatoes, salmon, soybeans, steak, sweet potatoes, tempeh, trout, wheat germ

Amount: 1.1 to 1.7 milligrams daily

B₁₂ (Cobalamin)

Vitamin B₁₂ is necessary for red blood cell production; helps build and maintain myelin, the protective coating around the nerves; and is needed for DNA synthesis.

Best sources: chicken, clams, crab, dairy products (except butter), eggs, herring, mackerel, salmon, steak, trout, yogurt

Amount: 1.0 to 1.4 micrograms daily

Biotin

Biotin is needed for fatty acid, carbohydrate, and protein metabolism; it maintains hair, skin, nerves, bone marrow, and sweat glands.

Best sources: cauliflower, egg yolks, milk, nuts, sweet potatoes, whole grains, whole wheat

Amount: 25 to 50 micrograms daily

Folic Acid

Folic acid is necessary for protein metabolism, production of DNA and RNA, red blood cell production, nervous system function, and healthy hair and nails.

Best sources: artichokes, asparagus, avocados, beets, black beans, blackberries, broccoli, chickpeas, eggs, green leafy vegetables, kidney beans, lentils, pinto beans, oranges, tofu, whole wheat

Amount: 75 to 150 micrograms daily

Vitamin C

Vitamin C builds and maintains connective tissue; aids wound healing and burn repair; maintains health of blood vessels; is an antioxidant, enhances immunity; increases iron absorption; is involved in the production of neurotransmitters; is necessary for adrenal hormone production and for healthy teeth, bones, gums, and ligaments; and aids in cholesterol metabolism.

Best sources: broccoli, brussels sprouts, cantaloupe, citrus fruits, green and red peppers, kale, kiwi, strawberries, tomatoes

Amount: 45 to 60 milligrams daily

FAT-SOLUBLE VITAMINS

Vitamin A (Beta-carotene)

Vitamin A is essential for proper functioning of the immune system; the mucus membranes of the digestive, respiratory, and urinary tracts; eyesight; and the adrenal glands.

Best sources: apricots, avocados, butter, butternut squash, cantaloupe, carrots, dandelion greens, dark green leafy vegetables, egg yolk, mangoes, nectarines, sweet potatoes

Amounts: up to 5,000 international units daily

Vitamin D

Vitamin D is needed for bone and tooth development and muscle function and is also essential for the absorption of calcium, phosphorus, magnesium, and zinc, and for healthy thyroid function.

Best sources: sunshine, butter, eggs, fish liver oil, fortified milk, herring, salmon, sardines, shiitake mushrooms, Swiss cheese

Amount: 10 micrograms daily (400 international units)

Vitamin E

Vitamin E protects cell membranes from free-radical damage from pollution and oxidation of fats, protects arteries, and is involved in red blood cell formation and normal enzyme function.

Best sources: almonds and almond oil, avocados, canola oil, egg yolks, green leafy vegetables, nuts, whole-wheat flour, wheat germ

Amount: 7 to 10 milligrams daily

Vitamin K

Vitamin K is essential for proper blood clotting and bone formation.

Best sources: dark green leafy vegetables, vegetable oils

Amount: 20 to 45 micrograms daily

MAJOR MINERALS

Calcium

Calcium builds strong teeth and bones and is necessary for transmission of nerve impulses, blood clotting, heart rhythm, and smooth muscle contraction.

Best sources: beans, broccoli, cheddar cheese, collard greens, dairy products, kale, tofu

Amount: 800 to 1,000 milligrams daily

Magnesium

Magnesium is important for muscle relaxation, blood sugar balance, carbohydrate and protein metabolism, the function of more than three hundred enzymes, the metabolism of vitamin C and calcium, and the genetic structure of DNA and RNA.

Best sources: almonds, bananas, cashews, avocados, black beans, butternut squash, corn, green vegetables, mackerel, milk, molasses, peas, potatoes, salmon, shellfish, tofu, whole grains

Amount: 120 to 280 milligrams daily

Phosphorous

Phosphorous is involved in the building of bones and teeth, DNA and RNA, cell growth and repair, heart muscle contraction, kidney functioning, muscle and nervous system health, carbohydrate and fat metabolism, and the synthesis of proteins and vitamins.

Best sources: almonds, artichokes, beans, cheddar cheese, chicken, corn, eggs, ham, lentils, peas, pumpkin seeds, quinoa, ricotta cheese, sesame seeds, Swiss cheese, tofu, trout, tuna, turkey, whole grains, and yogurt

Amount: 800 to 1,400 milligrams daily

Potassium

Potassium maintains the body's sodium-fluid balance; helps to transmit nerve impulses; supports nervous system function; supports heart, muscles, kidneys, and blood; and assists in the synthesis of proteins.

Best sources: acorn squash, avocados, bananas, broccoli, butternut squash, cantaloupe, Chinese cabbage, citrus fruits, cod, dried apricots, grouper, halibut, herring, honeydew, lentils, lima beans, milk, papaya, peanut butter, pinto beans, quinoa, soybeans, tomatoes, trout, wheat germ, yogurt

Amount: 1,400 to 2,000 milligrams daily

Sodium

Sodium maintains normal fluid balance and is needed for proper muscle functioning and for the blood and lymph system.

Best sources: most foods, particularly salty foods, cheese, milk, seafood, and tamari

Amount: 300 to 500 milligrams daily

SOME TRACE MINERALS

Chromium

Chromium maintains balanced blood sugar levels and promotes healthy circulation.

Best sources: cheese, legumes, molasses, whole grains

Amounts: 30 to 150 micrograms daily

Copper

Copper is needed for bone formation, healing, red blood cell production, iron transport, and neurological functions.

Best sources: Alaska king crab, Brazil nuts, cashews, cherries, chickpeas, clams, cocoa, eggs, lentils, legumes, lobster, nuts, peas, shiitake mushrooms, soybeans, tempeh, whole grains

Amount: 1 to 2 micrograms daily

Selenium

Selenium prevents free-radical damage to cell membranes, increases cancer resistance, helps the body utilize vitamin E, supports pancreatic function, and eliminates certain heavy metals from the body.

Best sources: Brazil nuts, barley, brown rice, couscous, eggs, ground beef, mackerel, pineapple, shiitake mushrooms, shrimp, sunflowers seeds, tofu, tuna, wheat germ, yogurt

Amount: 20 to 50 micrograms daily

Zinc

Zinc enhances immunity, is necessary for energy production, promotes burn and wound healing, is involved in carbohydrate and protein metabolism, is important for the growth and function of the reproductive organs, maintains normal insulin activity, helps maintain healthy skin, and is needed for DNA and RNA synthesis.

Best sources: oysters; black beans, brewer's yeast, carrots, chicken, chickpeas, lentils, lobster, oatmeal, nuts, peanuts, peas, pumpkin seeds, quinoa, sesame seeds, steak, sunflower seeds, tempeh, turkey, wheat germ, wild rice, yogurt

Amount: 10 to 15 milligrams daily

A Word about Sugar and Immunity

It is so common for children to get sick after a few days of holiday parties or birthday parties that I don't know why the connection between sugar and childhood illness isn't better recognized. A number of laboratory studies have confirmed the role of sugar in reducing immune activity. One study used one hundred grams (twenty teaspoons) each of glucose, fructose, sucrose, honey, and orange juice to evaluate the effects of sugar on immune function. Each one impaired immune activity by 50 percent for two to five hours after consumption.[65] Twenty teaspoons of orange juice is just over half a cup. If your child eats a lot of sweets, begin to reduce them by substituting healthful alternatives. Sugar also actually leaches minerals out of your body and causes you to excrete calcium through your urine.

Many kids reach for sweets because they are available, convenient, and quickly filling. Sweet cravings can indicate underlying nutritional deficiencies. Keep other snack options on hand, such as fresh vegetables and dip, bean burritos, roll-up sandwiches, and homemade treats that are nutritious but not too sweet. Let your child help you shop, and look through cookbooks together for ideas. If your child has been eating more sweets than usual, such as at holiday time, be sure to return to a balanced diet as quickly as possible. Natural sugars are still sugar, so supersweet foods from the health food store aren't necessarily a healthy choice (though they may contain fewer additives).

An interesting story exists demonstrating the connection between sugar consumption and polio outbreaks. It is well known that most polio outbreaks in the United States in the 1940s and 1950s occurred in late summer and early autumn. To this day no medical explanation for this has been given. But back in the late 1940s, Dr. Benjamin Sadler of Asheville, North Carolina, alerted the local public to the relationship between poliomyelitis and the consumption of large amounts of sugar products (including large quantities of fruit and fruit juices) and refined flour products.

Sadler, in the summer of 1949, undertook a statewide polio campaign and advocated that children be given a high-protein diet with low-starch vegetables and no sugar, sugar-laden foods, and processed foods. During that same summer, the polio rates in North Carolina numbered 214, compared with the 2,402 cases of the previous summer. Simultaneously, rates in thirty-nine other states showed an increase in cases.[66]

A Word about Dairy Products

Although dairy products provide a convenient source of protein, carbohydrates, and minerals, they are also strongly associated with increased susceptibility to upper respiratory congestion. Children who drink milk regularly are particularly prone to colds, allergies, earaches, and related health problems. Children can grow perfectly well without ever drinking a cup of milk—and they'll have fewer respiratory and digestive problems. Consider using dairy as a complement to meals, such as cheddar cheese on a bean and rice burrito, or yogurt in a bowl of granola.

Yogurt and hard cheese such as cheddar are the best dairy choices. Yogurt should contain live, active cultures and should not be loaded with sugar. Occasionally, if your child tolerates dairy well, a smoothie or milk in cereal can be fine. If your child is highly reactive to dairy products, learn about alternative sources of calcium, protein, and other nutrients. Soy milk is not a healthful alternative to milk; it is highly processed and predisposes children to allergies and digestive and respiratory weaknesses.

Refined Flour Products

Refined flour products, such as the white flour that composes so many baked goods and breads, are not only denatured—meaning they've had most of their nutrients removed—but they, like sugar, also leach minerals out of the body. Learn to use whole grains as your staple foods, using white flour only occasionally or on special occasions. The same goes for rice—brown rice is full of nutrients that have been removed from white rice in the refining process.

Highly Allergenic Foods

Certain foods are known contributors to allergies, which means that regularly eating them if one is sensitive to them keeps the immune system on the defensive. This can leave the child susceptible to infections. The most common problematic foods are dairy, eggs, peanuts, citrus fruits, chocolate, soy, and fish. If you suspect that your child is experiencing problems because of food sensitivities, refer to my books *Naturally Healthy Babies and Children* and *ADHD Alternatives* for a more complete discussion and treatment recommendations. Dr. Bove's, Dr. Zand's, and Dr. Galland's books are also especially informative (see Recommended Reading).

EIGHT

Herbal Medicines and Childhood Diseases

Natural medicine, in this case the use of herbs and nutrition, is more than just replacing drugs with natural substances. Natural medicine incorporates a different way of looking at health and disease than has been maintained for the past one hundred or so years through the lens of Western conventional medicine. Natural medicine is sometimes referred to as holistic medicine because it steps beyond the one-dimensional construct of the disease-treatment model into a multidimensional, multifactorial approach to healing the human being. The totality of the person and the person's circumstances are considered. In addition to the nature and severity of the disease (also considered by the allopathic doctor), the natural practitioner considers diet, body type and inherited qualities (constitution), individual manifestation of symptoms, environment, psycho-emotional factors, and sometimes even spiritual influences, depending upon the practitioner's background and the patient's spiritual orientation.

Natural medicine has also been referred to recently as complementary medicine, a somewhat Western medicocentric view of healing, around which all other modalities are perceived to pivot. Various systems of herbal and nutritional medicine, however, both predate allopathic medicine and stand alone as independent healing practices. Nonetheless, natural medicine and allopathic medicine do complement each other well, and ideally a new paradigm is emerging that represents a synthesis of models in which all models are respected.

Fortunately for parents trying to incorporate natural-healing approaches for their kids, most of the common childhood diseases have similar symptom patterns, so a lot of the same remedies can be applied for a wide range of different kids. You don't have to figure out body type, psycho-emotional issues, or complicated individual patterns. You can just jump right in and use the remedies accompanying the conditions, varying formulas only to meet your child's obvious symptoms. Another fortunate aspect of herbal and nutritional therapies for kids is that they tend to be quickly effective in acute conditions. Kids' bodies are highly receptive to these treatments, probably owing to their quick metabolism and general vigor and vitality; you don't have to wait around too long to see if something is going to work. If something doesn't give you results within a designated time, you can try another approach.

The recommendations in this chapter are based on traditional use and the clinical experiences of modern herbal practitioners. They are not intended to substitute for medical care when needed. You must use your common sense and discretion when treating your children with alternative therapies, and do not hesitate to use conventional medical treatments.

Using Herbal Medicines

Human beings have used herbs as food and medicine from early on in our existence on this planet. Only recently has the American public returned to an awareness of how beneficial herbs can be in preventing and treating illness and promoting excellent health. While much research is going on to find the active chemical constituents in plants, and doctors, pharmacists, and drug manufacturers are scrambling to get in on the "herbal craze," the most reliable information on herbal medicines tends to come from herbalists in clinical practice. Much of their knowledge is gleaned from the study of traditional plant uses, often a highly reliable source of information, which research scientists turn to when looking for new plant drugs. Herbalists also learn from each other, from scientific literature, and from clinical practice. Many naturopathic physicians are also well versed in the use of herbal treatments, as are acupuncturists who have studied Chinese herbal medicine. Some physicians may be knowledgeable in the use of herbal remedies. Interestingly, science frequently verifies that what the herbalists and traditional folk healers know—and have known for centuries—is entirely accurate.

Always ascertain a practitioner's training and experience before beginning a professional relationship, and make sure the practitioner has experience with pediatric herbal medicine.

182

HOW HERBS DIFFER FROM DRUGS

In some ways herbs and drugs are not that different—they are both used for treating the human body, and both contain a variety of chemical components that have specific bioactivity. However, there are differences in how they are prescribed and how they work in the body. Here is an example: It is well known that even in epidemic outbreaks of colds and flu, some people are more susceptible to infection than others. While conventional medicine might treat colds or influenza with antibiotics and decongestants, herbalists would suggest not only the palliative treatments but a look at why that particular person became ill. Is the person under stress, eating a nutritionally inadequate diet, not sleeping well? Herbalists would seek to reduce tendencies to manifest certain problems in people who are more susceptible by helping the people strengthen overall wellness. Furthermore, herbalists honor both the acute phase and the convalescent phase of illness, recognizing that the body needs to heal, not just get over symptoms. Finally, herbs frequently work synergistically with the body's natural functions, promoting and assisting them rather than overriding them. Many herbs and drugs can be used together, but caution should be exercised, as they can also interact with each other. If your child is already on medications, contact your doctor or a qualified herbalist to make sure that a potentially harmful interaction doesn't exist.

HEALTH IS MORE THAN THE ABSENCE OF ILLNESS

One of the central tenets of herbal healing is that health is more than the absence of illness—it is an active state of physical, emotional, and social well-being. Health is an inner spark that glows from the core of a being outward. The underlying philosophy of traditional medicine strives to help individuals achieve true health, not just cover up symptoms. Keep this in mind when your child is ill by paying attention to his or her overall state of mind, comfort, and surroundings. Keep the child comfortable, engage the child with stories read aloud (or books on tape) and gentle games that can be played in bed (cards, board games, hangman, ticktacktoe, and so on), and keep the environment fresh and pleasant. In some conditions (measles, for example), bright light may be disturbing to your child, so a dim environment is preferable. However, fresh flowers, an occasional light misting of refreshing essential oil into the air, soft music, and freshly plumped pillows can bring cheer and relief.

ARE HERBS SAFE?

It would be too simplistic to say that herbs are safe just because they are natural. There are a number of herbs that, taken even in small amounts, can prove fatal. However, few poisonings come from herbal medicines, and rarely do any occur from properly applied herbal medicines. Investigating the rates of human poisoning from herbs, researchers at the Herb Research Foundation in Boulder, Colorado, studied reports from the American Association of Poison Control Centers and discovered that almost all reported adverse effects from plants were due to accidental poisoning from toxic household plants and ornamental shrubs. Herbs have an excellent historical track record for safety, particularly those used for treating childhood illnesses and discomforts.

ARE PHARMACEUTICAL DRUGS SAFE?

Many of the medications that we take for granted as safe may carry more risk than we assume. Aspirin causes vast numbers of accidental poisonings in children annually, and when given to children with viral infections, it is the leading cause of Reye's syndrome. Prescription drugs are the fifth leading cause of death in the United States. Many of the drugs that are routinely used for children are actually adult medications that have not been proven safe for use in children. According to the author of the textbook *A Pediatric Dosage Handbook*, between 60 and 80 percent of the prescription drugs sold in the United States and used for children are not approved for such use. (These statistics appeared in the September 1994 issue of the *Annals of Pharmacotherapy* and the December 1994 issue of the *Wall Street Journal*. The articles are titled, respectively, "The Need for Conducting Research on Medications Unlabeled for Use in Pediatric Patients," [Nahata] and "F.D.A. to Make It Easier for Drug Makers to Give Pediatric Data to Doctors" [Kessler].)

While prescription drugs should certainly not be avoided when needed, caution should be exercised in using them needlessly or to suppress symptoms, such as rash or moderate fever, that are healthier to express fully.

USING HERBS

To maximize herbal safety and minimize adverse reactions, use only those herbs that have historical or clinical efficacy and safety for children. The ones mentioned in this book meet those criteria. Used appropriately and within recommended guidelines, they are known to be gentle, safe, and effective. Begin with lower doses, increasing as necessary (within the safe range of the dosage), and decreasing the dose any time you can achieve results at a lower rate. It is important, however, not to be afraid of using even a moderately effective (therapeutic) dose of an herb or herbs, as long as the dose remains within guidelines.

BOTANICAL NAMES OF HERBS

All the herbs listed in this chapter can be found listed with their botanical names, also known as the Latin name or scientific name, at the end of this book. The botanical name is the binomial (two names) that tells the genus and species of the plant. Any plant may have a number of common names—and totally different plant species may even share a common name. However, the botanical name is universal, used by scientists, botanists, and herbalists internationally. When using herbs medicinally, you want to know that you have the species and genus recommended as a medicinal herb. When purchasing, wildcrafting (harvesting from the wild), or growing your herbal medicines, it is essential that you are able to verify the botanical name of the plant.

EDUCATE YOURSELF

Feel free to do further research by consulting other books on children's herbal health. Review articles in scientific journals. Consult with knowledgeable herbal professionals. In these times of information mania, it is wise to be cautious and skeptical, and I applaud you for your good common sense.

DETERMINING DOSAGE

The herbal recommendations in this book include a dose range for babies one year and older to adolescents. This assumes a weight range of anywhere from 18 to 150 pounds. While the dosage range can be decreased for younger babies, for those under a year old seek professional care from a qualified practitioner. Doses are described in drops, teaspoon measures, or cups, as appropriate. The lowest dose range is for younger children in the lower weight range, the higher dose for older children in the upper weight range. You will have to fit your child into this range accordingly. Frequency of dosage is also provided in a range, going from mild symptoms to more severe problems. Again, you will need to fit your child into the appropriate range.

CREATING YOUR OWN FORMULA

While I provide formulas for each condition in this chapter, you may want to modify these or even create your own recipes. Developing a formula is fairly simple. The herbs in this book can be used singly or mixed compatibly together in teas, tinctures, and other preparations. To prepare a formula, select the herbs that you want to use and combine them either in equal parts or in varying amounts to achieve the effects you want. For example, if you want the herbal tea to be strongly relaxing and mildly decongestant, you would put more relaxing herbs into the blend, adding a lesser amount of decongestant herbs. Study the formulas in this book to get an idea of how formulation is done.

HERBAL PREPARATIONS

Making basic teas, syrups, herbal steam baths, and even topical preparations at home is not difficult. Preparing herbs at home is rewarding and is an activity in which children love to participate. It is magical to see how different herbs turn water, alcohol, and oils into lovely shades of gold, red, orange, green, and brown. Home preparation of herbs also reduces the expense of remedies. I feel that preparing one's own remedies adds a special potency to the medicines, that of love and care.

Only common supplies are required for making everything from teas to salves in your kitchen. Glass jars of varying sizes with lids, glass or stainless steel pots, a sharp knife, a small funnel, a mesh strainer, a vegetable grater, measuring spoons, and a cutting board are useful to have on hand. Water, vegetable oil, vodka, and beeswax complete the list once you have the herbs you need. Some preparations, such as tinctures, can be made at home but may be easier to purchase, unless you plan in advance and keep a variety of them on hand. The following discussion explains the different types of preparations used in this book, along with directions for preparing some of them. Many health food stores carry a large selection of herbal products. Quality varies, so shop selectively. For tinctures, look for brands listed in Resources. For bulk herbs, make sure the store has a regular turnover of products, or order from the mail-order companies found in Resources.

Teas

Teas are lightly medicinal, generally pleasant-tasting beverage preparations made by steeping one teaspoon to two tablespoons of fresh or dried herbs in one cup of boiling water for ten to twenty minutes. After this time strain out the liquid, discard the herb material (great for the compost pile), and drink the tea. When steeping strongly aromatic herbs (such as lemon balm, lavender, or chamomile), it is necessary to cover the cup or pot in which you are steeping the herbs. This retains the essential oil content of the plant and thus the medicinal quality of the tea. The dosage for tea is anywhere from one-quarter cup to one cup taken two to eight times daily, or sipped throughout the day as needed.

Infusions

Infusions are more concentrated than teas. They are generally made by steeping one-half to one ounce of herbs in one quart of boiling water for thirty minutes to two hours, depending on the strength desired. Infusions are used for extracting constituents from herbs that can't be extracted effectively by making tea, or when a more concentrated herbal preparation is needed. Dosage range of infusions is slightly less than or comparable to that of teas. The following are general guidelines for preparing infusions from different plant parts:

Roots. One ounce of dried root to one quart of boiling water; steep for eight hours.

Bark. Prepare as for roots.

Leaves. Delicate leaves and those rich in essential oils are generally prepared one-half to one ounce of dried leaves or one to two ounces of fresh leaves to one quart of boiling water, steeped one to two hours. Thick leaves require steeping up to four hours. When preparing leaves for nutritional purposes (such as nettle), steeping up to two hours is advisable.

Flowers. As they are delicate, steep one ounce of dried flowers in one quart of boiling water for a maximum of thirty minutes.

Seeds. Aromatic seeds such as anise or fennel are generally prepared by first gently crushing the seeds (about one teaspoon) with a mortar and pestle, then steeping for ten to fifteen minutes in one cup of boiling water, with a lid on the vessel.

Decoctions

Decoctions are made by gently simmering one ounce of herbs in one quart of water for up to thirty minutes. The herbs are first put in a pot of cool water and slowly brought to a simmer. This technique works best for extracting water-soluble constituents out of tough leaves, roots, and barks. It is usually not used with more delicate plant parts such as aromatic flowers, leaves, and seeds. Dose is one teaspoon to two tablespoons, or up to one-half cup, two to six times daily or as needed.

Syrups

Syrups are easy once you have made your decoction. Simply sweeten your decoction by adding an equal amount (by volume) of sweetener. One cup of decoction is eight ounces, so a decoction of this amount would require eight ounces of sweetener. I use one-fourth to one-half cup of honey per cup of liquid and find this adequate; honey is considered to be twice as sweet as sugar. Add the sweetener to your hot decoction, bring it to the boiling point while stirring, then immediately pour it into clean jars. Cool the syrup to room temperature, label, and refrigerate. Syrups can last for many months like this. Dosage is similar to a decoction but of course will vary from herb to herb. Do not give honey to children under one year of age because it may cause severe food poisoning; honey contains *botulinus* spores that young children cannot digest.

Herbal Baths

Herbal baths are tremendously useful for soothing children. They are prepared by adding two quarts of infusion to the bath, or by adding several drops of essential oils to the bath water, or a combination of both. If you keep the door to the bathroom closed, the aroma of the herbs will fill the air, as will any volatile oils. This adds to the relaxing effect of the bath. Herb baths are a nourishing gift that children especially appreciate. Floating herbs directly in the tub makes for a fun bath, if your plumbing can handle it.

Steam Baths

Steam baths can be used therapeutically for upper respiratory congestion and fevers. Saunas and sweat lodges are similarly used in many parts of the world. This is a simplified version for your home. Children should always be accompanied by an adult in a steam bath and should be allowed to leave at any point when they have had enough. Hot water and steam can result in serious burns, so take extra precautions. Fill a pot with a few quarts of water and bring it to a boil. Remove the water from the stove and add a handful of herbs rich in volatile oils (mint, sage, and thyme work well) or up to three drops of essential oil (any of the above or eucalyptus). Cover immediately. Gather a couple of chairs, a large warm blanket—preferably wool—and your pot of hot water. Wearing only underclothes, sit in the chairs and put the covered pot near your feet, being careful not to touch the pot. Make a tent over yourself and your child with the blanket. When you are fully in, uncover the pot and breathe in the steam. When you have had enough, quickly dress the child and bundle him or her into bed.

Poultices and Compresses

Poultices and compresses are ways of applying herbs externally to specific areas of the body. Poultices can be made quickly by mashing, bruising, or even chewing fresh herbs into a pulpy mass and applying as is to the affected area.

They can also be made by taking fresh or dried herbs (dried herbs will need to be moistened with warm water first), mashing them, and spreading them on a thin cotton cloth, which is then applied. A hot water bottle can be placed over the herbs or cloth to retain the warmth. Poultices are used for stings, bites, localized infections, wounds, boils, abscesses, swellings, and tumors.

Compresses are made by soaking a cloth in a hot infusion or decoction, wringing out the excess liquid, and applying the cloth to the needy area. The compress is replaced when it cools. As with a poultice, a hot water bottle over the preparation retains heat.

Washes

Washes are just what they sound like; you wash the area with an infusion or decoction. This can be done as an eyewash, for example, in treating conjunctivitis, or as a wash over a skin rash. It is an effective and simple external remedy.

Tinctures

Tinctures are alcohol-and-water extractions of plants. The combination of solvents allows for maximum extraction of a number of plant constituents that are not highly soluble in either the water or the alcohol alone. Because of their concentrated nature they allow the user to take small quantities—often as little as five drops to as much as a teaspoon. Owing to their alcohol content, they also have a very long shelf life and are easily absorbed.

As you read the information on tincture bottles you will notice that along with the recommended tincture dose there might be a ratio symbol that says 1:2, 1:3, or the like. This relates to the ratio of herb to solvent used in making the tincture. In a 1:1 tincture, one measure of herb was extracted with an equivalent weight of solvent (alcohol). In a 1:2 tincture, one part herb is used to two parts alcohol. The lower the ratio, the stronger the tincture. Therefore a 1:2 tincture is considerably stronger than a 1:5 tincture. This is significant in dosing, particularly when using potent medicinal plants. Ten drops of a 1:5 tincture would equal only two drops of a 1:1 tincture.

To avoid accidental overdose of medicinal herbs when treating children, it is generally recommended to use plants extracted in a 1:3, 1:4, or 1:5 ratio. This allows a greater margin of safety in your dosing. Exceptions are those plants in which a higher ratio is required for medicinal effectiveness. In this chapter it is assumed that you are using a 1:3 or 1:4 ratio of tincture. To determine the ratio of purchased tincture, look for this information on the bottle. Avoid buying from tincture companies that don't provide this information, as it is impossible to know the strength of the preparation.

Instruction in tincture preparation is beyond the scope of this book, but interested readers can consult general herbals or purchase their tinctures at health food stores or through sources listed in Resources.

Glycerites

Tinctures made by using glycerin as a solvent are called glycerites. Their advantage is that they are incredibly sweet and are therefore quite palatable. The disadvantage is that glycerin is not always a highly effective solvent and it has a very high sugar content. It is therefore best reserved for the worst-tasting herbs or for use in combination with alcohol extracts as a sweetener. Glycerite production is also beyond the scope of this book, but any alcohol tincture can be sweetened with glycerin by adding 25 to 50 percent of the tincture's volume in glycerin to the tincture. The dose of the tincture will need to be increased to compensate for the dilution of the remedy.

Oils

Massage can be a useful and effective stress-reduction practice and is enhanced by the use of herbal massage oils. Relaxing herbs and essential oil scents can be added to a base of almond oil. Two methods of preparation follow:

Method 1: Infuse one-half ounce of dried herbs such as chamomile or lavender blossoms in one-half cup of almond oil for five days. Strain and store in a clean jar or squeeze bottle.

Method 2: Add five to fifteen drops of essential oil to four ounces of almond oil depending on desired strength of scent, and shake well. Store in a clean jar or squeeze bottle.

Essential Oils

Essential oils are highly concentrated extracts of the volatile oils of plants. They are almost always for external use only and are applied to the skin, used in baths, or used for aromatherapy in amounts as small as two to three drops. They are not easily prepared at home without sophisticated equipment. Their effect is both transdermal and olfactory, acting on the limbic system of the brain.

Herbal Oils

Sometimes called medicated oils, herbal oils are vegetable oils in which herbs have been infused for a week or more. They are used for sore muscles, sprains, aches, infections, and irritated skin, and for massage.

To make an herbal oil, fill a clean and totally dry jar with dry herbs. Now fill the jar to the brim with oil. Almond, olive, and sesame oils are the most commonly used, but any vegetable oil is acceptable. Store at room temperature in indirect sunlight for two to six weeks. Direct light and heat should be avoided. Infuse and store the oil on a surface that will not be damaged by seepage, which may occur. At the end of the given time period, strain the oil well and store it in a fairly cool and dark place or refrigerate it. Oils will keep for up to a year and are considered good as long as the oil has not turned rancid.

Salves

Salves are used for healing skin injuries. They can be made a few different ways, all of which are effective. This first method is preferable because it requires the least cooking of the herbs and oil, thereby retaining more of the subtle properties of the herbs.

Method 1: Prepare an herbal oil using your chosen salve ingredients. Then pour the herbal oil into a small pot. To this add one tablespoon of grated beeswax per ounce of oil. Heat over a low flame until the wax is melted. To test for readiness, put a small amount on a teaspoon and place it in the refrigerator. After a minute it will harden to its finished consistency. Salve should be firm and solid without being so hard that it can't be melted upon contact with your skin. If the consistency is correct, then pour your salve into small jars, cool to room temperature, cover, and store. If your salve is too soft, add more beeswax; if it is too hard, add more oil.

Method 2: Place about an ounce of herbs and one-third cup of oil in a small pot. Simmer for two hours on a *very low* flame, with the pot covered. Add a bit of oil if necessary and watch carefully to avoid scorching. Strain the herbs well through a cotton cloth or cheesecloth, squeezing as much of the oil as possible out of the plant material. You may need to let the oil cool before this can be done. Clean the pot and dry it (discarding the used plant material), then pour your oil back in, adding a couple of tablespoons of grated beeswax. Melt this over a low flame, stirring constantly. Check for readiness as in the first method, then bottle and store.

Method 3: This method requires less watching. Mix four ounces of oil, one ounce of herb, and one-half ounce of beeswax in an ovenproof pot with a cover. Bake at 250 degrees Fahrenheit for about three hours. Strain the mixture through cheesecloth, then bottle and store it.

Salves will keep for about a year, sometimes longer if kept refrigerated. To extend the life of your salve, you can add one teaspoon of vitamin E oil or one to two teaspoons of an herbal tincture such as echinacea or calendula per four ounces of salve (while still warm, before bottling).

PREPARING CHINESE HERBAL DECOCTIONS INTO SYRUP

Chinese herbs are often strong and strange tasting. An effective method of preparing bulk Chinese herbs for children is to decoct the formula in two quarts of water for one hour and then strain. Simmer the liquid down to two cups, then add one-fourth cup of honey and one-fourth cup of vegetable glycerine to make a syrup. The dose is one to two tablespoons, two to three times daily, though this will vary with different formulas. Syrups prepared with this method generally store well for several weeks if kept in the refrigerator.

Boosting Immunity

Some children get sick more easily or more often than others. Most children live in an environment replete with air pollution, stress, and other factors that naturally burden the immune system. All children will benefit from the use of herbs and foods to enhance immunity, especially during those times of year when colds, flu, and infections are more prevalent. In the previous chapter we looked at the use of nutrition to enhance immunity. Combining those simple concepts with the herbal hints in this chapter, you can virtually assure improved health for your child. Some of my favorite immune-enhancing recipes are prepared as foods that most children will enjoy.

IMMUNE-ENHANCING SOUP

This is a simple miso soup that is very tasty. The optional variation, which includes Chinese herbs to boost immunity, can be prepared in the autumn and winter months. It has a slightly unusual taste, but children hardly seem to notice the difference.

1 yellow onion, sliced
Toasted sesame or olive oil, for sautéing
6 shiitake mushrooms
4 garlic cloves, chopped
2 large carrots, thinly sliced
$1/_2$-inch piece ginger

1 pound firm tofu, cubed
6 four-inch slices alaria (wakame) seaweed
6 inches fresh burdock (gobo) root, thinly sliced (optional; available in
    natural foods stores, some farmer's markets, and Chinese grocery stores)
Miso paste, to taste

Sauté onion in a small amount of toasted sesame or olive oil until slightly
golden. Add remaining ingredients and 6 to 8 cups of water. Bring to a boil,
reduce to a simmer, and cook covered for 30 minutes. Remove the ginger. Add
miso paste (I prefer red barley miso) to taste, up to several tablespoons. Noodles
or cooked rice can be added to the soup for extra body and flavor.

Optional Variation
When adding the vegetables to the recipe above, also add:

3 (3-inch) pieces of codonopsis
2 (4- to 6-inch) pieces of astragalus root
1 teaspoon of Chinese red ginseng

Cook the soup as above and remove the herbs before serving. The red ginseng
can be placed in a stainless steel tea ball and tossed into the pot, or it can be
scooped out after cooking. The herbs can be obtained in Chinese herb shops
or through mail order sources (see Resources).

Serve either soup one to three times each week, using the greater frequency for kids who have a tendency to be chilly and get colds frequently.

GRANDMA IDA'S CHICKEN SOUP

This is my grandma's recipe. It's called "Jewish penicillin" for a good reason!

1 four-pound chicken
Vegetables: carrots, celery, parsnips, onion
Parsley
Salt and pepper to taste
Noodles (optional)

Buy a whole chicken (organic, though that's not my grandma's idea) and have
it cut into quarters if possible, or cut it at home. To wash the chicken before
cooking: Put it into a pot of boiling water for a minute, remove and then scrub
the skin to get the dirt off.

Fill a pot with enough water to cover the chicken (Grandma recommends
about four pounds of chicken for a medium-sized pot of soup) and bring the

water to a boil. Put in the chicken and generous amounts of carrots, celery, parsnips, and onion. Cook until the chicken is soft. Skim off any foam that comes to the surface. Toward the end, tie up a small bunch of parsley and put it into the pot. Cook a bit longer ("the soup gets the flavor, but people don't all like parsley in their bowls," she says). It should cook for at least an hour and a half. Add salt and pepper to taste. When done, let it cool, then remove the chicken. Put the chicken on a plate and separate the meat from the bones (the meat will fall away from the bones). Put the chicken into bowls and pour the soup over the chicken, or serve the chicken separately. On the side, cook noodles and add to the soup. Grandma said to be sure to use a lot of vegetables to make it taste sweet.

This can be made weekly, and leftovers can be eaten throughout the week as a complement to meals or as a snack.

VEGETABLE-BARLEY STEW

$1/2$ yellow onion, chopped
2 celery stalks
10 small mushrooms, chopped
2 medium carrots, diced
2 tablespoons olive oil
1 cup barley

Sauté all the vegetables in the olive oil. Add the barley and 6 cups of water. Cook for 1 hour or until the barley is done. Add salt to taste. This is simple, delicious, and nourishing as an accompaniment to a meal.

GARLIC LEMONADE

Okay, it sounds weird, but my kids love this, and frankly, I do too. It's sweet, sour, and a bit spicy—but not overly spicy if made properly.

3 medium-sized garlic cloves, chopped
Juice of 1 lemon
Maple syrup or honey to taste

Place the garlic in a 1-quart jar and fill the jar with boiling water. Let the garlic steep for 20 minutes and then strain it out. Add the lemon juice and sweeten with the maple syrup or honey.

Give $1/2$ to 2 cups daily, the lower dose to prevent illness and for younger children and the greater quantity for older kids who feel like they are coming down with a cold.

Don't give the lemonade every day; just use it periodically as needed.

Immune-Boosting Herbs

There is a Chinese proverb that says "A man is not sick because he has an illness; he has an illness because he is sick." Immune-building herbs can be given periodically during cold and flu season, more often to kids who are susceptible to infections and illnesses, or to kids who have been exposed to or are "coming down" with an illness. Remember, the goal is not to never have a cold or infection. However, healthy children should not succumb to every "bug" that crosses their paths or be sick seemingly all the time with a chronic runny nose, ear infection, and so on. As you will recall, many people remain healthy in spite of exposure even to serious illness. Your goal is to help your child to achieve or maintain overall strength and vitality. This can be accomplished by using herbs that directly boost immunity, as well as by promoting the health of individual organ systems, such as the lymphatic, digestive, and respiratory systems. Constipation is a significant contributor to chronic illness and susceptibility to inflammatory, infectious conditions and must be addressed. Similarly, lymphatic congestion and chronic swollen glands can decrease the body's ability to rid itself of infection and maintain health, and must therefore be treated. Furthermore, stress is a significant contributor to immune dysfunction; therefore, the nervous system must be treated if there is stress and a tendency to immune weakness. The following herbs can be used regularly or periodically to tonify the immune system, and some can also be used as antimicrobial agents should illness occur.

ASTRAGALUS *(Astragalus membranaceous)*

Astragalus, a member of the pea family, possesses a long fibrous root that, when cut and prepared for commercial purposes, resembles tongue depressors in size, shape, and color. It is a primary herb of traditional Chinese medicine (it also grows here in the United States) that, owing to its effectiveness, has become widely used in the United States as an immune tonic. Astragalus is one of the most respected herbs in the Chinese herbal repertoire for strengthening general resistance against illness. Modern clinical trials have reinforced its reliability in this area.[1] Astragalus has been shown to stimulate macrophage activity, promote antibody formation, activate complement, and increase T-lymphocyte proliferation.[2]

The easiest way to give astragalus regularly is in Immune-Enhancing Soup (see page 193). The flavorful broth can be taken several times weekly.

Astragalus can also be made into a decoction by simmering three root pieces in three cups of water for one hour. Discard the root and save the liquid. Bouillon flavor or miso paste can be added to create a quick broth. Give one-fourth to one cup daily for several weeks or even months.

Tincture is also acceptable. Give one-fourth to one teaspoon twice daily. Astragalus is best avoided during acute febrile conditions and eruptive diseases. It can, however, be used after an illness has passed to restore energy and immunity.

CALENDULA *(Calendula officinalis)*

Calendula blossoms look like little tufts of sunshine. They are a reliable herb to use internally in the treatment of many infectious illnesses as well as topically to treat skin rashes and sores. Calendula has the ability to stimulate the functioning of the lymphatic system, is responsible for removing waste from organs and blood, and is instrumental in maintaining strong immunity.[3] In days of old in Europe, women threw a handful of the blossoms into the family soup pot to prevent sickness. While the role of this herb in treating infection is widely recognized, its use as an immune tonic is often overlooked. Nonetheless, calendula blossoms may well be used in this capacity. It is especially good for children who have swollen glands, either in the throat or around the neck, at the base of the head, and behind the ears.

Because the herb has a bitter taste, it is best given in tincture form to children. Being a potent (though entirely safe and gentle) herb, I prefer to give it in small doses, five to twenty drops two or three times daily as needed for a couple of weeks at a time.

CHAMOMILE *(Matricaria recutita)*

Chamomile has long been used as a gentle and reliable children's herb for soothing all manner of aches and discomforts. It is also a mild bitter, digestive tonic, and nervous system support. Chamomile has been shown in studies to have immunoregulating effects on the blood, increasing the sensitivity of helper cells, and it may also be directly immunostimulating.[4] As chamomile tea has a lovely taste when steeped for a short time, it may easily be given to children in this form, plain or lightly sweetened with honey or maple syrup. Steep one teaspoon to one tablespoon of the blossoms in boiling water for ten minutes. Cover the vessel while steeping. Strain the liquid and serve warm. Chamomile tincture can also be given, and it is lovely tasting as a glycerite. Give one-fourth to one teaspoon of glycerite up to three times daily.

CLEAVERS *(Galium aparine)*

Cleavers, like calendula, though not typically considered a strong immune-enhancing herb, effectively reduces lymphatic congestion (swollen glands). Indeed, the two are quite compatible in formulas, though not interchangeable. Cleavers is hardy in the wild, but once picked and dried it loses effectiveness quickly. Therefore, fresh tincture is preferable to other forms. I give it when there is lymphatic congestion (as described under calendula) but find it has more of an affinity for inflammation and lymphatic congestion that occurs in the spring and summer. It is also useful when there are swollen glands or sore throat, as will be discussed under specific conditions. Give tincture, one-fourth to one teaspoon up to four times daily, for swollen lymph nodes or glands.

ECHINACEA *(Echinacea angustifolia, E. purpurea, E. pallida)*

Almost unheard of ten years ago in the United States except by herbalists and their clients, echinacea is now practically a household herb, and rightly so. Echinacea (I prefer *E. angustifolia*) is a very reliable antiviral and mild antibacterial herb that has proven its mettle in preventing infection and enhancing immune activity. Some of the components of this plant have shown immunomodulating activity, including enhanced nonspecific action on cell-mediated immunity and enhanced natural killer cell function, both in healthy individuals and in those with depressed cellular immunity.[5] Good echinacea causes a buzzing, cold sensation on the tongue. Infusion can be made using one ounce of the dried root to one quart of boiling water, letting the herb steep for two hours. Strain and give one-fourth to one cup up to twice daily. Tincture can be given in a dose of ten drops to one teaspoon twice daily to boost immunity and prevent illness. It can be used for several weeks at a time but should not be continued indefinitely. Use of echinacea for acute care will be discussed under specific illnesses.

ELDER *(Sambucus nigra, S. canadensis)*

Elder is known for its ability to reduce the symptoms and duration of flu, and I find elder blossoms to be a fine, gentle immune enhancer for children. Elder gently stimulates the body to resist infection, and I prefer to reserve this herb for the very early and subtle signs of illness, such as mild tickly throat, increased urination, achiness, and chill. Give as a hot tea, made by steeping one to two teaspoons of the blossoms and one-fourth teaspoon of spearmint leaf in boiling water for ten minutes. Steep with a cover on the cup. Serve one-fourth to three cups daily, hot and lightly sweetened with honey or maple syrup, or sipped hot as needed. Essential oils found in mint are also considered to have mild immunostimulating properties, but here it is used to ease the tummy, as elder alone can be very mildly irritating.[6]

GARLIC *(Allium sativum)*

Garlic has a longtime reputation for warding off "evil spirits" and diseases. It is said that during the Great Plague in Europe, those who regularly ate large amounts of garlic avoided the disease. It is currently widely recognized to enhance various aspects of immunity, such as enhancing macrophage activity and T-lymphocyte function, while also being directly antimicrobial.[7]

Garlic is best for children who have generally good digestion and are not too frail but who may still have a tendency to catch colds, have cold hands and feet, and have sluggish circulation. It can be added raw in small amounts to grains and vegetables or soup, or added at the end of cooking to lessen its "bite." Garlic Lemonade (see page 194) is most palatable to many children (especially those who are accustomed to it at a young age), or garlic perles (soft capsules), available at natural foods stores, may be substituted. Give no more than one small clove daily throughout the winter to children over seven years old. Raw garlic is too strong for younger children, though Garlic Lemonade may be taken by those as young as two years old.

RAITA

Raita (known as tzaziki in Greece) is a condiment from Indian cuisine that is healthful and delicious. Older children (five or six years and older) will often enjoy it thoroughly.

1 medium-sized cucumber, skinned and grated
2 to 3 garlic cloves, crushed in a garlic press
1 cup plain, unsweetened, organic yogurt
$^1/_4$ to $^1/_2$ teaspoon salt

Mix the cucumber and garlic together with the yogurt. Add salt to taste. Stir well and serve. Delicious with meals including lentils, rice, and pita bread. Keeps well overnight in the refrigerator.

GINSENG *(Panax ginseng, P. quinquefolium, Eleutherococcus senticosus)*

There are three herbs on the market known as ginseng: Chinese red ginseng, American ginseng, and Siberian ginseng. All of these herbs have a significantly beneficial impact on immunity.[8] Red ginseng, an ingredient in Immune-Enhancing Soup page 193, is an excellent immune tonic but is overly heating and stimulating for use with most children and is therefore not recommended for general use other than in the soup. It has, however, been proven to enhance macrophage production, as well as B- and T-cells, natural killer cells, and activity in the bone marrow. American ginseng is gentler and more appropriate for children, serving as a reliable medicine for gently boosting immunity and vital energy. Siberian ginseng has also been demonstrated to have immunostimulating qualities and can be used on a regular basis.[9] I generally do not recommend these herbs for children under five years old. Red ginseng is best reserved for adults or occasionally used in food. American and Siberian ginseng both increase stamina while reducing stress and fatigue.[10]

American ginseng and Siberian ginseng can be given as tinctures; give either one in a dose of five to thirty drops, up to three times daily. They can be used on a regular basis and combine well with licorice root and ginger root. Children with hypertension or kidney or adrenal disease should not take licorice root. Ginger is a mild antimicrobial and anti-inflammatory herb that is warming and stimulating to the immune system.[11] Compounds in licorice have similarly exhibited immunomodulatory effects.[12]

SHIITAKE MUSHROOMS *(Lentinus edodes)*

Shiitake mushrooms, among other medicinal mushrooms such as reishi and maitake, have long been known in traditional Chinese medicine to have immunomodulating properties. These immunity-enhancing qualities are now well recognized by Western herbalists as well. While most of the research on medicinal mushrooms and immunity relates to their use as anticancer agents, they make an excellent addition to the repertoire of herbs for general immunity. And because they are delicious in soups, stir-fries, and any number of dishes, they can easily be added to the diet. They can also be made into a decoction by simmering six shiitake mushrooms in one and one-half cups of water for thirty minutes. Strain and season with miso or vegetable broth powder. The mushrooms can be eaten, discarded (boo hoo), or added to a food dish. Give one-half to one cup up to four times per week, or serve in meals two to three times a week.

THYME *(Thymus vulgarus)*

Though I am sure it is purely coincidental, it is interesting to me that thyme, so beneficial in the treatment of a wide variety of infections, should bear the name of the thymus gland, essential for immune function. While thyme is generally used by herbalists for the treatment of active infections, I find it to be most reliable, used occasionally as a tea, in preventing infections during the autumn and winter months. Steeped for a short time, it is most palatable, and clearly beneficial to the circulation and immune system.

To prepare thyme as a beverage, steep 1 teaspoon of thyme along with 1 tablespoon of raisins in 1 cup of boiling water for 10 minutes. Strain the liquid and lightly sweeten it with honey or maple syrup if desired. Give one-half to one cup once a week or so, more often if your child loves it. Five to seven drops of thyme essential oil can be added to a bath for children with a tendency to catch upper respiratory infections. Inhaling the vapors bathes the lungs in the antimicrobial volatile oils. Repeat once weekly throughout the cooler months.

Body System Tonics

Promoting immunity may require more than immune-enhancing herbs for children who have weaknesses in specific body systems. The following formulas are specific to those systems that when blocked or inhibited from optimal functioning may decrease the efficiency of the immune system.

BOWEL HEALTH

Our intestines are our first line of immune defense, and thus bowel health is an important factor in optimal immune function. Constipation (meaning less than a bowel movement daily; sometimes every other day for children under one year) reduces resistance to infections and also interferes with optimal nutrient absorption. The following preparation can be used daily for children with constipation or bowel troubles. For persistent bowel problems, seek the help of a qualified care provider.

CHILDREN'S GENTLE LAX

$1/2$ ounce dandelion root tincture
$1/2$ ounce yellow dock root tincture
$1/4$ ounce licorice root tincture
$1/4$ ounce fennel tincture
$1/2$ ounce vegetable glycerin

Mix all the ingredients together. Store in an amber glass jar. Give one-half to one teaspoon up to four times daily until healthy bowel movements are achieved. Discontinue if no results are seen after two days.

This can also be made into an infusion, using the same measures of dry herbs and steeping $^1/_2$ ounce of herbs in 1 pint of boiling water for 2 hours. Omit the glycerin and sweeten with 4 tablespoons of honey, rice syrup, or barley malt. Give one teaspoon to one tablespoon up to four times daily and continue as directed above. Avoid licorice for children with hypertension or kidney or adrenal disorders. For these children substitute marshmallow or slippery elm root.

LYMPH SYSTEM TONIC

Consider this for children with chronically swollen glands, which may or may not be tender, as well as for children with chronic skin problems or recurrent sore throats. A healthy lymph system will allow the body to rid itself of infections quickly and effectively. Constipation may also be present and should be treated as discussed above.

CLEAR CHANNELS LYMPH SYSTEM TONIC

$^1/_2$ ounce cleavers tincture
$^1/_2$ ounce echinacea root tincture
$^1/_2$ ounce calendula blossom tincture
$^1/_2$ ounce burdock tincture

Mix the tinctures together. Give one-fourth teaspoon to one teaspoon up to three times daily for up to three months for chronic swollen lymph nodes, or up to four times daily in acute conditions.

RESPIRATORY TONIC

Children with chronically clogged, congested, or inflamed respiratory passages are unable to fight infection as easily as those with healthy respiratory mucosa. If your child has chronic respiratory congestion (cough, allergies, earaches, runny nose, sinus infections, and the like), then consider one of the following formulas to improve strength and immunity.

The following tea is a pleasant-tasting formula by herbalist Rosemary Gladstar and is modified and reprinted from my book *Naturally Healthy Babies and Children*.

EASY BREATHING RESPIRATORY TONIC

$^1/_2$ ounce red clover blossoms
$^1/_2$ ounce dried mullein leaves
$^1/_4$ ounce calendula flowers

$^1/_4$ ounce elder flowers

$^1/_4$ ounce dried marshmallow root, finely chopped

$^1/_4$ ounce dried lemongrass

$^1/_4$ ounce dried rose hips

$^1/_4$ ounce anise seeds

Combine all the herbs and place 4 tablespoons of the mixture in a quart jar. Fill with boiling water, cover, and steep for 20 minutes. Stir and give one-fourth to one cup twice daily for three weeks, then use periodically as needed.

You may alternatively use the following elixir.

RESPIRATORY STRENGTH ELIXIR

1 ounce astragalus tincture

1 ounce angelica tincture

$^1/_4$ ounce mullein leaf tincture

$^1/_4$ ounce elder flower tincture

$^1/_4$ ounce thyme tincture

$^1/_4$ ounce anise seed tincture

$^1/_2$ ounce black cherry concentrate

$^1/_2$ ounce glycerin

Combine all the ingredients and shake well before use. Give one-half to two teaspoons twice daily for three weeks, then as needed, especially during seasons of greater susceptibility.

NERVOUS SYSTEM

Stress and sickness certainly go hand in hand, and even kids can have significant enough stress to decrease immunity. The following tea and tonic formulas can be given as needed to tonify the nervous system and during times of acute stress to promote relaxation.

Perhaps the best preparation for toning children's nervous systems, called Calm Child Formula, comes to me through my teacher, friend, and colleague, herbalist Michael Tierra, O.M.D. Here is a version that you can prepare at home, reprinted from my book *ADHD Alternatives:*

CHILD SOOTHER

$^1/_2$ ounce angelica tincture

$^1/_2$ ounce catnip tincture

$^1/_2$ ounce chamomile tincture

$^1/_2$ ounce hawthorn tincture

$1/_2$ ounce lemon balm tincture

$1/_2$ ounce licorice tincture

$1/_2$ ounce zizyphus tincture

1 ounce glycerin

Combine all the ingredients and shake well before each use. Give one-fourth to one teaspoon as needed, not to exceed six doses daily. Omit the licorice for children with hypertension.

EASY GOING NERVE TONIC TEA

$1/_2$ ounce chamomile blossoms

$1/_2$ ounce lemon balm

$1/_4$ ounce catnip

$1/_8$ ounce lavender blossoms

Combine all the herbs and place1 teaspoon to 1 tablespoon of the herb blend in 1 cup of boiling water. Place a lid on the cup. Steep for 10 minutes, strain, and sweeten with honey or maple syrup if desired. Serve warm, one-fourth to one cup up to three times daily.

Herbal Approaches to the Childhood Diseases

This chapter is a guide to how herbalists approach childhood diseases in clinical practice. The herbalist's approach includes not only herbal protocol but also attention to nutrition, hygiene, and the patient's surroundings. Everything has been explained in a clear and concise manner, so that you can apply these approaches at your own discretion. Common sense and safety are guiding principles for herbalists and should be for parents as well. Natural medicine is highly effective and reliable, but there are times when medical care is needed and should be sought.

Because the symptoms and complications associated with each disease were discussed thoroughly in previous chapters, this section provides only a brief review of primary symptoms of the given illness, then discusses in detail the treatment options and warning signs. At the end of each section describing the appropriate herbs to use, I offer selections from traditional Chinese medicine. Many of these formulas have deep and strong actions and can be brought into use as a part of the overall treatment program, as alternatives to the Western herbs, or in more difficult cases. The traditional Chinese formulas are especially useful for convalescence from illness. My primary experience with children's ailments is with Western herbs, but I do use traditional Chinese medicine a great deal in my practice, and with convincing results. Chinese herbs are available at some larger natural food stores, at herb shops in the Chinatown section of many cities, and through companies listed in Resources. For convenience, I recommend the granulated preparations, as these are easy to reconstitute in water. For children who don't like the taste of the liquid, the granules can be placed directly on the tongue and chased with water or a small amount of fruit juice, hidden in food, or mixed with honey on a spoon and licked off the spoon (for children over the age of eighteen months). However, the herbs may also be purchased in bulk and prepared as directed in Preparing Chinese Herbal Decoctions into Syrups (see page 192).

SEEKING MEDICAL CARE

Many parents wonder how to know when to treat naturally and when to seek medical care. When a situation is beyond the scope of natural medicine or home health care, you will see a warning such as SEEK MEDICAL CARE IMMEDIATELY if it is an emergency or SEEK MEDICAL CARE PROMPTLY when medical care is required but it is not an immediate emergency. If the situation requires expert advice, you might see a warning that says "Seek the advise of an experienced care provider."

SIX STEPS OF HEALING

Herbalist Susun Weed has defined a system that parents I have taught have found eminently useful for sorting through health care options and decision making. Following are the "Six Steps of Healing," as discussed in my book *Naturally Healthy Babies and Children:*

Step 0: Do nothing to interfere; observe. This is naturally the first step regardless of the magnitude of any situation, even if the observation step takes place in a split second. It gives you time to gather your wits, take a deep breath, and respond wisely.

Step 1: Gather information. This is a natural extension of the previous step. You may have plenty of time to gather information by doing research, calling a friend or practitioner, or doing an on-line search. The situation may be more serious, leaving you only moments to gather information about what is happening. For example, let's pretend you come upon an unconscious child. You have only seconds to try to sort through what might be going on as you call for emergency help. Did the child choke on something? Is she having an allergic reaction to something? Did he fall and hurt his head? Clear information is an important part of finding the best solution.

Step 2: *Work with the energy.* This is about keeping or moving the energy in a healing direction. It can entail working with the person directly or working with the environment. For example, a bored and irritable child might benefit from having stories read aloud, having a window open for a while and a mist of lavender blossom air freshener spritzed in the air, or watching a comedy movie while propped up on freshly plumped pillows. Working with the energy merely requires that you be perceptive about how the environment might be influencing or interfering with healing. Flower essences, aromatherapy, homeopathy, prayer, color therapy, music, and laughter (and crying), are all examples of working with the energy.

Step 3: *Nourish and tonify.* In this step one uses herbs, nutrition, massage, baths, and so on, to build or support the child's overall vitality. Herbs are most likely to be used as foods or gentle tonics, such as the examples given earlier for building immunity. In fact, this may be one of the most significant steps in fostering a healthy immune system, regardless of vaccination choices.

Step 4: *Stimulate or sedate.* Here one might be using stronger remedies to stimulate the immune system to fight an active infection. Headaches, high fevers, itching, or nausea might all be sedated with the use of herbs to reduce (sedate) those symptoms, as appropriate.

Step 5: *Use pharmaceutical medications.* This might include over-the-counter medications, prescription drugs, and even standardized herbal extracts or extremely strong herbs in some cases. This step generally requires the involvement of a skilled practitioner and is usually necessary only in complicated or unresponsive cases.

Step 6: *Physically invade.* This includes X-rays, use of enemas or colonics, surgery, or other invasive procedures. Clearly this is the most forceful approach and would be a last resort. However, should a situation become severe very quickly (for example, a child cuts herself badly and requires stitches), one might proceed to this step almost automatically.

SETTING TIME LIMITS

Another technique many parents have found helpful is setting time limits. Let's say your child has a fever of 104 degrees Fahrenheit. You've worked with natural medicine before, and you know that sometimes a child can run a high fever and still be perfectly fine. Furthermore, your child displays no symptoms of a more serious and acute disease such as meningitis. Yet you feel a little nervous about such a high temperature. You decide to set a time limit before calling the pediatrician's office. You say to yourself, if my child is no better and no worse in four (you pick the time) hours, I will reevaluate. If at any time in the next four hours he gets worse, that's it, I'm going to see the doctor. If in four hours the fever has begun to come down a little, I'll keep working with the herbs, baths, and so on. During that time you work closely with the remedies, perhaps giving a tepid bath, and helping the child to rest if he is able to sleep.

The time limit gives you a comfortable frame of reference and helps you to feel active rather than that you are just sitting around waiting and wondering if you should be doing something different. Time limits are flexible, can be reevaluated at any point, and can really help you keep a diligent eye on a situation.

The Herbal

Rarely do herbal medicines have any side effects, but it is always possible for a child to have an unusual reaction to any new substance. Always give a small initial dose of an herb to make certain it is well tolerated. Many herbs and pharmaceutical medications can be used together. For example, it is perfectly fine to drink chamomile tea while taking antibiotics. However, not all herbs and drugs mix. Children on antidepressant medications should not take antidepressant herbs, for example, and children on stimulant drugs should not take ephedra or other stimulant herbs. Therefore, consult with a qualified practitioner before giving herbs to a child already on medications, or when introducing medications to a child using herbs.

GENERAL DIETARY ADVICE

Give foods rich in vitamin A and vitamin C, particularly vegetables, during infection. Vitamin C can be supplemented, 250 to 500 milligrams every two to four hours, during an infectious disease, depending upon the severity of the condition. Vitamin A can be obtained from fresh carrot-apple juice, by eating a sweet potato or carrots, or by a supplement, up to 5,000 international units daily of beta-carotene.

Natural Measles Infection

Measles is an infection associated with internal heat and dampness. The initial symptoms are coldlike, with a runny nose, cough, and fever. The eyes are sore and sensitive, and the fever gets progressively higher, often as high as 105 degrees Fahrenheit. A rash appears around the hairline and spreads progressively over the rest of the body. The rash may itch considerably. There may also be a sore throat, cough, diarrhea, and listlessness. After a week or so, all the symptoms begin to fade. Should your child at any time exhibit symptoms of secondary infection, such as painful cough with difficulty breathing (possibly pneumonia), severe headache or convulsions (possibly encephalitis), or any other behavior that indicates that your child is seriously ill, SEEK MEDICAL CARE IMMEDIATELY. Prompt medical care or professional help is advisable if your child seems generally healthy but is extremely uncomfortable, or if you feel you need assistance handling the situation. Remember, for most children, measles is a lengthy and very uncomfortable but relatively minor illness that allows for a complete recovery with lifelong immunity.

GENERAL RECOMMENDATIONS

Keep your child home from school and other engagements. Encourage rest and quiet activities from the time of exposure or onset of the illness until the rash begins to fade.

Other susceptible family members may also have been exposed to measles. Keeping them at home may also be advisable, as it avoids spreading the illness to others.

Comfort measures for rash, aches and pains, sore eyes, and other symptoms are important. Try to keep the environment pleasant and relaxed, avoid bright lights if this bothers the child, and keep loud noise to a minimum.

DIETARY RECOMMENDATIONS

Keep the diet light and nourishing. Give simple whole grains and steamed vegetables with small amounts of protein (beans, fish, and poultry only), seasonal fruits in small amounts, and soups.

Fluids are critically important for preventing dehydration. Give water frequently—as often as every hour. A squeeze of lemon or lime in the water is refreshing. Also give herb teas freely (see below) or as recommended. *Avoid* all sodas, bottled fruit juices (except for occasionally, and then only diluted), orange juice, and milk.

HERBAL RECOMMENDATIONS

Your goals will be to support the body in expressing the fever, bringing the fever down only enough to preserve your peace of mind, if you get worried, and to keep it from getting out of control; encouraging the rash to come out while reducing the attendant discomfort; reducing the overall discomforts of accompanying symptoms; and providing immune-boosting, heat-clearing, inflammation-reducing herbs that are also antiviral.

Fever

Fever itself is not an illness; it is the body's healthy and active response to illness. Fever, therefore, is to be encouraged, within reason. What is within reason? Well, that really depends on the comfort level of individual parents and physicians, but my comfort zone is up to about 104.3 degrees Fahrenheit. Up to that point I am very assertive in giving fluids, providing tepid baths or sponge baths, and letting the child sleep—which is what they generally do when a temperature runs that high. I also stay close to the child and very watchful. If the fever is higher than that, I start to bring it down slightly so it stays at an effective range but one that I feel safe within. You will have to decide for yourself what your comfort zone is. However, suppressing fevers with acetaminophen does not allow the body to do what it is specifically attempting to do. Fever plays an important role in the immune response, stimulating the production of antiviral chemicals such as interferon. Inhibiting the fever may drive the illness deeper into the body rather than allowing a full-blown manifestation that naturally and spontaneously resolves. If you must try to bring the fever down, try herbal infusions and tepid baths first. Never give cold baths, cold water, or cold enemas to feverish children—this can cause shock.

Many of the herbs that can be used to keep children comfortable during fevers, and which are mildly antimicrobial, also keep the fever from soaring too high. These include lemon balm, catnip, elder, spearmint, and chamomile. These are best used singly or combined as a tea. Following is a formula for a delicious tea.

COOL DOWN TEA

$1/2$ ounce lemon balm
$1/2$ ounce catnip
$1/2$ ounce chamomile.
$1/4$ ounce elder blossoms
$1/4$ ounce spearmint leaf

Combine the herbs and steep 1 tablespoon of this herbal mixture in 2 cups of water for 15 minutes. Strain and lightly sweeten the tea with honey or maple syrup. Serve hot to promote perspiration and reduce achiness. Give as often as needed throughout the course of illness, up to two quarts daily. It is very pleasant tasting.

Measles Tincture

Here is a good general blend for reducing inflammation, fighting viral infection, relieving cough and aches, reducing swollen glands, and bringing out the rash.

CLEAR HEAT FORMULA FOR SKIN INFLAMMATION

1 ounce echinacea tincture
$^1/_2$ ounce cleavers tincture
$^1/_2$ ounce burdock root tincture
$^1/_2$ ounce dandelion root tincture
$^1/_2$ ounce licorice root tincture (omit if the child has hypertension or kidney or adrenal disease)
$^1/_2$ ounce Chinese skullcap
$^1/_2$ ounce catnip
$^1/_2$ ounce black cohosh tincture
$^1/_4$ ounce anise seed tincture
$^1/_2$ ounce vegetable glycerin

Combine all the ingredients. Give one-fourth to one teaspoon up to every three hours during the acute phase of the illness, and every four hours as the illness begins to subside.

A secondary formula for children with high fever and more severe symptoms is echinacea and goldenseal in combination. Combine $^1/_2$ ounce of the tincture of each of these herbs and give ten to thirty drops every two hours if needed. Do not use for children under two years old without professional guidance. As goldenseal is endangered in the wild because of overharvesting, use only cultivated goldenseal, not the wild-crafted herb. It is extremely bitter, so offer a spoonful of applesauce or a sip of diluted juice for children who are resistant to the taste. It is also available in glycerite form, which is slightly more pleasant.

Cough Syrup

For more severe and persistent coughing, you can add the following cough syrup to the daily herbs, giving one teaspoon to one tablespoon as needed.

AUNTY AVIVA'S COUGH SYRUP BLEND

$^1/_2$ ounce angelica root
$^1/_2$ ounce elecampane
$^1/_2$ ounce dried mullein leaves
$^1/_2$ ounce marshmallow root
$^1/_2$ ounce licorice root
$^1/_2$ ounce thyme
$^1/_2$ ounce anise seed
$^1/_4$ ounce wild cherry bark
$^1/_4$ ounce burdock root
$^1/_4$ ounce lobelia
$^1/_4$ ounce slippery elm bark

Prepare a syrup as described on page 192, using 1 ounce of the herb blend per 1 quart of water and reducing it to 1 cup prior to adding sweetener.

Skin Soother

To reduce the itching and inflammation associated with measles rash, bathe the child daily or as needed in infusions of any one or a combination of the following herbs: calendula flowers, burdock root, red clover blossoms, chamomile blossoms, chickweed, violet leaves, or lavender flowers.

An excellent combination is calendula blossoms, lavender blossoms, chamomile blossoms, and peppermint leaf. Combine all the herbs in equal parts and place a handful of the blend in a quart of boiling water. Cover and steep for twenty minutes. Strain and use warm or slightly cool as a wash, or add the entire quart of liquid to a tepid bath.

An oatmeal bath is also soothing and easy to prepare. Take a handful of rolled oats (the same kind one uses to make oatmeal for breakfast) and put them into a white sock. Tie the sock closed with a rubber band and place it in warm water in the bathtub. Squeeze the sock under water until the oats start to release a milky liquid, and gently rub this over your child's skin. It is emollient and really relieves the itching for a while.

Sore Eyes

Chamomile compresses are reliable for soothing sore eyes. Simply make a cup of chamomile tea, strain well, and apply to the closed eyelids with a cloth, warm or slightly cool as preferred by your child. Repeat as often as needed.

A small silk pillow filled with flaxseed is very soothing for older children when placed against the closed eyes. These can be purchased in some larger health food stores and even department stores.

Sore Throat

The two best remedies I have found for sore throat are echinacea and chlorophyll. They may be used alternately every hour or two as needed. Squirt a dropperful of echinacea tincture directly on the back of the throat, or have the child gargle lightly or swallow one teaspoon of liquid chlorophyll diluted in two tablespoons of water.

Sucking on chewable vitamin C can help to relieve throat inflammation and may be combined with the recommendations above.

Earache or Infection

If there is ear involvement, give the Clear Heat Formula for Skin Inflammation (see page 209) or use Garlic-Mullein Eardrops (below) made in an olive oil base up to every three hours. This is reliable for eliminating middle-ear infections. The drops can be made at home or purchased in a health food store or by mail order (see Resources).

To prepare Garlic-Mullein Eardrops at home, place 1 peeled, chopped whole bulb of garlic and $1/2$ ounce of mullein flowers into a pint jar. Fill the jar entirely with olive oil and stir the ingredients lightly with a chopstick or butter knife to release air bubbles. Cap and store in a cool, dark place for 1 week. Strain and place in a clean bottle. Label and store for use.

To apply the eardrops, have the child lie on his or her side with the affected ear facing the ceiling. Pull back gently on the earlobe and drip five drops of slightly warmed oil into the ear canal. (Warm the oil by placing the bottle in hot water. Test the oil on the inside of your wrist to avoid burning the child.) Do not insert the dropper into the ear canal, just the drops. Have the child lie in this position for five to ten minutes. Repeat every few hours, treating both ears if necessary.

Convalescence

It is important to allow a full recovery from measles, which can be an exhausting and demanding illness. The child should be allowed to remain home from school and free from activities for at least several days after the symptoms have abated. The diet should be healthy and nourishing but still light. Avoid heavy foods, fried foods, baked goods, and packaged foods. Keep the diet simple and natural, primarily based around whole grains, cooked vegetables, soups, and good protein sources. Fruit can be used sparingly. Keep dairy products to a minimum for a couple of weeks after the illness. Have the child continue to rest, take it easy, bathe regularly, avoid chill, and avoid undue strain or excitement. This will prevent further illness and will rebuild energy and strength.

Following is an excellent convalescent formula that helps restore energy while gently nourishing the immune system.

RESTORE ENERGY FORMULA

$^1/_2$ ounce American ginseng tincture
$^1/_2$ ounce Siberian ginseng tincture
$^1/_2$ ounce skullcap tincture
$^1/_4$ ounce shiitake mushroom tincture
$^1/_4$ ounce licorice root tincture

Combine ingredients in a glass jar (preferably amber glass with a dropper top—see Resources) and store away from direct heat and light. Give one-half to one teaspoon three times daily to children over five years old. Omit licorice and children with hypertension.

TRADITIONAL CHINESE MEDICINE

In Chinese medicine, the herbal treatment of measles is divided into the three stages of the illness. The overall approach is to "clear heat and dampness" (infection, inflammation) using herbs.

Early stage. In the early, "coldlike," preeruptive stage of the illness, the following remedy can be used to relieve tension, fever, chills, and aches. This can be used for colds and flu as well. To prepare Cimicifuga and Pueraria Decoction *(Sheng Ma Ge Gen Tang)*, mix the following:
3 to 6 grams radix cimicifuga
3 to 9 grams radix pueraria
3 grams honey-fried radix *Glycyrrhiza uralensis*
6 to 9 grams radix *Paeonia rubra*

If there is a great deal of heat, add 6 grams honeysuckle, 6 grams burdock seed, 3 grams mentha, and 3 grams scrophularia. This is especially beneficial if there is a lot of redness to the skin, sore throat, or high fever. Prepare as a decoction using 9 grams of the herbs in 4 cups of water, and do not simmer for more than 20 minutes. Add $^1/_4$ cup each of honey and vegetable glycerin to form a syrup and give one to two tablespoons three to four times daily. Or take it in prepared form, 2 grams, two to three times daily.

Second stage. In the second stage of the illness, the eruptive stage, the goal is to clear out heat and toxins and bring out the rash fully. Give Clear Heat and Resolve Toxins Decoction *(Qing Re Jie Du Tang)* with Lonicera and Forsythia

6 to 9 grams honeysuckle

6 to 9 grams forsythia

3 to 6 grams burdock seed

6 to 9 grams *Morus albi* leaf

Prepare as above, or take it in prepared form, three to six grams daily.

Third stage. In the third stage, when the illness is starting to resolve and the rash is beginning to fade, the goal is to clear any remnant of heat and to nourish the body's fluids, which may have been damaged by the heat. This modified formula is called Glehnia and Ophiopogon Decoction, and it contains the following:

6 to 9 grams glehnia

6 to 9 grams ophiopogon

6 grams *Polygonatum odorati*

4.5 grams *Morus albi* leaf

4.5 grams honeysuckle

3 grams *Glycyrrhiza uralensis*

Prepare as a syrup or take three to six grams daily in prepared form. Omit licorice for children with hypertension.

Mumps Infection

Mumps may go entirely undetected, but typical symptoms include moderate to high fever, headache, appetite loss, malaise, neck pain, and swelling of the glands under the ear, appearing on one side and then the other. Swallowing and even talking can be extremely painful.

Although complications are rare, they include testicular or ovarian swelling (sometimes painful), and in rare cases, encephalitis or meningitis and several other problems. If you suspect complications, CONSULT A PHYSICIAN IMMEDIATELY. Review other possible complications of mumps discussed in chapter 4. Most children will need antiviral, immunomodulating herbs and herbs to relieve discomfort and swelling.

GENERAL RECOMMENDATIONS

As with measles, comfort measures and activities to occupy the time are needed.

DIETARY RECOMMENDATIONS

Foods that are easy to swallow are essential for children with significant parotid gland swelling, as swallowing will be quite painful for them.

Do not give cold, sweet, dairy-based items such as ice cream or yogurt, which will only aggravate the illness and weaken immunity. Instead, provide light soups, potatoes, sweet potatoes, or cooked squash, soft cooked cereals, stewed fruits, blended stews, and freshly made fruit and vegetable juices.

Herbalist and naturopathic physician Mary Bove suggests that acidic foods (vinegar, lemons, orange juice, tomatoes) should be avoided during the mumps. They are likely to make swallowing additionally painful.

Give plenty of fluids to drink. Avoid juice, soda, and milk (including soy milk and rice milk). Give water, tea, and broth.

HERBAL RECOMMENDATIONS

Viral-Lymph Formula

To address fever, viral infection, glandular inflammation, and immunity, prepare the following formula.

VIRAL-LYMPH FORMULA

2 ounces echinacea tincture

$1/_2$ ounce calendula tincture

$1/_2$ ounce licorice tincture (replace with lemon balm if desired or for children with hypertension or kidney or adrenal disease)

$1/_4$ ounce thyme tincture

$1/_4$ ounce cleavers tincture

$1/_2$ ounce vegetable glycerin

Store in an amber glass jar and give one-fourth to one teaspoon every two hours for two to three days, then reduce to every four hours until symptoms are gone.

Give a soothing and tasty tea, either warm or at room temperature, made from any combination of the following herbs: red clover, chamomile, lemon balm, spearmint, licorice, elder, or yarrow.

Fever

For high and persistent fever, give Cool Down Tea (see page 208) as needed.

Achiness

Fever Tea can also be given to reduce aches and pain.

For more severe achiness, the following tincture can also be given, or even added directly to the tea.

ACHE RELIEF

$^1/_4$ ounce cramp bark
$^1/_4$ ounce passionflower
$^1/_4$ ounce skullcap
$^1/_4$ ounce black cohosh
1 ounce vegetable glycerin

Combine the herbs and make a tincture as instructed on pages 189 to 190. Give one-fourth to one teaspoon as often as every two hours.

Another excellent preparation for achiness and fever, especially if there are chills, or if there is neck and shoulder ache, is Kudzu-Apple Juice. It is delicious, and even very young children will ask for it again. To prepare it, dilute $^1/_2$ cup of pure unfiltered apple or pear juice with $^1/_2$ cup of water and bring to a very light simmer. In a cup, dissolve one-half teaspoon of kudzu starch in $^1/_4$ cup of juice. When well dissolved, add it to the pot and stir well for two minutes, or until the juice begins to thicken very slightly. Serve warm or at room temperature. This can be given freely and is very beneficial and nutritive.

Swollen Parotid Gland, Swollen Testicles or Ovaries

Give Viral-Lymph Formula frequently, up to every two hours.

Apply warm compresses to the affected area(s) every two hours, or apply continuously with a hot water bottle to retain the warmth of the herbs. Herbal compresses may also be used to reduce inflammation. A combination of cramp bark, violet leaves, and lobelia can be made either as an infusion or by diluting the tinctures (1 teaspoon of each per $^1/_2$ cup of water) and then applying.

Grated potato poultices are very effective at drawing inflammation and swelling out of glands. Take a raw white potato of any variety and grate it. Apply the grated potato directly to the affected area and cover with a clean gauze or piece of fabric. Replace with fresh potato when the poultice becomes warm. Repeat as often as every two hours until inflammation is reduced. Lobelia tincture may be added to the grated potato material to reduce local pain. Use $^1/_4$ teaspoon lobelia tincture per 1 tablespoon of potato, and be certain that the tincture is applied to the skin.

Poke root is potentially toxic when taken internally and should be avoided with children. However, it is a very effective topical application for drawing inflammation out of the glands. The fresh root may be grated and applied directly, or poke root tincture may be applied to the raw grated potato and placed over the affected area. Add 1 teaspoon of fresh poke root or $^1/_4$ teaspoon poke root tincture per 1 tablespoon of potato. It maybe combined with the lobelia as well. Do not apply the poke root to broken skin.

TRADITIONAL CHINESE MEDICINE

The treatment principles of Chinese medicine are to dispel wind and clear heat, as well as to disperse the glandular swelling. A standard formula for this is Lonicera and Forsythia (Clear Heat and Resolve Toxins), which can be obtained as a prepared formula. Another formula for high fever; hard, swollen, painful glands; and sore throat is called Universal Benefit Decoction to Eliminate Toxin. It was developed in China during widespread epidemics, and it contains the following herbs:

15 grams *Scutellaria baicalensis*
15 grams coptis
3 grams burdock seed
3 grams forsythia
3 grams mentha
1.5 grams scrophularia
3 grams isatidis
6 grams platycodon
6 grams *Glycyrrhiza uralensis*
6 grams citrus peel
6 grams bupleurum
1.5 grams cimicifuga

This formula is available in prepared form, which is the advisable way to take it. Give two to six grams daily. The herb coptis in this formula is very similar in action to our Western herb goldenseal. Use this formula for children over the age of seven. Omit the licorice *(Glycyrrhiza uralensis)* for children with hypertension.

Rubella

Rubella is generally so mild a disease that is goes unnoticed or is entirely asymptomatic. When symptoms do appear they include initial coldlike symptoms with swollen lymph nodes around the neck and base of the head and a low-grade fever, appetite loss, fatigue or malaise, and a rash that begins on the face and spreads over the body. The rash, which generally lasts only a few days, may itch. The treatment for rubella consists mainly of providing comfort measures and herbs that support immunity, are antiviral, and promote healthy lymph node activity.

GENERAL RECOMMENDATIONS

Keep your child at home until past the contagious stages (see chapter 4) to avoid exposing susceptible pregnant women to the virus. Encourage the child to rest more than usual.

DIETARY RECOMMENDATIONS

Provide a light, healthful diet that is easy to swallow, if there is sore throat, and easy to digest. Give plenty of fluids to drink.

HERBAL RECOMMENDATIONS

Give either Clear Heat Formula for Skin Inflammation (page 209) or Viral-Lymph Formula (page 214) as directed, or simply give one-half to one teaspoon of echinacea tincture along with 250 milligrams of vitamin C every two hours.

Use skin treatments described under Skin Soother to relieve itching. Another excellent formula can be made by adding 1 tablespoon each of calendula, echinacea, lavender, and peppermint tinctures to 1 cup of witch hazel, available at any pharmacy. Apply to rashy areas as needed. For external use only.

TRADITIONAL CHINESE MEDICINE

The Clear Heat and Resolve Toxins formula mentioned for treating measles is the specific formula for rubella as well, and may be taken in the prepared form.

Diphtheria

Owing to the potentially severe and life-threatening nature of diphtheria, it is not recommended that you attempt to care for a child with this illness at home. Therefore, though recommendations do exist, I have chosen not to include them. If you suspect your child has diphtheria SEEK IMMEDIATE MEDICAL CARE. Convalescent care with herbal medicines can be done after the child has safely recovered from the disease.

Pertussis

The initial symptoms of pertussis, a demanding childhood illness, are a cold and cough. The cough progresses to a severe nature within a few weeks of the initial symptoms and may persist for many weeks. The coughing, which often causes the child to turn blue, appearing as if he or she will suffocate, and then to vomit, is the most serious symptom. In severe cases, the coughing spells can cause oxygen loss to the brain, seizures, and choking. Furthermore, pertussis can cause encephalitis and permanent brain damage, although these problems are rare among healthy, well-nourished children.

Once the severe coughing has set in, there is no medication that can treat the disease, as it is no longer directly caused by a microorganism but by irritants from the *Bordetella pertussis* bacterium. Comfort measures should be taken, including giving herbal remedies to minimize coughing and maximize rest, as well as herbs to prevent secondary infections (for example, pneumonia).

Caution:

- For children under two, seek the assistance of a qualified health care provider. Children under one year are especially prone to complications.

- Seek medical care when dealing with very young children. In a known outbreak or if there is known exposure, a course of prophylactic antibiotics is advisable and may prevent severe illness in very young children.

- Any child exhibiting symptoms of complications, including high unrelenting fever, seizures, difficulty breathing, or persistent cyanosis (blueness around the mouth), should be seen by a medical doctor immediately.

GENERAL RECOMMENDATIONS

Begin treating the child for whooping cough as soon as you suspect exposure, in order to minimize the severity of the illness.

If your child has whooping cough, you will need to be available for him or her for as long as several weeks. Because it is such a demanding illness, you will also need to arrange for times when you can replenish yourself, even if just to get out for some fresh air or a cup of tea.

Rest is critically important for you as well as your child if your child is fretful and wakeful at night, or if there are severe coughing spells at night, which there frequently are. Take naps each day, and get to sleep at a reasonable hour. If morning is the time when the coughing fits are the least frequent, sleep in.

Minimize the child's contact with others until your child's strength has begun to return, in order to avoid exposure to additional infections while your child is recovering.

Massage, particularly over the back and chest, can be helpful in preventing respiratory spasms and is relaxing for children. Foot massage as the child is going to sleep can also be highly relaxing. You do not have to be a massage therapist to give someone a relaxing massage. Trust your hands and your instincts, or pick up a book on infant and child massage at your local bookstore. A small amount of massage oil can make your job easier, and if it is lightly scented with herbs that promote relaxation, such as lavender or sandalwood, that can add to the beneficial effects.

DIETARY RECOMMENDATIONS

Simplify the diet, paying extra attention to avoiding heavily mucus-producing foods such as dairy, orange juice, and wheat products. Also avoid cold foods and sweets, focusing on a more bland and nourishing diet. Soups, protein foods (fish, poultry, lentils and other legumes), and steamed vegetables are excellent. All vegetables rich in vitamin C and vitamin A are excellent, especially dark leafy green vegetables, potatoes, and sweet potatoes.

If your child has appetite loss, this is normal. Eating can also trigger coughing fits, so your child might be naturally reluctant to eat. However, ample nourishment is essential for optimal immunity. Continue to provide light fare that is easily digestible and nutrient rich. Soups and stews can be very beneficial in such cases. Appetite can be stimulated by making Bitters Soda. Take 1 cup of lemon-flavored carbonated water and add 5 to 10 drops of Angostura bitters (Swedish bitters), available from the natural foods store, or add 5 drops of gentian tincture and 5 drops of dandelion tincture if you are unable to find the bitters. Give one-half cup thirty minutes before meals to stimulate digestive juices.

Both fever and excessive coughing cause the body to use up enormous amounts of fluids. It is essential to replace these to avoid dehydration and to promote wellness on a cellular level. Give your child plenty of water (plain or with a squeeze of lemon), herbal tea, garlic lemonade, soup broth, and occasionally fresh fruit or vegetable juice. Avoid milk, soy and rice milk, orange juice, excessive fruit juice consumption, sodas, and all caffeinated beverages.

HERBAL RECOMMENDATIONS

Begin treating as soon as you suspect whooping cough in order to minimize the severity of the illness.

For initial coldlike symptoms, prepare the following syrup.

CHILDREN'S COLD AND FLU SYRUP

1 ounce echinacea tincture
$^1/_2$ ounce thyme tincture
$^1/_2$ ounce lemon balm tincture
$^1/_2$ ounce elder tincture
$^1/_2$ ounce licorice tincture
$^1/_4$ ounce calendula tincture
$^1/_4$ ounce anise seed tincture
1 ounce vegetable glycerin

Combine all the ingredients and shake well. Give one-fourth to one teaspoon up to every hour during the initial stage, and every two to four hours after that.

These herbs can also be made into an infusion using the same measurement of dry herbs (not tincture) and omitting the glycerin. Give one-fourth to one cup up to every hour initially, then every two to four hours thereafter, served hot or at room temperature and lightly sweetened if preferred. It is pleasant tasting and generally palatable to children.

A second excellent formula that can be used alternately with the above if your child feels achy or has nausea or chills was developed by my daughter Naomi and is very reliable.

NAOMI'S MAGICAL HERBAL FORMULA

1 ounce echinacea tincture
$^1/_2$ ounce angelica tincture
$^1/_4$ ounce anise seed tincture
$^1/_4$ ounce orange peel tincture
$^1/_4$ ounce cinnamon tincture
$^1/_2$ ounce vegetable glycerin

Combine all the ingredients and shake well. Give one-fourth to one-half teaspoon as needed, up to every hour, to reduce chills, aching, and discomforts. This preparation is also gently antimicrobial, particularly for respiratory conditions.

Garlic Lemonade (see page 194) is indispensable for the treatment of respiratory infections, especially those accompanied by copious amounts of mucus. Give freely throughout the day as a beverage.

Whoop-Ease tea is specific for children with pertussis, easing irritated and inflamed respiratory passages, while being gently antispasmodic and expectorant.

WHOOP-EASE

$1/_2$ ounce dried thyme
$1/_2$ ounce dried red clover blossoms
$1/_2$ ounce marshmallow root

Combine the herbs. Bring 1 quart of water to a boil. Put herbs into a one-quart jar, add the boiling water, and let steep for 1 hour. Strain, sweeten with honey, and give one-fourth to one-half cup every two hours. This can be used along with any of the other herbal suggestions.

Aunty Aviva's Cough Syrup Blend (see page 210) can be used, and is excellent for thinning and promoting expectoration of mucus while soothing and relaxing the respiratory passages. It is important to help the body expel the mucus, not just quiet the cough. This syrup may be given as often as needed, either in teaspoon or tablespoon doses. It should be used in addition to the other tincture choices given above but can substitute for Whoop-Ease, as those ingredients, except the red clover, are included in the syrup. Red clover ($1/_2$ ounce of dried blossoms) may be added to the cough syrup blend prior to preparation of the syrup.

If your child is irritable, nervine teas and tinctures can relieve stress and promote relaxation. Consider using Child Soother (pages 202–03) or Nerve Tonic Tea (page 203). Either of these can be given freely in addition to the other respiratory remedies.

Long ago, mustard plasters were popular for bringing circulation to the chest and reducing serious coughs. My great-grandmother, who died when I was very young, employed this technique for her children, though it was not until I had been doing them for many years that I was aware of this. Mustard plasters are simple to administer and very effective, but there are several precautions, as mustard powder is an extremely caustic and irritating substance, which can cause burns if left on for too long.

Caution:

- Never use a mustard plaster on a child under four years old.

- Never use a mustard plaster on a sleeping patient.

- Always apply some salve or petroleum jelly to the nipples before applying a mustard plaster to protect this sensitive tissue.

- Never leave a patient wearing a mustard plaster unattended.

- Remove a mustard plaster as soon as (preferably before) the patient complains of any irritation.

- Have a bowl of cool water and a washcloth on hand to sponge off any mustard powder residue.

MUSTARD PLASTER

Supplies:
2 glass bowls
$^1/_4$ cup mustard powder (the type used for cooking is adequate)
1 old dish towel
1 large bath towel
1 washcloth
Salve or petroleum jelly

To prepare the mustard plaster:

1. Lay the dish towel out on a flat surface.

2. Leaving a one-inch border around the towel, spread the mustard powder over the center of the towel.

3. Fold the border of the towel over the edges of the mustard.

4. Beginning at each end and working toward the center, roll the towel over the mustard as if rolling a jelly roll or strudel.

5. Fill a medium-sized glass bowl with very hot water.

6. Place the roll in the water.

7. Have the patient in bed with the large bath towel spread underneath his back.

8. Apply a liberal amount of salve or petroleum jelly to the nipples.

9. Remove the mustard roll from the water and wring out thoroughly. The fumes might sting your eyes or nose, so don't breathe in the steam directly.

10. Place the roll on the center of the patient's chest and begin to unroll each side, mustard side down, extending as far toward the child's sides as the towel will reach.

11. Wrap the large bath towel over the child's chest and the mustard plaster, to keep the heat in, and tuck the child into the covers.

12. Leave the plaster on for no longer than ten minutes. Young children or fair-skinned children may be able to tolerate only two to three minutes.

Remove the plaster the moment the child begins to describe any stinging or burning sensation.

13. Quickly remove the towels and plaster, sponging the child with tepid water to remove any remaining particles of powder. It is normal for the chest to be slightly red.

14. Tuck the child back into the covers to maintain warmth.

15. Discard the mustard powder and clean the towels.

A mustard plaster can be reserved for cases with severe coughing. It is remarkable in its ability to reduce coughing fits and to promote rest. Do not apply more than once daily, and not for more than several days in a row.

CONVALESCENCE

Convalescence is critical to prevent secondary infections that often come after a lengthy illness because of the body's exhaustion. Allow extra rest before a return to school and provide excellent foods high in protein and nutrients. Protein is very important for restoring any damaged tissue, as are the antioxidant nutrients. Give Restore Energy Formula in addition, as described on page 213.

TRADITIONAL CHINESE MEDICINE

Chinese medicine divides whooping cough into three distinct treatment phases, corresponding with the three phases of the illness also recognized in Western medicine, the initial stage lasting seven to ten days, the paroxysmal coughing stage lasting forty to sixty days, and the decline or convalescence lasting twenty to thirty days. The duration of the illness is decreased with prompt and effective herbal and dietary treatment. Whooping cough is seen as an accumulation of phlegm in the body, owing particularly to poor assimilation. The diet must be free of dairy products and cold-natured and cold-temperature foods, and should include warming, nourishing foods that are easy to digest.

Stage 1. The major treatment principles of this stage are to warm the lungs and reduce phlegm while strengthening the protective energy of the body. The primary formula for this stage is Minor Bluegreen Dragon Decoction, which contains the following ingredients:

6 grams ephedra
3 grams pinellia
9 grams white peony
9 grams cinnamon

9 grams schisandra

3 grams perilla

3 grams licorice

6 grams ginger

This formula is available in a prepared powder that is mixed with a small amount of honey and taken off a spoon or hidden in juice or tea. Alternatively, a decoction can be made from the whole herbs using 10 grams per 4 cups of boiling water, simmering for 30 minutes, and giving from one to two tablespoons every two to four hours. It can be turned into a syrup by adding ¼ cup each of honey and vegetable glycerin.

Note: Ephedra has received a lot of bad publicity in recent years due to side effects associated with its use. However, serious reactions that have occurred have been mainly due to misuse of ephedra as a diet aid or stimulant drug. When it is used properly and in moderation in traditional Chinese formulas, these side effects are not expected to occur. For precaution, avoid use of ephedra in formulas for children under seven years old, and do not exceed two tablespoons of the formula every two hours. In addition, do not take after five o'clock in the evening because it may cause restlessness or insomnia. Discontinue if it causes irritability or sleep disturbance.

Another approach is to clear heat, reduce coughing, and "resolve the exterior," meaning to relieve symptoms such as chills, headache, thirst, and sore throat. A primary herbal formula is Morus and Chrysanthemum Decoction, which contains:

7.5 grams mulberry leaf *(Morus albi)*

3 grams chrysanthemum

4.5 grams forsythia

2.4 grams mentha (add near end of cooking)

6 grams platycodon

4 grams apricot seed

6 grams phragmitis

2.4 grams *Glycyrrhiza uralensis*

Decoct 10 grams in 3 cups of water for no longer than 20 minutes. This can be turned into a syrup by adding ¼ cup each of honey and vegetable glycerin. Also available in prepared form. Omit licorice *(Glycyrrhiza uralensis)* for children with hypertension.

Stage 2. In this stage the coughing is most severe and the primary therapeutic objective is to clear heat, drain the lungs, and reduce coughing. Morus Bark

Decoction is the traditional general formula for this. Modified for children, the formula contains mulberry root, Chinese skullcap, coptis, gardenia, perilla, apricot seed, and phragmitis, and is available in prepared form.

Stage 3. In the decline stage, the cough has diminished and the child may be weak and exhausted. The goal here is to replenish and rebuild the vital energy, nourish the lungs, and support healthy digestion and assimilation. The recommended general formula for this is called Ginseng and Schisandra Decoction, which contains *Panax ginseng*, schisandra, atractylodes, hoelen, licorice, ophiopogon, citrus peel, and pinellia. (Omit licorice for children with hypertension.) It is available in prepared form and is highly recommended during convalescence for pertussis.

Tetanus

Tetanus is a deadly infection. Unvaccinated children must receive medical attention for any suspicious or extensive wounds. IF TETANUS IS SUSPECTED, THIS IS A MEDICAL EMERGENCY.

Natural approaches to treating tetanus will not be discussed. Remember, tetanus infection can take several weeks to appear after the time of injury, and the injury may have gone unnoticed. Therefore, any symptoms of tetanus require immediate evaluation and should be well recognized by parents who do not vaccinate against it.

Unvaccinated children possibly exposed to tetanus must receive Tetanus Human Immune Globulin (THIG) after injury. This differs from a tetanus booster shot and must be requested from the doctor or hospital at the medical visit. Vaccinated children who sustain a questionable injury should receive only a booster unless their last booster was more than five years previous, in which case THIG may be recommended.

The following discussion explains how to keep wounds clean and reduce the likelihood of tetanus infection in unvaccinated children.

GENERAL RECOMMENDATIONS

Allow wounds to bleed (of course not severely), as the blood flow cleans the site and removes debris.

Clean all wounds thoroughly, removing dirt and particulate matter or splinters carefully.

Wash wounds thoroughly, holding the injured part under running water for as long as ten minutes.

Clean cuts and minor wounds with hydrogen peroxide solution. The bubbling action brings oxygen to the area and helps remove dirt and debris. Remember, tetanus is anaerobic; hydrogen peroxide is an aerobic agent.

Wounds should be encouraged to heal from the inside out, not quickly on the surface, as infection can be harbored in pockets beneath the healed skin. Keeping puncture wounds moist will encourage them to heal from below without sealing over on the surface first.

Have children wear shoes and be extra cautious in high-risk areas, such as around horses and other livestock, in pastures where horses have grazed, and when handling knives, such as on camping trips.

Observe excellent hygiene with wounds so that they stay clean.

Seek medical care for extensive wounds, wounds sustained in high-risk areas, serious burns, deep puncture wounds, and any wounds in which foreign matter is retained.

DIETARY RECOMMENDATIONS

Keep nutrition high and sugar and processed flours to a minimum when trying to prevent infection.

HERBAL RECOMMENDATIONS

Clean all wounds thoroughly with an antimicrobial herbal solution. The following wash is an effective wound cleaner.

ANTIMICROBIAL HERBAL WASH

1 ounce echinacea tincture
1 ounce calendula tincture
1 ounce thyme tincture
$^1/_2$ ounce goldenseal tincture (from cultivated sources only)

To make a wash, dilute 1 tablespoon of tincture in $^1/_4$ cup of water and apply directly to the affected area as often as every two hours. During the first twenty-four hours after injury, tincture may be applied directly and undiluted. However, this stings, and it is contraindicated for burns. Burns must always be rinsed with dilute solution.

This same tincture may be taken internally, ten to thirty drops every two hours for forty-eight hours, then every four hours until danger of infection has passed.

Never apply oil-based preparations such as salve to a fresh wound or puncture wound, as they can trap dirt in the wound and create an anaerobic environment. Always use washes, tinctures, baths, or compresses until you are sure there is no infection and the wound has begun to heal—at least several days.

Polio

It is highly unlikely that a child would contract paralytic polio while living in the United States, or even in the Americas. However, it *is* possible, particularly with travel abroad. Again, most cases of polio are nonparalytic, mild, self-limiting illnesses, some so mild you'd never imagine your child had polio. If you child should truly contract polio, medical care is advisable, and in severe cases, necessary. PARALYTIC POLIOMYELITIS REQUIRES MEDICAL ATTENTION.

Because polio is so rare in Western developed nations, little has been written about natural treatment for this illness. I have never treated polio infection. However, recommended therapies would include physical therapy and massage with oil containing St. John's wort to treat the nervous system. St. John's wort tincture can be used internally, in combination with the Viral-Lymph Formula described on page 214. Add one ounce of St. John's wort to the preparation and shake well to mix. High doses of vitamin C and vitamin A in a highly nourishing diet, as well as complete avoidance of sugar, are important to keep immunity high. Herbal medicines can be used in conjunction with conventional therapies. Consider the formulas used for convalescence in the recuperative phases of this disease. Use Restore Energy Formula on page 212 or the Ginseng and Schisandra Decoction described on page 225.

TRADITIONAL CHINESE MEDICINE

In the early stages of illness, which in mild cases manifests simply as a cold, or with flulike symptoms, one can give the formula known as Ginseng Powder to Overcome Pathogenic Influences, also known as Ginseng and Mentha Formula. Available as a prepared formula, it contains:

10 grams notopterygii
10 grams *Angelica pubescentis*
10 grams cnidium
10 grams bupleurum
10 grams platycodon
10 grams citrus peel
10 grams peucedanum
10 grams ginseng

10 grams hoelen
5 grams *Glycyrrhiza uralensis*

This should be given in the first coldlike stage of the illness. Omit licorice (*Glycyrrhiza uralensi*) for children with hypertension.

Traditional Chinese medicine also offers several formulas to be used in recovering from the paralytic and debilitating aspects of poliomyelitis. Such formulas, however, are beyond the scope of this book; a doctor of traditional Chinese medicine should be consulted.

Chicken Pox

Generally a common childhood illness of little consequence that confers permanent immunity, chicken pox rarely requires more than comfort measures, a healthy and simple diet, and perhaps herbs to maintain strong immunity or bring out the rash fully. Should your child exhibit any signs of complication, including neurological involvement (for example, seizures), severe unrelenting headache, or persistent nausea and vomiting, or should any of the pox appear infected or develop in the eyes, SEEK IMMEDIATE MEDICAL CARE. Newborns exposed to chicken pox may require medical attention; consult with your pediatrician, obstetrician, or midwife.

It is particularly important to prevent chicken pox from becoming infected. Use proper hygiene and keep your child's fingernails short and clean. Mild infection can be treated at home if tended to promptly and assertively, but if boils develop owing to staphylococcal infection (or other organisms, such as strep), or if the infection appears to be spreading, SEEK MEDICAL CARE.

The following recommendations are for uncomplicated chicken pox. For more severe cases, increase the frequency and dosage of remedies as well as the frequency of topical applications and consult with a qualified health professional.

Shingles is also caused by the chicken pox virus; children with chicken pox can transmit shingles to susceptible adults.

GENERAL RECOMMENDATIONS

Follow general hygiene by washing your hands before touching any sores and keeping the child's hands clean and nails short. In most cases this will prevent the chicken pox from getting infected from the child's scratching them.

Keep the child in light clothing that prevents excessive heat from building up near the skin. However, lightweight long-sleeved shirts and long pants may be necessary to prevent the child from scratching excessively.

Encourage the child to rest each day and provide quiet activities to keep your child occupied, and even distracted, if the child is quite uncomfortable.

DIETARY RECOMMENDATIONS

Keep the diet simple and light, offering generally bland and easy-to-digest foods.

Give plenty of fluids, including water, herbal teas, and freshly made vegetable or fruit juices such as carrot-apple juice in moderation.

HERBAL RECOMMENDATIONS

Give echinacea tincture, one-fourth to one-half teaspoon every two to four hours, depending on the severity of the infection, or give Viral-Lymph Formula as directed on page 214, but add one ounce of St. John's wort tincture to the preparation, as this herb is specifically active against the varicella-zoster virus. These are good general immune tonics that fight viral infections and promote healthy lymphatic activity.

Clear Channels Lymph System Tonic (page 201), with one ounce of St. John's wort added to the preparation, is an excellent choice for children with a great deal of itching and skin redness, and it helps bring out the rash fully and effectively. St. John's wort is also an effective herb for supporting the nervous system.

Both Child Soother (page 202) and Easy Going Nerve Tonic Tea (page 203) are good choices for irritable, uncomfortable children and either can be used in conjunction with any of the above-mentioned treatments.

Lemon balm tea is an excellent nervine, prevents fever from getting out of control, and is specifically antiviral for the chicken pox virus. Lemon balm makes a delicious tea and may be given liberally during chicken pox infection.

Cool Down Tea (page 208) can be used if needed.

Use Clear Heat for Skin Inflammation (page 209) if the child has a very bad case of chicken pox.

Topically, the external applications described for measles may be applied to the chicken pox rash. Or use any of the following applications:

Skin spritzer. Combine calendula blossoms, lavender blossoms, chamomile blossoms, and peppermint leaf in equal parts and place a handful of the blend in 1 quart of boiling water. Cover and steep for 20 minutes. Strain and use warm or slightly cool as a wash, or add the entire quart of liquid to a tepid bath. Alternatively, you can dilute the tinctures of these herbs, 1 teaspoon to $1/4$ cup of witch hazel extract (from any pharmacy), and use a spray bottle to apply.

Oatmeal bath. Take a handful of rolled oats (the same kind one uses to make oatmeal for breakfast) and put them into a white sock. Tie the sock closed with a rubber band and place it in warm water in the bathtub. Squeeze the sock under water until the oats start to release a milky liquid, and gently rub this over your child's skin. It is emollient and really relieves the itching for a while.

Salve. When the sores start to scab over, apply salve made of plantain, calendula, and comfrey to heal the skin. Salve can easily be purchased at a natural foods store or made at home.

If any of the chicken pox appear to be infected, apply a tincture combination of goldenseal, calendula, and myrrh directly to the sores every few hours, or dilute one teaspoon in one-quarter cup of water and rinse every two hours. If infection worsens or persists, seek medical care.

TRADITIONAL CHINESE MEDICINE

Chicken pox is seen as a condition of heat and dampness, and the primary therapeutic goals are to clear and dispel them. For a typical mild-to-moderate case of chicken pox, the standard formula is Lonicera and Forsythia Combination, containing

9 to 15 grams honeysuckle
9 to 15 grams forsythia
3 to 6 grams platycodon
9 to 12 grams burdock seed
3 to 6 grams soja (prepared soybeans)
6 to 9 grams schizonepeta
3 to 6 grams lopatherum
15 to 30 grams phragmitis
3 to 6 grams *Glycyrrhiza uralensis*
3 to 6 grams mentha

Mix all the ingredients except the mentha and prepare as a decoction using 10 grams of the mixed herbs and cooking for 30 minutes. Add the mentha 5 minutes before the end. Give one-fourth to one-half cup up to four times daily or prepare as a syrup and give one to two tablespoons up to four times daily. Omit the licorice *(Glycyrrhiza uralensis)* for children with hypertension.

Hib

While general infections caused by Hib, such as ear infections, may be treated with herbal alternatives, Hib meningitis requires IMMEDIATE MEDICAL ATTENTION. Any child with severe unremitting headache, nausea, or vomiting, severe malaise, or stiff neck should be seen by a medical doctor immediately. However, much can be done to prevent Hib infection, most notably to breast-feed and practice excellent nutrition. Children in day care are the most prone to exposure and should be given herbal immune-enhancing herbs periodically, much as one would give a vitamin supplement, but in this case, don't give daily. Several times weekly should be adequate. Give a combination or variety of the herbs discussed under Immune-Boosting Herbs.

Hepatitis B

Hepatitis B infection should be treated by a qualified health care provider or team of providers knowledgeable about both the disease and natural alternatives that are safe for use in children. While Western medicine offers few cures for hepatitis B, traditional Chinese medicine may offer significant opportunity for improvement and cure. In traditional Chinese medicine, hepatitis B is considered a disease of excessive dampness and heat accumulated in the body, primarily affecting the liver. Therapeutic goals, therefore, are to reduce heat and dampness, support the liver, and encourage the healthy flow of bile. In addition, it is important to support the immune system and to use antiviral herbs. According to herbalist Alan Tillotson, examples of herbs that a practitioner might consider using to treat hepatitis B in children include the medicinal mushrooms (reishi, shiitake, maitake), turmeric, chrysanthemum, dandelion root, Chinese skullcap, elderberry, schisandra, milk thistle, prunella, bupleurum, baptisia, licorice, and *Artemesia capillaris.* Do not use these herbs for children under two years old and omit the licorice for children with hypertension. Seek the guidance of a qualified health care provider before attempting to treat hepatitis B in children, and be certain that appropriate medical tests for liver enzymes are being followed.

Herbal and natural medicine offers a range of options for preventing and treating illness. Using a healthy dose of common sense and caution, you can help your child to achieve optimal levels of immunity. A child with a healthy immune system has many advantages for enjoying a long and healthy life. Whether or not you choose to vaccinate, the value of investing in your child's health cannot be overstated. It is a special gift, one that should be the birthright of every child on this planet.

NINE

Homeopathy and Childhood Diseases

Much as public interest in herbal medicine has grown, so too has attention to homeopathic medicine. In fact, many people make the mistaken assumption that homeopathy and herbal medicine are the same discipline, when really they are quite dissimilar. While both make use of some of the same substances, in general they have widely differing principles. There are a few philosophies, however, that homeopaths and herbalists share. A significant shared belief is that the body possesses the inherent capacity to heal itself and is, indeed, constantly striving for balance. There is also the common recognition that there is an underlying vital essence that infuses life. Both homeopaths and herbalists also believe that the elements needed for restoring health can be found in the natural environment. However, homeopaths use plants very differently than herbalists. They also use nonherbal substances such as animal parts and heavy metals. Homeopaths, like herbalists, believe in allowing the disease process to follow a natural course, while supporting the patient's well-being, rather than simply suppressing symptoms. This chapter will explain some of the foundational principles of homeopathic medicines and how homeopathic remedies are typically applied for childhood infectious diseases.

As a clinical herbalist, I use homeopathic remedies only on occasion, and primarily for substances that are too toxic to use in crude plant form. My preference for herbal remedies over homeopathic remedies is based on the fact that I am more comfortable with the use of crude plant substances that have measurable chemical constituents than with relying on the unmeasurable and energetic qualities of homeopathic remedies. I am inclined toward the tangible in clinical practice, particularly when it comes to acute and potentially danger-ous conditions. I prefer the variety of scents, textures, and tastes of leaves, flowers, and roots of herbs to the homogenous pills and liquids of homeo-pathy, which all taste, smell, and look the same. Furthermore, I find that herbal remedies are easier to apply than homeopathic remedies, the latter being al-most entirely specific to the individual. For example, most people with an upper respiratory infection will benefit from a small selection of respiratory system–specific herbs, whereas there may be only one homeopathic remedy that will be of benefit to a given individual. This can make homeopathic remedies a bit impractical and inaccessible if a parent calls me in the middle of the night with a sick child and doesn't happen to have hundreds of homeopathic remedies to choose from. A parent will, however, be likely to have some ginger root, honey, and lemon on hand, or at least a yellow onion or some fresh garlic. The ho-meopathic information in this chapter is based on my research, rather than on direct clinical experience, and is included for those readers who prefer this option or who may be trying to make sense of it.

Why People Choose Homeopathic Remedies

People choose homeopathic medicines for many of the same reasons they choose herbs and other alternative medicines: They are looking for a safe and natural alternative to conventional medical therapies. Homeopathic medicines are highly diluted forms of a variety of substances, so dilute, in fact, that they are entirely benign (although some homeopaths believe that taking the incor-rect remedy can drive symptoms deeper into the body). It is the very fact that they are harmless that leads many people to question whether they could pos-sibly even work. But homeopaths and many patients of homeopaths are con-vinced of their efficacy, based on clinical practice and personal use.

Not only are homeopathic remedies safe to use (it would be virtually im-possible to poison someone with a properly prepared homeopathic remedy, for example), but the forms in which they are delivered—a few drops of ex-tremely dilute liquid, or three to five lactose-based pellets that dissolve in the mouth—make administration convenient, even for use with small children.

Finally, homeopathic remedies appeal to those whose interest in illness extends beyond the physical into the emotional and spiritual realms, as the remedies often provide instruction for use that is descriptive not only of physi-cal ailments but of personality types and tendencies that may also manifest. So the remedy chamomila is not only for the child who is teething but also for the child who is displaying whining, fretful behavior; pulsatilla is not only for running eyes or nose but also for the weepy, sensitive person possibly also displaying these physical symptoms. Homeopaths, much like herbalists, look to the circumstances of the person's life and to the person's emotions, not just to physical symptoms.

Disadvantages of Homeopathic Remedies

Convenience and safety, when combined with efficacy, are advantages to using homeopathic preparations. However, there may be several disadvantages as well. Perhaps one of the greatest disadvantages to homeopathy is that it is very hard to find the right remedies.

As mentioned earlier, homeopathic remedies are highly specific to individuals. While this may make certain remedies, when carefully chosen for specific patients by a skilled homeopath, almost miraculously successful, it also leaves a very wide margin for error. It requires that one keep on hand a tremendous variety of remedies and have an extensive knowledge of the materia medica from which to make a choice. While herbal medicine is a very broad field with a vast materia medica, choosing an appropriate and effective remedy does not necessarily require as detailed a life assessment, particularly for acute disease conditions.

Homeopathic remedies are considered to be highly sensitive, with many factors that can render them entirely ineffective. For example, strong scents such as perfumes, spices, or even the scent or flavor of mint toothpaste can cause them to have no effect. Because of their sensitivity to strong scents, they should not be stored in the bathroom or kitchen. Nor should the remedies ever be touched by hand; they need to be placed in the mouth directly from the package. This is so even with pills and pellets. Unlike herbal remedies, which can be combined with homeopathic remedies or pharmaceuticals, homeopaths consider it best not to use other remedies along with homeopathic remedies, even herbal medicines, because they believe this interferes with the effectiveness of the homeopathic remedies. This can be extremely limiting when there is a complex health condition occurring, requiring several modalities to be used at once.

Principles of Homeopathic Medicine

Homeopathic medicine is based on the principle that like cures like. So, for example, coffee, which in high doses causes excessive nervous stimulation, is used to treat hyperactivity in the form of the homeopathic remedy coffea. Samuel Hahnemann, the founder of homeopathy as a formal healing system, "proved" hundreds of substances by ingesting them in doses sufficient to cause side effects. He cataloged these side effects and used the remedies based on these side effects to treat diseases whose symptoms were similar to the reactions to the substances. It is believed that Pasteur and other early modern vaccine researchers may have been influenced by the principles of homeopathy, evidenced in part by the fact that modern vaccination principles are to some extent similar to those of homeopathic principles. One may use a substance that causes certain symptoms to prevent or treat a disease with those same symptoms. It is believed that the curative substance stimulates a subtle cellular response that enables the body to change the disease pattern. Therefore, actual dilutions of disease organisms are sometimes used in homeopathy to treat the same diseases; vaccines employ the use of weakened, diluted, or attenuated disease organisms to prevent those diseases.

While homeopathic preparations are not in and of themselves dangerous, avoiding medical attention in favor of homeopathy, if the former is needed, *is* dangerous. It is therefore important that parents choose what is most effective for their children, not just what is philosophically more appealing.

Homeopathic medicines are prepared by making an initial preparation called the "mother tincture," much like an herbal tincture. However, this mother tincture is then progressively diluted and "succussed" (vigorously shaken a certain number of times in a repetitive fashion). This pattern of dilution and succussion is thought to render the substance harmless while sending the energy pattern or wavelength of the substance throughout the preparation. It is these wavelengths or energy patterns that are believed to be capable of altering and curing unhealthy patterns present during disease states.

The degree to which a remedy is diluted and succussed is expressed in a numerical symbol, which reveals the strength of the remedy. The numbers 6, 10, 30, and 200 are commonly seen on remedies available in the marketplace. The letters X, C, and M are found in combination with the numbers and refer respectively to dilutions to the tenth, hundredth, and thousandth. The greater the dilution, the stronger the remedy is considered to be. So a 200C remedy is thought to be much stronger than a 6X remedy. Taking two 100C pills does not equal a 200C remedy, and so on. In general, one begins by using a low potency, such as a 6C dose, and moves progressively to higher potencies if needed. The exception to this is when the illness or complaint has a strong emotional component. For such conditions, one might begin with a 30C dose.

Homeopathic Remedies for Childhood Illnesses

As stated earlier, I do not particularly advocate the use of homeopathic remedies for addressing serious health conditions. However, they may be a first line of response to early and mild signs of illness, if parents wish to try these safe and easy-to-administer treatments. It will require that you find the remedy that is absolutely specific to your child. Therefore, the remedies provided in the following sections on specific illnesses are only generalizations. They may be applicable to a wide variety of children manifesting similar symptom patterns, or they may not match your child's constitutional type at all. Therefore, it is best for parents who want to use this system of healing with the greatest chance of effectiveness to consult other books specific to homeopathy and to consult a qualified homeopath.

The material that follows provides the reader with introductory information on the homeopathic remedies commonly used during childhood infections, with brief descriptions of the indications for the remedies. Please consult books specifically on homeopathic medicine for more detailed information on its use and on the particulars of the medicines. Following this information is a section on the childhood illnesses, with lists of the remedies most frequently prescribed for them. Refer back to the materia medica for the prescriptive indications.

MATERIA MEDICA

Aconite is considered a highly toxic plant in crude form, but as a homeopathic remedy it is used in the early, acute stages of illness when there is a sudden onset of burning fever, thirst, and tremendous restlessness. It is primarily used for children with a hearty constitution and rosy cheeks. The child may exhibit symptoms of anxiety or fearfulness. Children may begin to exhibit "aconite" symptoms after exposure to cold, dry, windy weather. These children are extremely hot and dry, and heat and touch worsen their condition.

Antimonium tartaricum is the remedy commonly given when there is a lot of mucus in the chest, or when there is cough or damp, pus-filled eruptions. The child is generally whiny or cries a lot and may be irritable. The lips, nostrils, or eyes may possess a bluish or blackish discoloration around the edges, and the tongue generally has a thick white coating, though there may be red edges. Dampness, motion, and the seasons of spring and autumn often aggravate the symptoms. This remedy if often prescribed in the later stages of a cough.

Apis is generally prescribed for bites, stings, and puncture wounds, or any time there are puffy, watery swellings or blisters. There may be restlessness or dullness, and heat and touch aggravate, though pressure to the head may relieve some symptoms. There is frequently a burning sensation, and the child has little thirst.

Arsenicum album is appropriate when there is vomiting, diarrhea, and extreme weakness. There is generally extreme anxiety, extreme pallor, dry skin, and aversion to cold. There may be very strong thirst, but the child is unable to drink more than small sips at a time. There may be extreme restlessness and a strong desire for cold air in spite of being chilled.

Belladonna is recommended when there are illnesses that arise suddenly after exposure to cold, wet weather, and from chills after being overheated. Overexposure to the sun is also an indication. The illnesses manifest as acute inflammations, often accompanied by fever and cough. Heat and bright redness are cardinal signs for the use of this remedy, as are dilated pupils and red eyes. There is frequently sweat under the hair at the back of the head. The personality ranges from irritable to angry, there may even be violent outbursts, and there may be throbbing or spasmodic pain. Though the child is apt to be very restless, motion, noise, and touch often aggravate symptoms. Hypersensitivity is evident. Cold is also extremely aggravating, particularly drafts.

Bryonia is indicated when there has been exposure to cold, dry, windy weather resulting in dryness and inflammation of the mucous membranes. There tends to be irritability, facial redness, dry and cracked lips, and extreme thirst for warm drinks. Usually there is little sweating and eruptions may appear to be suppressed. There may be pain even from slight movement. Cool, fresh air improves the disposition, as does firm touch. Symptoms generally come on slowly.

Drosera is particularly indicated where there is unrelenting, spasmodic coughing aggravated by heat and reclining positions.

Eupatorium is called for in cases where there is severe aching of the limbs and extreme chills with shaking. It is indicated in the early stages of illness and may prevent severe cases from developing.

Euphrasia is primarily used when the eyes are red, irritated, inflamed, or sore, or when there is sensitivity to light. There may also be clear nasal discharge.

Gelsemium is indicated when there is anxiety, aching limbs, extreme weakness, and a hot head with a cold body. There may be fever but little thirst, chills, a desire to be held close, and headache. The condition often has a slow onset and may be precipitated by exposure to dampness, heat, and humidity.

Ipecachuana (ipecac) has long been used as a remedy for coughing with copious mucus that is hard to cough up. The child may be irritable or moody, and the condition may be more prevalent in damp weather.

Lachesis is used when there is a painful throat that affects the left side first, then the right; when swallowing is difficult; when the throat appears reddish purple; and when there is a tickly, croupy cough. There is often extreme chill with a cool, damp sweat, and there may be excessive chatter and a suspicious aspect to the personality. Cool drinks improve the discomfort.

Ledum is primarily indicated for puncture wounds. It is also indicated for splinters, bites, and stings. The body may feel cold to the touch, though the child feels hot, there may be shooting pains or prickling sensations, and cool air provides comfort. Touch and heat are extremely aggravating.

Lycopodium is specifically indicated for painful throat that affects the right side first, then the left. The patient is often cross and irritable when awaking from sleep, there is often gas and scanty urination, and the tongue is swollen and dry. Warm drinks improve the discomfort.

Phytolacca is used when there is sore throat that is very painful and feels as if there is a lump in the throat. The throat is dark and puffy, the tip of the tongue is red, and there may be headache, sore back and extremities, nausea, vertigo, faintness, and pain in the ears upon swallowing. Hot beverages may be aggravating to swallow.

Phytostigma is indicated when there is muscle weakness or tremors or twitching eyes, and when symptoms are aggravated by anything that is cold. There may be paralysis and uncoordinated gait.

Pilocarpine is specific for treatment of symptoms of mumps and is used to reduce the severity of the illness.

Pulsatilla is indicated when there is extreme moodiness, which can range from laughter to tears. There are pains that move from place to place, digestive discomfort, and thick discharges. Changeable symptoms are a clear call for pulsatilla. Stuffy environments aggravate, and symptoms are more common in those with a tendency to overheat easily. The child is often worse in the evening and is clingy and wants to be held and cuddled a great deal.

Rhus tox is used for symptoms that arise after exposure to cold, damp weather, chills, and drafts. There may be itchy skin eruptions, muscle aches and pains, and extreme restlessness and forgetfulness. Cold drinks may be desired, but warmth improves symptoms. Rubbing painful parts may also improve symptoms. Symptoms are more characteristically slow to appear, reappear at the same time each day, and are often more concentrated on the left side of the body.

Sulphur is specifically indicated for itchy rashes that are worst just around noon. It may be especially beneficial when rashes don't erupt easily and when symptoms linger after the infection has begun to clear up. It is commonly used to treat measles symptoms.

SPECIFIC CHILDHOOD ILLNESSES

Refer to the above materia medica when choosing the appropriate remedy for your child.

The remedies listed first may be the most specific to the condition, but any of these choices may have a role in treatment and should be considered as options.

Measles

Consider using aconite, apis, arsenicum album, belladonna, bryonia, euphrasia, gelsemium, ipecac, pulsatilla, or sulphur.

Mumps

Consider using belladonna, lachesis, lycopodium, pilocarpine, or rhus tox.

RUBELLA

Consider using aconite, coffea, or pulsatilla.

DIPHTHERIA

While apis, arsenicum album, lachesis, lycopodium, phytolacca, or other remedies may have a place in treatment, appropriate medical care is imperative in caring for children suspected of having diphtheria.

PERTUSSIS

Consider bryonia, drosera, or ipecac.

TETANUS

While ledum and hypericum may be used as adjunct therapies, medical care must be sought immediately if tetanus is suspected.

POLIO

Belladonna, eupatorium, gelsemium, and phytostigma are all remedies that may be considered in the prevention and treatment of polio, but if paralytic polio is suspected, medical care is also essential.

CHICKEN POX

Consider antimonium tartaricum, rhus tox, and sulphur.

HIB

If meningitis is suspected, immediate medical care must be sought. Consider the following for adjunct therapy: aconite, apis, arnica, belladonna, bryonia, gelsemium, or rhus tox.

In all situations, appropriate therapies should be used. Necessary medical care should not be abandoned or avoided for homeopathic remedies. If homeopathic remedies don't work after a single dose, the dose may be repeated another time, but no time should be wasted in getting the child onto the appropriate treatment plan, whether this be herbs or conventional therapies.

Again, there are many books that deal with homeopathy in a much more comprehensive fashion. For those of you primarily interested in homeopathic medicines, please refer to such references for guidance.

TEN

Late-Breaking News

Since the completion of this manuscript, I have received updates on the latest news in the vaccine world. This new information is significant and interesting, so I feel it is worth adding here.

Global Polio Eradication

Although the objective of global poliomyelitis eradication by the year 2000 was not achieved, the Western Pacific region of the World Health Organization certified on October 29, 2000, that that region is "free of indigenous wild poliovirus transmission."[1] This area includes thirty-seven countries and 27 percent of the global population. The Americas were declared free of polio in 1994. The European region is expected to be declared polio-free soon, because it has been free of indigenous cases since 1998.[2]

Thimerosol Use on the Wane?

Perhaps vaccine manufacturers are catching on to the risks of thimerosol, a mercury preservative used in many pediatric vaccinations. The FDA approved a formulation of the DTaP vaccine by Aventis Pasteur called Tripediaa. This new product contains no preservatives and only trace amounts of thimerosol, representing a 95 percent reduction in the quantity in the original product.[3] The removal of thimerosol from vaccines is a result of pressure from the American Academy of Pediatrics and the United States Public Health Service to limit pediatric exposure to mercury, particularly from vaccines. The initial recommendation to reduce the thimerosol content of vaccines occurred on July

241

8, 1999. According to Buck in the article "2001 Pediatric Vaccine Update," all recommended pediatric vaccines are currently available in at least one thimerosol-free or reduced-thimerosol form.[4]

New Vaccine "Cocktails"

In response to concern from parents and health care providers that the average child will receive more than twenty injections by age six, vaccine manufacturers are seeking to develop ever new combinations of vaccinations, thus reducing the actual number of shots children receive. However, the safety of such immunologic combinations has not been determined, and on March 7, 2001, the FDA Vaccines and Related Biologic Products Advisory Committee voted to recommend that a combination of DTaP and hepatitis B not be approved at that time. In fact, when standard vaccines had the pneumoccocal vaccine added, the rate of fever in recipients rose from 26 percent in the standard vaccine group to 43 percent in the conjugate pneuomoccal vaccine group.[5] Parents should therefore be wary of new vaccine combinations until conclusive research is available demonstrating their safety and efficacy.

APPENDIX A

Botanical Names

In order to be sure of the herbs you are using, you need to know the proper scientific name of the plant, as many plants share common names. The list below provides the most common name of the herb, which is the name used in this book, along with the correct botanical name.

Common Name	Botanical Name
American ginseng	*Panax quinquefolium*
Angelica	*Angelica archangelica*
Apricot seed	*Prunus armeniaca*
Arnica	*Arnica montana*
Asarum	*Asarum sieboldi*
Anise	*Pimpinella anisum*
Astragalus	*Astragalus membranaceous*
Black cohosh	*Cimicifuga racemosa*
Burdock	*Arctium lappa*
Bupleurum	*Bupleurum falcatum*
Calendula	*Calendula officinalis*
Carthamus	*Carthamus tinctorius*
Catnip	*Nepeta cataria*
Chamomile	*Matricaria recutita*
Chickweed	*Stellaria media*
Chinese red ginseng	See *Ginseng*
Chinese skullcap	*Scutellaria baicalensis*
Chinese licorice	*Glycyrrhiza uralensis*

Cinnamon	*Cinnamomum cassia*
Citrus peel	*Citrus aurantii*
Cleavers	*Galium aparine*
Cnidium	*Ligusticum walichii*
Codonopsis	*Codonopsis pilosula*
Comfrey	*Symphytum officinale*
Coptis	*Coptis chinensis*
Cramp bark	*Viburnum opulus*
Dandelion	*Taraxacum officinale*
Dang gui	*Angelica sinensis*
Dolichos	*Dolichos lablab*
Echinacea	*Echinacea* spp.
Elder	*Sambucus nigra; S. canadensis*
Elecampane	*Inula helenium*
Ephedra	*Ephedra sinica*
Eucommia	*Eucommia ulmoides*
Fennel	*Foeniculum vulgare*
Forsythia	*Forsythia suspensa*
Gentian	*Gentiana lutea*
Garlic	*Allium sativum*
Ginger	*Zingiber officinale*
Ginseng	*Panax ginseng*
Glehnia	*Glehnia littoralis*
Goldenseal	*Hydrastis canadensis*
Hawthorn	*Crataegus laevigata*
Hoelen	*Poria cocos*
Honeysuckle	*Lonicera japonica*
Isatis	*Isatis tinctoria*
Kudzu	*Pueraria lobata*
Lavender	*Lavendula officinalis*
Lemon balm	*Melissa officinalis*
Licorice	*Glycyrrhiza glabra*
Lobelia	*Lobelia inflata*
Marshmallow	*Althea officinale*

Milk thistle	*Silybum marianum*
Mint	*Mentha piperita*
Mulberry	*Morus alba*
Mullein	*Verbascum thapsus*
Myrrh	*Commiphora molmol*
Ophiopogon	*Ophiopogon japonicus*
Passionflower	*Passiflora incarnata*
Peony	*Paeonia rubra*
Peppermint	*Mentha piperita*
Pinellia	*Pinellia ternata*
Plantain	*Plantago* spp.
Platycodon	*Platycodon grandiflorum*
Poke	*Phytolacca* spp.
Polygonatum	*Polygonatum odorati*
Red clover	*Trifolium pratense*
Rehmannia	*Rehmannia glutinosa*
Rose hips	*Rosa canina*
Sage	*Salvia officinalis*
Schisandra	*Schisandra chinensis*
Scrophularia	*Scrophularia ningpoensis*
Shiitake mushrooms	*Lentinus edodes*
Siberian ginseng	*Eleutherococcus senticosus*
Slippery elm	*Ulmus rubra*
Spearmint	*Mentha spicata*
St. John's wort	*Hypericum perforatum*
Trichosanthes	*Trichosanthes kirowilii*
Tumeric	*Curcuma longa*
Thyme	*Thymus vulgaris*
Violet	*Viola odorata*
Wild cherry	*Prunus serotina*
Yarrow	*Achillea millefolium*
Yellow dock	*Rumex crispus*
Zizyphus	*Zizyphus spinosa*

APPENDIX B

Resources

The resources listed below will enable you to find vaccine information, vaccine information groups, information on herbal medicine, and herbal products.

Vaccine Resources

Many states have their own vaccine-information organizations run by concerned parents and professionals. Contact the National Vaccine Information Center for information on a group in your area.

National Vaccine Information Center (NVIC)
421 Church Street, Suite E
Vienna, VA 22180
800-909-SHOT
Web site: www.909shot.com

New Atlantean Press
P.O. Box 9638
Santa Fe, NM 87504
505-983-1856
Web site: www.new-atlantean.com

Vaccine Information

Centers for Disease Control and Prevention
National Immunization Hotline: 800-232-2522
Spanish: 800-232-0233
Web site: www.cdc.gov/nip/recs/contraindications.htm (enter here and search the entire site)

Alternative Medicine

To find information on botanical medicine, homeopathy, or traditional Chinese medicine, or to locate a practitioner in your area, contact the following organizations:

American Herbalists Guild
1931 Gaddis Rd.
Canton, GA 30115
770-751-6021
Web site: www.americanherbalist.com
This is the only peer-reviewed organization for professional herbalists in the United States. Offers a variety of resources on herbal medicine and practitioners. Nonprofit membership organization that publishes a peer-reviewed academic journal of botanical medicine, *The Journal of the American Herbalists Guild*, offers an annual symposium, and has a variety of other publications. Sets the standard for botanical practitioners in the United States.

American Association of Naturopathic Physicians
8201 Greensboro Drive, Suite 300
Mclean, VA 22102
703-610-9037
Web site: www.naturopathic.org

American Association of Oriental Medicine
433 Front Street
Catasanqua, PA 18032
888-500-7999

National Center for Homeopathy
801 N. Fairfax Street, Suite 306
Alexandria, VA 22314
703-548-7790

Botanical and Homeopathic Products

The author personally purchases from the following companies and knows them to be highly reliable and to offer top-quality products and services.

LifeCycles Midwifery and Center for Herbal Medicine
1931 Gaddis Rd.
Canton, GA 30115
770-751-7548
Run by herbalist, midwife, and author Aviva Romm, this company specializes in the herbal needs of mothers and children. Offers organically grown products that are hand-prepared in small batches to ensure quality and care. For the convenience of readers trying to obtain these and other hard-to-find herbal products, we supply the Chinese herbal ingredients mentioned in this book. Aviva also offers herbal consultations, both in her office and by phone.

Avena Botanicals
219 Mill Street
Rockport, ME 04856
207-594-0694
Bulk herbs, tinctures, and other organic herbal products.

Blessed Herbs
109 Barre Plains Rd.
Oakham, MA 01068
800-489-4372
A wide variety of organic, bulk herbal products.

Cascade Health Care Products
141 Commercial St. NE
Salem, OR 97301
800-443-9942
Specializing in the needs of pregnant women, offers books and products for natural care and home birth preparation.

Frontier Cooperative Herbs
P.O. Box 299
Norway, IA 52318
800-669-3275
Bulk herbal products, tinctures, supplements, as well as oils and other materials for preparing herbal products.

Herb Pharm
P.O. Box 116
Williams, OR 97544

800-348-4372
Excellent, high-quality, reliable organic and ethically wild-crafted tinctures.

Herbalist and Alchemist
P.O. Box 553
Broadway, NJ 08808
908-689-9092
Excellent tincture products, including hard-to-find Chinese herbal tinctures; high quality and high integrity.

Homeopathic Educational Services
2124 Kittredge St.
Berkeley, CA 94794
800-359-9051
Homeopathic books and products; reliable company with high-quality products.

Maine Seaweed Company
P.O. Box 57
Steuben, ME 04680
207-546-2875
A variety of seaweeds, very high quality, ethically harvested with good nutrition and environmental sensibility in mind.

Mayway Chinese Herbs and Herbal Products
780 Broadway
San Francisco, CA 94133
415-433-3765
Web site: www.mayway.com
An established supplier of quality Chinese herbal products, Mayway sells bulk Chinese herbs to the general public.

Redwing/Meridian Books
44 Linden St.
Brookline, MA 02146
800-873-3946
Books and products for those interested in learning more about traditional Chinese medicine.

Notes

Introduction

1. Stanley Plotkin and Edward Mortimer, *Vaccines* (Philadelphia: W. B. Saunders, 1988).

2. Barbara Loe Fisher, *The Consumer's Guide to Childhood Vaccines* (Vienna, Va.: National Vaccine Information Center, 1997), 66.

1. A Curious History

1. Stanley Plotkin and Edward Mortimer, introduction to *Vaccines* (Philadelphia: W. B. Saunders, 1988).

2. Harris Coulter and Barbara Loe Fisher, *DPT: A Shot in the Dark* (New York: Warner Books, 1985), 335. Catherine J. M. Diodati, *Immunization: History, Ethics, Law, and Health* (Windsor, Ontario: Integral Aspects, 1999), 3.

3. Coulter and Fisher, 335.

4. Diodati, 3.

5. Plotkin and Mortimer, introduction to *Vaccines*.

6. Ibid.

7. Ibid.

8. Ibid., Diodati, 3.

9. Leon Chaitow, *Vaccination and Immunisation: Dangers, Delusions, and Alternatives* (Essex, England: C. W. Daniel, 1987), 4. Harris Coulter, *Divided Legacy: Twentieth-Century Medicine: The Bacteriological Era* (Berkeley, Calif.: North Atlantic Books, 1994), 56. Coulter provided a thorough discussion of the history of isopathic medicine, its relationship to homeopathic medicine, and the possible relationship of the two to the development of vaccines by Pasteur and his contemporaries.

10. Ibid.

11. Plotkin and Mortimer, introduction to *Vaccines*.

12. Diodati, 4.

13. Neil Miller, *Immunization: Theory vs. Reality* (Sante Fe, N. Mex.: New Atlantean Press, 1999), 23.

14. Diodati, 4.

15. Ibid., Miller, 24.

16. Diodati, 4.

17. Plotkin and Mortimer, introduction to *Vaccines*. Chaitow, 4.

18. Plotkin and Mortimer, introduction to *Vaccines*.

19. Miller, 24.

20. Ibid.

21. Ibid., 28.

22. Diodati, 5.

23. Ibid., 28. Chaitow, 5.

24. Chaitow, 6. Miller, 28.

25. Coulter, 45.

26. Chaitow, 6.

27. Ibid.

28. Chaitow, 6. Coulter, 385.

29. Coulter, 385.

30. Ibid.

31. Plotkin and Mortimer, introduction to *Vaccines*.

32. Diodati, 7. Plotkin and Mortimer, introduction to *Vaccines*.

33. Walene James, *Immunization: The Reality behind the Myth* (Westport, Conn.: Bergin and Garvey, 1995), 70.

34. Jill Stansbury, "From Morbid Matter to Modern Microbiology: A Discussion of Toxemia, Morbid Matter, and the Germ Theory," *Medicines from the Earth: Official Proceedings* (Black Mountain, N.C., 2000), 164. James, 72. Chaitow, 11. Miller, 29.

35. Coulter, 358.

36. Chaitow, 6.

37. Coulter and Fisher, 24.

38. Stephen Preblud and Samuel Katz, "Measles Vaccine," in Plotkin and Mortimer, *Vaccines*, 182.

39. Robert Weibel, "Mumps Vaccine," in Plotkin and Mortimer, *Vaccines*, 223.

40. Stanley Plotkin, "Rubella Vaccine," in Plotkin and Mortimer, *Vaccines*, 235.

41. Frederick C. Robbins, "Polio-Historica," in Plotkin and Mortimer, *Vaccines*, 98.

42. Ibid., 98. The issue of the seasonal appearance of polio will be discussed in chapter 4, under polio, and in later chapters when nutrition and Traditional Chinese Medicine are discussed.

43. Ibid.

44. Jonas Salk and Jacques Drucker, "Noninfectious Poliovirus Vaccine," in Plotkin and Mortimer, *Vaccines*, 159.

45. Diodati, 16.

46. Diodati, 12.

47. Ibid.

48. Ibid., 13.

2. Declining Disease Rates and Vaccine Efficacy

1. Walene James, *Immunization: The Reality behind the Myth* (Westport, Conn.: Bergin and Garvey, 1995), 32.

2. Stanley Plotkin and Edward Mortimer, introduction to *Vaccines* (Philadelphia: W. B. Saunders, 1988). Robert Koch developed Koch's Postulates of Disease. His work led to the production of pure strains of anthrax bacillus, proving it to be the cause of anthrax disease.

3. Leon Chaitow, *Vaccination and Immunisation: Dangers, Delusions, and Alternatives* (Essex, England: C. W. Daniel, 1987), 6.

4. Plotkin and Mortimer, introduction to *Vaccines*.

5. Richard Moskowitz, "Immunizations: The Other Side," *Mothering*, no. 31 (spring 1984): 32. See also James, 26; Chaitow, 53–58; and Barbara Loe Fisher, *The Consumer's Guide to Childhood Vaccines* (Vienna, Va.: National Vaccine Information Center, 1997), 26.

6. Moskowitz, 32.

7. Catherine J. M. Diodati, *Immunization: History, Ethics, Law, and Health* (Windsor, Ontario: Integral Aspects, 1999), 99–102.

8. Alan Hinman, "The Pertussis Vaccine Controversy," *Public Health Reports* 99, no. 3 (May-June 1984): 258.

9. Edward J. Mortimer, "Immunization against Infectious Disease," *Science* 200 (May 26, 1978): 904. Mortimer cites the following sources for his statistics: Bureau of the Census, *Historical Times to 1970*, part 1 (Washington, D.C.:

Department of Commerce, Government Printing Office, 1975); Bureau of the Census, *Special Reports, Mortality Statistics 1900–1904* (Washington, D.C.: Departments of Commerce and Labor, Government Printing Office, 1906); National Center for Health Statistics, *Vital Statistics of the United States, 1973*, vol. 2, *Mortality*, part A (Rockville, Md.: Department of Health, Education, and Welfare, Public Health Service, 1977).

10. Moskowitz, 33.

11. Chaitow, 54.

12. Diodati, 100.

13. Ibid., 255.

14. Ibid., 256.

15. Mortimer, "Immunization Against Infectious Disease," 256.

16. U.S. Department of Health and Human Services and the Centers for Disease Control and Prevention, *Six Common Misconceptions about Vaccination and How to Respond to Them* (Baltimore: U.S. Department of Health and Human Services and the Centers for Disease Control and Prevention, 1996), 14–15.

17. Robert Mendelsohn, *How to Raise a Healthy Child in Spite of Your Doctor* (New York: Ballantine, 1984), 230.

18. Ibid., 33.

19. Ibid.

20. Harris Coulter and Barbara Loe Fisher, *DPT: A Shot in the Dark* (New York: Warner Books, 1985), 16.

21. Ibid., 17.

22. Ibid., 18–19.

23. Ibid., 172.

24. Ibid.

25. Ibid., 173.

26. Mortimer, "Immunization against Infectious Disease," 256.

27. Celia D. C. Christie et al., "The Epidemic of Pertussis in Cincinnati: Resurgence of Disease in a Highly Immunized Population," *New England Journal of Medicine* 331, no. 1 (July 17, 1994): 16.

28. Ibid., 18.

29. Scott Halperin et al., "Persistence of Pertussis in an Immunized Population: Results of the Nova Scotia Enhanced Pertussis Surveillance Program," *Journal of Pediatrics* 115, no. 5 (November 1989): 686–93.

30. Ibid.

31. Alan Hinman and Jeffey Koplan, "Pertussis and Pertussis Vaccine: Reanalysis of Benefits, Risks, and Costs," *Journal of the American Medical Association* 251, no. 23 (June 15, 1984): 3109–13.

32. Gordon Stewart, "Pertussis Vaccine: Benefits and Risks," *New England Journal of Medicine* 302, no. 11 (March 13, 1980): 634.

33. Neil Miller, *Vaccines: Are They Really Safe and Effective?* (Sante Fe, N. Mex.: New Atlantean Press, 1999).

34. Neustaedter, R. *The Immunization Reason.* (Berkeley, Calif.: North Atlantic Books, 1990), 45.

35. Ibid.

36. Mortimer, 904. Mendelsohn, 236. Miller, 25–29.

37. Diodati, 105.

38. Ibid.

39. Ibid., 108.

40. James, 38. Chaitow, 69.

41. Neustaedter, 54.

42. James, 38.

43. Neustaedter, 54.

44. Ibid.

45. Miller, 25–29.

46. Diodati, 108.

47. Diodati, 109–10.

48. Ibid., 39.

49. Miller, 25–29.

50. Joseph L. Melnick, "Live Attenuated Poliovaccines," in Plotkin and Mortimer, *Vaccines*, 115.

51. Diodati, 115.

52. Melnick, 119.

53. Ibid., 115. Neustaedter, 37.

54. Peter Strebel et al., "Epidemiology of Poliomyelitis in the United States One Decade after the Last Reported Case of Indigenous Wild Virus-Associated Disease," *Clinical Infectious Disease* 114 (February 1992): 570.

55. Ibid.

56. *Washington Post*, September 24, 1976, cited in Miller, 21.

57. Miller, 11–23.

58. Melnick, 138. Miller, 11–23. Diodati, 118. James, 36. Strebel et al., 569.

59. James, 36.

60. Michael Lawless et al., "Rubella Susceptibility in Sixth Graders: Effectiveness of Current Immunization Practice," *Pediatrics* 65, no. 6 (June 1980), 1087.

61. Ibid., 1089.

62. Miller, 29.

63. Lawless et al., 1088.

64. Ibid. Neustaedter, 64. Moskowitz, 35.

65. Mortimer, 904.

66. Chaitow, 54.

67. Neustaedter, 51.

68. Chaitow, 58.

69. Ibid.

70. Neustaedter, 51.

71. Ibid. Mendelsohn, 223.

72. Miller, 24–25.

3. The Marvelous Immune System

1. Walene James, *Immunization: The Reality Behind the Myth* (Westport, Conn.: Bergin and Garvey, 1995), 105.

2. James, 106.

3. Richard Moskowitz, "The Case against Immunizations," *Mothering* (spring 1984): 31–37. James, 39–40.

4. Robert Wallace, *Biology: The World of Life* (New York: Addison Wesley Longman, 1997), 200.

5. Jill Stansbury, "From Morbid Matter to Modern Microbiology: A Discussion of Toxemia, Morbid Matter, and the Germ Theory," *Medicines from the Earth: Official Proceedings* (Black Mountain, N.C., 2000), 165.

6. Cedric Mims et al., *Medical Microbiology* (Boston: Mosby, 1993), 32–37.

7. Edward Mortimer, "Immunization against Infectious Disease," *Science* 200 (May 26, 1978): 902.

8. Joseph Bellanti, "Basic Immunologic Principles Underlying Vaccination Procedures," Pediatric Vaccinations: Update 1990 (special edition), *Pediatric Clinics of North America* 37, no. 3 (June 1990): 515.

9. Harold Buttram and John Chris Hoffman, "Bringing Vaccines into Perspective," *Mothering* (winter 1985): 29.

10. Bellanti, "Basic Immunologic Principles," 515.

11. Ibid., 514.

12. Ibid., 515.

13. The author directly contacted the major vaccine manufacturers to obtain package inserts. Companies whose material I have drawn from include Pasteur Merieux Connaught, Merck and Company, Lederle, Wyeth-Ayerst, and Smith Kline Beecham. All material was obtained in the year 2000 and most is copyrighted 1999.

14. "Use of Human Cell Cultures in Vaccine Manufacturing," Centers for Disease Control and Prevention National Immunization Program, www.cdc.gov/nip/vacsafe/concerns/gen/humancell.htm, 1.

15. Catherine J. M. Diodati, *Immunization: History, Ethics, Law, and Health* (Windsor, Ontario: Integral Aspects, 1999), 71.

16. Ibid.

17. E. L. Hurwitz and H. Morgenstern, "Effects of Diphtheria-Tetanus-Pertussis or Tetanus Vaccination on Allergies and Allergy-Related Respiratory Symptoms among Children and Adolescents in the United States," *Journal of Manipulative Physiologic Therapy* 23, no. 2 (February 2000): 81-90.

18. N. P. Thompson et al., "Is Measles Vaccination a Risk Factor for Inflammatory Bowel Disease?" *Lancet* 29, no. 345 (April 2000) (8957):1071–74.

19. Margaret B. Rennels, "Reinstitute Hepatitis B Vaccine for All Infants," *American Academy of Pediatric News* 15, no. 11 (November 1999), 6.

4. The Childhood Illnesses and "Vaccine-Preventable Diseases"

1. Centers for Disease Control. "Morbidity and Mortality Weekly Report" 2000; 49: 35–47. *Journal of the American Medical Association* 283, no. 7 (February 16, 2000): 876.

2. Ibid.

3. Ibid. In the mid 1990s, the OPV (oral poliovirus) vaccine was given for two doses, followed by two doses of IPV (inactivated poliovirus). Prior to that, and into the first half of the 1990s, OPV was given for all four doses. After 1996, in recognition that OPV can cause poliomyelitis, and in the effort to eliminate the possibility of vaccine-associated paralytic poliomyelitis (VAPP), IPV is recommended for all four doses. OPV, if available, may be given in the following circumstances only: In the case of mass vaccination campaigns to

control polio outbreaks; for unvaccinated children traveling within four weeks to areas where polio is endemic or epidemic; for children of parents who won't accept the recommended number of IPV injections. They should be given OPV for the third and fourth doses only, and only after risks of VAPP have been discussed.

4. Edward Mortimer, "Immunization against Infectious Disease," *Science* 200 (May 26, 1978): 904.

5. "Morbidity and Mortality Weekly Report," 35–47. *Journal of the American Medical Association*, 876.

6. Robert L. Davis, "Vaccine Extraimmunization—Too Much of a Good Thing?" *Journal of the American Medical Association* 283, no. 10 (March 8, 2000): 1339. Suzanne M. Feikema et al., "Extraimmunization among U.S. Children," *Journal of the American Medical Association* 283, no. 10 (March 8, 2000): 1311.

7. Feikema et al., 1311–12.

8. Davis, 1340.

9. Stanley Preblud and Samuel Katz, "Measles Vaccine," in Stanley Plotkin and Edward Mortimer, *Vaccines* (Philadelphia: W. B. Saunders, 1988), 182.

10. James Cherry, "The 'New' Epidemiology of Measles and Rubella," *Hospital Practice* (July 1980): 49. Preblud and Katz, 183.

11. Barbara Loe Fisher, *The Consumer's Guide to Childhood Vaccines* (Vienna, Va.: National Vaccine Information Center, 1997), 16.

12. Preblud and Katz, 188.

13. Ibid.

14. Cherry, 54.

15. Ibid., 9.

16. Ibid., 50.

17. Ibid., 51.

18. Ibid.

19. Robert E. Weibel, "Mumps Vaccine," in Plotkin and Mortimer, *Vaccines*, 223.

20. Ibid.

21. Ibid., 224.

22. Stanley Plotkin, "Rubella Vaccine," in Plotkin and Mortimer, *Vaccines*, 235.

23. Fisher, 19.

24. Michael Lawless et al., "Rubella Susceptibility in Sixth Graders: Effectiveness of Current Immunization Practice," *Pediatrics* 65, no. 6 (June 1980): 1086–89.

25. Walter Orenstein et al., "Rubella Vaccine and Susceptible Hospital Employees: Poor Physician Participation," *Journal of the American Medical Association* 245, no. 7 (February 20, 1981): 711–13.

26. Stanley Plotkin and Edward Mortimer, "Diphtheria Toxoid," in Plotkin and Mortimer, *Vaccines* (Philadelphia: W. B. Saunders, 1988).

27. Ibid.

28. Michael Alderson, "International Mortality Statistics," Washington, D.C., Facts on File, 1981, 177–78.

29. Leon Chaitow, *Vaccination and Immunisation: Dangers, Delusions, and Alternatives* (Essex, England: C. W. Daniel, 1987), 53.

30. Chaitow, 58. Neil Miller, *Vaccines: Are They Really Safe and Effective?* (Santa Fe, N. Mex.: New Atlantean Press, 1999), 24–25.

31. *Taber's Cyclopedic Medical Dictionary*, 15th ed. (Philadelphia: F. A. Davis, 1985), 470.

32. Plotkin and Mortimer, "Diphtheria Toxoid."

33. Ibid.

34. Ibid.

35. Alan Hinman and Jeffrey Koplan, "Pertussis and Pertussis Vaccine: Reanalysis of Benefits, Risks, and Costs," *Journal of the American Medical Association* 251, no. 23 (June 15, 1984): 3109.

36. Fisher, 10.

37. Hinman and Koplan, "Pertussis and Pertussis Vaccine," 3109–10.

38. Edward Mortimer, "Pertussis Vaccine," in Plotkin and Mortimer, *Vaccines*, 78.

39. Mortimer, "Pertussis Vaccine," 78.

40. Fisher, 11.

41. Mortimer, "Pertussis Vaccine," 82.

42. Ibid.

43. Stanley Plotkin and Edward Mortimer, "Tetanus," in Plotkin and Mortimer, *Vaccines*.

44. Plotkin and Mortimer, "Tetanus."

45. Mortimer, "Immunization against Infectious Disease," 902.

46. Plotkin and Mortimer, "Tetanus."

47. Ibid.

48. Ibid.

49. Neustaedter, R. *The Immunization Reason* (Berkeley, Calif.: North Atlantic Books, 1990), 31. Richard Moskowitz, "Immunizations: The Other Side," *Mothering*, no. 31 (spring 1984): 33–37.

50. Joseph L. Melnick, "Live Attenuated Poliovaccines," in Plotkin and Mortimer, *Vaccines*, 115. Frederick Robbins, "Polio—Historical," in Plotkin and Mortimer, *Vaccines*, 98.

51. Melnick, 115.

52. Fisher, 15.

53. *Taber's Cyclopedic Medical Dictionary*, 1337.

54. Ibid.

55. Melnick, 116.

56. *Taber's Cyclopedic Medical Dictionary*, 1337.

57. Merck and Company, "Varivax, Varicella Live Virus Vaccine" (package insert for chicken pox vaccine from Merck and Company), 1995.

58. Michiaki Takahashi, "Varicella Vaccine," in Plotkin and Mortimer, *Vaccines*, 526.

59. Ibid., 527.

60. Fisher, 24–25.

61. *Taber's Cyclopedic Medical Dictionary*, 1835–36.

62. Fisher, 20. Joel Ward and Sephen Cochi, "*Haemophilus influenzae* Vaccines," in Plotkin and Mortimer, *Vaccines*, 303.

63. Ward and Cochi, 300.

64. Fisher, 21.

65. Ward and Cochi, 304.

66. Ibid.

67. Ibid., 301.

68. Ward and Cochi, 304. Merck and Company, "Liquid PedvaxHIB" (package insert for *Haemophilus* B conjugate vaccine), 1998.

69. Gary Freed et al., "Family Physician Acceptance of Universal Hepatitis B Immunization of Infants," *Journal of Family Practice* 36, no. 2 (February 1993): 153–57.

70. Ibid.

71. Catherine J. M. Diodati, *Immunization: History, Ethics, Law, and Health* (Windsor, Ontario: Integral Aspects, 1999), 122–23.

72. Merck and Company, "Recombivax HB" (package insert for hepatits B vaccine), 1998. Diodati, 122–23.

73. Diodati, 122–23.

74. Janet Zand et al., *Smart Medicine for a Healthier Child* (Garden City, N.Y.: Avery Publishing, 1994).

75. Fisher, 22.

76. Gary Freed et al., "Reactions of Pediatricians to a New Centers for Disease Control Recommendation for Universal Immunization of Infants with Hepatitis B Vaccine," *Pediatrics* 91, no. 4 (April 1993). Freed et al., "Family Physician Acceptance," 153–57.

5. What about the Risks?

1. Kathleen Stratton et al., *Adverse Events Associated with Childhood Vaccines: Evidence Bearing on Causality* (Washington, D.C.: National Academy Press, 1994), v.

2. Claudia Kalb and Donna Foote, "Necessary Shots?" *Newsweek*, September 13, 1999, 73–74.

3. Stratton et al., 73.

4. Stratton et al., 1.

5. Pharmaco-Epidemiology and Central Drug Monitoring and Medical Department, CIBA-GEIGY, Basel, Switzerland, *Bratisl Lek Litsy*, 1991, Nov.; 92 (11): 549–53.

6. Ibid.

7. Stratton et al., 2.

8. Ibid.

9. "A High-Priced Vaccine," *The Washington Post*, May 23, 1986.

10. Kalb and Foote, 73–74.

11. Ibid. Centers for Disease Control and Prevention, "Update: Vaccine Side Effects, Adverse Reactions, Contraindications, and Precautions: Recommendations of the Advisory Committee on Immunization Practices (ACIP)," *Morbidity and Mortality Weekly Report* 45, no. RR-12 (September 6, 1996).

12. Robert Chen and Beth Hibbs, "Vaccine Safety: Current and Future Challenges," *Pediatric Annals* 27, no. 7 (July 1998): 445.

13. Ibid., 446.

14. Leon Chaitow, *Vaccination and Immunisation: Dangers, Delusions, and Alternatives* (Essex, England: C. W. Daniel, 1987), 88.

15. Ibid., 74.

16. Stratton et al., 23.

17. Charles Marwick, "Clearing the Way for New Combination Vaccine Use," *Journal of the American Medical Association* 283, no. 10 (2000): 876–78. Chen and Hibbs, 447. Edward Mortimer, "Immunization against Infectious Disease," *Science* 200 (May 26, 1978): 906.

18. Chen and Hibbs, 447.

19. Mortimer, "Immunization against Infectious Disease," 906. Chen and Hibbs, 447.

20. Mortimer, "Immunization against Infectious Disease," 906.

21. Ibid.

22. Ibid.

23. Chen and Hibbs, 447.

24. Ibid.

25. Marwick, 876–78.

26. U.S. Department of Health and Human Services and the Centers for Disease Control and Prevention, *Six Common Misconceptions about Vaccination and How to Respond to Them* (Baltimore: U.S. Department of Health and Human Services and the Centers for Disease Control and Prevention, 1996), 14–15.

27. Stratton et al., 279.

28. M. M. Braun and S. S. Ellenberg, "Descriptive Epidemiology of Adverse Events after Immunization: Reports to the Vaccine Adverse Events Reporting System (VAERS), 1991–1994," *Journal of Pediatrics* 131, no. 4 (October 1997): 529–35.

29. Ibid.

30. Stratton et al., 274–83. Barbara Loe Fisher, *The Consumer's Guide to Childhood Vaccines* (Vienna, Va.: National Vaccine Information Center, 1997), 64–65.

31. Fisher, 64. Neil Miller, *Vaccines: Are They Really Safe and Effective?* (Santa Fe, N. Mex.: New Atlantean Press, 1999), 57.

32. Miller, 63.

33. Andrea Rock, "The Lethal Dangers of the Billion-Dollar Vaccine Business," *Money* 25, no. 12 (December 1996).

34. Ibid.

35. Chen and Hibbs, 448.

36. Rock, cited in Catherine J. M. Diodati, *Immunization: History, Ethics, Law, and Health* (Windsor, Ontario: Integral Aspects, 1999), 173.

37. Ibid.

38. Ibid.

39. Diodati, 173.

40. Chen and Hibbs, 449.

41. Ibid.

42. Chaitow, 82.

43. U.S. Department of Health and Human Services and the CDC, *What You Need to Know about Vaccine Information Statements* (U.S. Department of Health and Human Services and the CDC, 1999).

44. Miller, 31–32. Roland Sutter et al., "Attributable Risk of DTP Injection in Provoking Paralytic Poliomyelitis during a Large Outbreak in Oman," *Journal of Infectious Diseases* 165 (1992): 444–49. Personal conversation with Vance Dietz, M.D., specialist in infectious diseases, Centers for Disease Control, July 2000.

45. U.S. Department of Health and Human Services and the CDC, *What You Need to Know.*

46. Marwick, 876–78.

47. Ibid.

48. Ibid.

49. Stratton et al., 274–83.

50. C. Flavo and H. Horowitz, "Adverse Reactions Associated with Simultaneous Administration of Multiple Vaccines to Travelers," *Journal of General Internal Medicine* 9, no. 5 (May 1994): 255–60.

51. Fisher, 38.

52. Centers for Disease Control and Prevention, "Update: Vaccine Side Effects."

53. Stratton et al., 274–83. Fisher, 118.

54. Ibid.

55. Centers for Disease Control and Prevention, "Update: Vaccine Side Effects."

56. Fisher, 38. Stratton et al., 129.

57. Stratton et al., 122.

58. Ibid., 122–30.

59. Stratton et al., 163–65. Fisher, 38.

60. Stratton et al., 164, 176.

61. Ibid., 168.

62. Ibid., 141–46.

63. Ibid., 144.

64. Ibid., 148.

65. Kevin Morris and George Rylance, "Guillain-Barré Syndrome after Measles, Mumps, and Rubella Vaccine," *Lancet* 343 (January 1, 1994): 60.

66. Ibid.

67. Stratton et al., 135–42.

68. J. McEwen, "Early Onset Reaction after Measles Vaccination: Further Australian Reports," *Medical Journal of Australia* 110 (November 12, 1983): 503–505.

69. Central Drugs Laboratory, Central Research Institute (Himachal Pradesh, India), "Adverse Reactions after Measles Vaccination in India," *National Medical Journal of India* 8, no. 5 (September-October 1995): 208–10.

70. Diodati, 221–24. Wendy Pugh, "Australian Scientists Plan Measles-Modified Food," Reuters, February 2000. "Aerosol Administration of Measles Vaccine Superior to Subcutaneous Method," *Lancet* 355 (2000): 798–803.

71. Pugh, "Measles-Modified Food."

72. Diodati, 233.

73. Anne-Marie Plesner, "Gait Disturbances after Measles, Mumps, and Rubella Vaccine, *Lancet* 345 (February 4, 1995): 316.

74. Ibid.

75. V. Jayarjan and P. A. Sedler, "Hearing Loss Following Measles Vaccination," journal citation uncertain, (July 22, 1994), 184.

76. M. Feeney et al., "A Case-Control Study of Measles Vaccination and Inflammatory Bowel Disease: The East Dorset Gastroenterology Group," *Lancet* 350, no. 9080 (September 13, 1997): 764–66. N. P. Thompson et al., "Is Measles Vaccination a Risk Factor for Inflammatory Bowel Disease?" *Lancet* 345, no. 8957 (April 29, 1995): 1071–74.

77. Thompson et al., 1071–74. A. J. Wakefield et al., "Ileal-Lymphoid-Nodular Hyperplasia, Non-specific Colitis, and Pervasive Developmental Disorder in Children," *Lancet* 351 (February 28, 1998): 637–41.

78. Thompson et al., 1071.

79. Ibid., 1073.

80. Peter Patriarca and Judy Beeler, "Measles Vaccination and Inflammatory Bowel Disease," *Lancet* 345, no. 8957 (April 29, 1995): 1062–63.

81. A. Sugiura and A. Yamada, "Aseptic Meningitis as a Complication of Mumps Vaccination," *Pediatric Infectious Disease Journal* 10, no. 3 (March 1991): 209–13.

82. Norman Begg, "Reporting of Vaccine Associated Mumps Meningitis," *Archives of Disease in Childhood* 68 (1993): 526.

83. Stratton et al., 134.

84. "Mumps Meningitis and MMR Vaccination," *Lancet* (October 28, 1989): 1015.

85. Jane McDonald et al., "Clinical and Epidemiologic Features of Mumps Meningoencephalitis and Possible Vaccine Related Disease," *Pediatric Infectious Disease Journal* 8, no. 11 (November 1989): 751–55.

86. H. J. Schmitt et al., "Withdrawal of a Mumps Vaccine: Reasons and Impacts," *European Journal of Pediatrics* 152 (1993): 387–88.

87. Ibid. McDonald et al., 751–55.

88. "Mumps Meningitis Following Measles, Mumps, and Rubella Immunization," *Lancet* (August 12, 1989): 394.

89. Stratton et al., 154.

90. Ibid.

91. Ibid., 188.

92. Ibid., 176.

93. Mortimer, "Immunization against Infectious Disease," 905.

94. J. K. Chantler, et al., "Persistent Rubella Virus Infection Associated with Chronic Arthritis in Children," *New England Journal of Medicine* 131, no. 18 (October 31, 1985): 1117.

95. Walene James, *Immunization: The Reality Behind the Myth* (Westport, Conn.: Bergin and Garvey, 1995), 10.

96. Stanley Plotkin, "Rubella Vaccine," in Stanley Plotkin and Edward Mortimer, *Vaccines* (Philadelphia: W. B. Saunders, 1988), 247–48.

97. Ibid.

98. Ibid.

99. Walter Orenstein et al., "Rubella Vaccine and Susceptible Hospital Employees: Poor Physician Participation," *Journal of the American Medical Association* 245, no. 7 (February 20, 1981): 713.

100. Ibid.

101. Allen D. Allen, "Is RA27/3 Rubella Immunization a Cause of Chronic Fatigue?" *Medical Hypotheses* 27 (1988): 217–20.

102. A. P. Lieberman, "Rubella Virus in Chronic Fatigue Syndrome," *Clinical Ecology* 7, no. 3: 51–54.

103. Stratton et al., 156.

104. Plotkin, "Rubella Vaccine," 247–49.

105. Ibid.

106. Mary Megson, "Is Autism a G-Alpha Protein Defect Reversible with Natural Vitamin A?" (presentation proceeding from the 1999 Defeat Autism Now!

conference). Dr. Megson, a developmental pediatrician, can be reached at Highland II Office Park, 7229 Forest Avenue, Suite 11, Richmond, VA 23226. Her paper is available on-line at www.autism.com/ari/megson.html.

107. Deborah Hirtz, "The Challenges of Autism—Why the Increased Rates?" (presentation by the National Institute of Neurological Disorders and Stroke, NIH, before the Committee on Government Reform, April 6, 2000).

108. Dan Burton, Opening Statement, "Autism: Present Challenges, Future Needs—Why the Increased Rates?" (presentation to Committee on Government Reform, April 6, 2000). Available on-line at www.house.gov/reform/hearings/healthcare/oo.06.04/opening_statement.htm.

109. Stratton et al., 34–39.

110. Vijendra Singh, "Autism: Present Challenges, Future Needs—Why the Increased Rates?" (presentation to Committee on Government Reform, April 6, 2000). Available on-line at www.house.gov/reform/hearings/healthcare/oo.06.04/opening_statement.htm.

111. Wakefield et al., 637–41.

112. Ibid., 638.

113. Ibid., 639–40.

114. Ibid., 640. Andrew Wakefield, "Testimony before Congressional Oversight Committee on Autism and Immunization."

115. See n. 106 above.

116. Bernard Rimland, "The Autism Increase: Research Needed on the Vaccine Connection" (presentation to Committee on Government Reform, April 6, 2000).

117. Wakefield.

118. F. Edward Yazbak, "Autism: Is There a Vaccine Connection?" (1999). Available on-line at: http://garynull.com/Documents/autism99b.htm.

119. E. H. Relyveld et al., "Rational Approaches to Reduce Adverse Reactions in Man to Vaccines Containing Tetanus and Diphtheria Toxoids," *Vaccine* 16, no. 9-10 (May-June 1998): 1016–23.

120. Burton.

121. Shelley Hendrix Reynolds, "Autism: Present Challenges, Future Needs— Why the Increased Rates?" (presentation to Committee on Government Reform, April 6, 2000).

122. Relyveld et al., 1016–23. A. Mark and M. Granstrom, "The Role of Aluminum for Adverse Reactions and Immunogenicity of Diphtheria-Tetanus Booster Vaccine," *Acta Paediatrica* 83, no. 2 (February 1994): 159–63.

123. Stratton et al., 75–76.

124. Ibid., 97.

125. Ibid., 98.

126. Alan Hinman, "The Pertussis Vaccine Controversy," *Public Health Reports* 99, no. 3 (May-June 1984): 255.

127. Mortimer, "Pertussis Vaccine," 84.

128. Gordon Stewart, "Pertussis Vaccine: Benefits and Risks," *New England Journal of Medicine* 302, no. 11 (March 13, 1980): 634. Gordon Stewart, "Benefits and Risks of Pertussis Vaccine," *New England Journal of Medicine* 303, no. 17 (October 23, 1980): 1004.

129. Hinman, 255.

130. Ibid. Scott Halperin et al., "Persistence of Pertussis in an Immunized Population: Results of the Nova Scotia Enhanced Pertussis Surveillance Program," *Journal of Pediatrics* 115, no. 5 (November 1989): 687.

131. Hinman, 256.

132. Halperin et al., 690.

133. Ibid., 691.

134. Alan Hinman and Jeffrey Koplan, "Pertussis and Pertussis Vaccine: Reanalysis of Benefits, Risks, and Costs," *Journal of the American Medical Association* 251, no. 23 (June 15, 1984): 3110.

135. Roger Barkin and Michael Pichichero, "Diphtheria-Pertussis-Tetanus Vaccine: Reactogenicty of Commercial Products," *Pediatrics* 63, no. 2 (February 1979): 256–60.

136. U.S. Department of Health and Human Services and the CDC, *What You Need to Know.*

137. Barkin and Pichichero, 259.

138. Jeffrey Koplan et al., "Pertussis Vaccine: An Analysis of Benefits, Risks, and Costs," *New England Journal of Medicine* 30, no. 17 (October 25, 1979): 907.

139. Ibid.

140. Hinman and Koplan, 3113.

141. Barkin and Pichichero, 260.

142. Gordon Stewart, "Vaccination against Whooping Cough: Efficacy versus Risk," *Lancet* 1, no. 8005 (January 29, 1977): 234–37.

143. P. E. Fine and R. T. Chen, "Confounding Variables in Studies of Adverse Reactions to Vaccines," *American Journal of Epidemiology* 136, no. 2 (July 15, 1992): 121–35.

144. Barkin and Pichichero, 259.

145. Hinman, 257.

146. T. M. Pollock and J. Morris, "A Seven-Year Survey of Disorders Attributed to Vaccination in North West Thames Region, *Lancet* 1, no. 8327 (April 2, 1983): 753–57.

147. Hinman, 258.

148. G. S. Golden, "Pertussis Vaccine and Injury to the Brain," *Journal of Pediatrics* 116, no. 6 (June 1990): 854–61.

149. Mortimer, "Pertussis Vaccine," 85.

150. U.S. Department of Health and Human Services and the CDC, "Update: Vaccine Side Effects, Adverse Reactions, Contraindications, and Precautions: Recommendations of the Advisory Committee on Immunization Practices," *Morbidity and Mortality Weekly Report* 45, no. RR-12 (September 6, 1996): 22–23.

151. Ibid.

152. H. C. Stetler et al., "History of Convulsions and Use of Pertussis Vaccine," *Journal of Pediatrics* 107, no. 2 (August 1985): 175–79.

153. Ibid.

154. James Cherry et al., "Report of the Task Force on Pertussis and Pertussis Immunization," *Pediatrics* 81 (1988), 939–84.

155. L. J. Baraff et al., "Infants and Children with Convulsions and Hypotonic-Hyporesponsive Episodes Following Diphtheria-Tetanus-Pertussis Immunization: Follow-up Evaluation," *Pediatrics* 81, no. 6 (June 1988): 789–94. H. Goodwin et al., "Vaccination of Children Following a Previous Hypotonic-Hyporesponsive Episode," *Journal of Pediatric Child Health* 35, no. 6 (December 1999): 549–52. C. P. Howson and H. V. Fineberg, "Adverse Events Following Pertussis and Rubella Vaccines: Summary of a Report of the Institute of Medicine," *Journal of the American Medical Association* 267, no. 3 (January 15, 1992): 392–96.

156. R. M. Andrews et al., "Vaccinating Children with a History of a Serious Reaction after Vaccination or of Egg Allergy," *Medical Journal of Australia* 168, no. 10 (May 1998): 491–94.

157. U.S. Department of Health and Human Services and the CDC, "Update: Vaccine Side Effects."

158. R. K. Gupta and E. H. Relyveld, "Adverse Reactions after Injection of Adsorbed Diphtheria-Pertussis-Tetanus (DPT) Vaccine Are Not Only Due to Pertussis Organisms or Pertussis Components in the Vaccine," *Vaccine* 9, no. 10 (October 1991): 699–702.

159. E. L. Hurwitz and H. Morgenstern, "Effects of Diphtheria-Tetanus-Pertussis or Tetanus Vaccine on Allergies and Allergy-Related Respiratory Symptoms

among Children and Adolescents in the United States," *Journal of Manipulative Physiologic Therapy* 23, no. 2 (February 2000): 81–90. Michel Odent, "Pertussis Vaccination and Asthma: Is There a Link?" *Journal of the American Medical Association* 272, no. 8 (August 24-31, 1994): 592–93. E. Cserhati, "Current View on the Etiology of Childhood Bronchial Asthma," *Orv Hetil* 140, no. 48 (November 28, 1999): 2675–83.

160. Hurwitz and Morgenstern, 81–90.

161. Odent, 592–93.

162. S. M. Wintermeyer et al., "Whole-Cell and Acellular Pertussis Vaccines," *Annals of Pharmacotherapy* 28, no. 7-8 (July-August 1994): 925–39.

163. M. E. Pichichero et al., "Acellular Pertussis Vaccination of Two-Month-Old Infants in the United States," *Pediatrics* 89, no. 5, part 1 (May 1992): 882–87.

164. James Cherry, "Comparative Efficacy of Acellular Pertussis Vaccines: An Analysis of Recent Trials," *Pediatric Infectious Disease Journal* 16, supplement (April 1997): S90–96.

165. S. Meriste et al., "Safety and Immunogenicity of Combine DTaP-IPV Vaccine for Primary and Booster Vaccination," *Scandinavian Journal of Infectious Disease* 31, no. 6 (1993): 587–91.

166. Italian Institute of Health, "Pertussis Project 1992–1994," *Istisan Report*, 18.

167. Fisher, 35.

168. Ibid.

169. Harris Coulter and Barbara Loe Fisher, *DPT: A Shot in the Dark* (New York: Warner Books, 1985), 236.

170. Roger Bernier et al., "Diphtheria–Tetanus Toxoids–Pertussis Vaccination and Sudden Infant Deaths in Tennessee," *The Journal of Pediatrics* 101, no. 3 (September 1982), 419.

171. Ibid., 420–21.

172. Neustaedter, 45.

173. Stratton et al., 70.

174. Ibid., 107–8.

175. Ibid., 108.

176. Ibid., 107.

177. Ibid., 110.

178. Dan Vergano, "Oral Polio Vaccine Still Used Despite Risks," *USA Today*, November 9, 1999.

179. Stratton et al., 190.

180. Peter Strebel et al., "Epidemiology of Poliomyelitis in the United States One Decade after the Last Reported Case of Indigenous Wild Virus-Associated Disease," *Clinical Infectious Diseases* 114 (February 1992): 568–79.

181. Stratton et al., 200.

182. Ibid.

183. Debbie Bookchin and Jim Schumacher, "The Virus and the Vaccine, Parts 1– 3," *Atlantic Monthly* (January, February, and March 2000). Walter Kyle, "Simian Retroviruses, Poliovaccine, and Origin of AIDS," *Lancet* 339 (March 7, 1992): 600–601.

184. Centers for Disease Control, "Simian Virus 40 (SV40) and Cancer," March 28, 2000. Available on-line at www.cdc.gov/nip/vacsafe/concerns/Cancer/default.htm.

185. Ibid.

186. Ibid.

187. Kyle, 600–601.

188. Ibid.

189. B. L. Horvath and F. Fornosi, "Excretion of SV-40 Virus after Oral Administration of Contaminated Polio Vaccine," *Acta Biologica* (June 1964), 11–12.

190. Centers for Disease Control, "Simian Virus 40."

191. Ibid.

192. Bookchin and Schumacher.

193. Ibid.

194. Ibid.

195. Centers for Disease Control, "Simian Virus 40."

196. Fisher, 7.

197. Merck and Company, "Varivax, Varicella Live Virus Vaccine" (package insert for chicken pox vaccine from Merck and Company), 1995.

198. Fisher, 45.

199. Merck and Company, "Varivax, Varicella Live Virus Vaccine."

200. M. Brisson, et al., "Analysis of Varicella Vaccine Breakthrough Rates," *Vaccine* 18, no. 25 (2000): 2775–78.

201. Merck and Company, "Varivax, Varicella Live Virus Vaccine."

202. Michiaki Takahashi, "Varicella Vaccine," in Plotkin and Mortimer, *Vaccines*.

203. Smith Kline Beecham, "OmniHIB Haemophilus B Conjugate Vaccine (Tetanus Toxoid Conjugate)," (package insert for Hib vaccine from Smith Kline Beecham), 2000.

204. Stratton et al., 239.

205. Ibid., 250–53.

206. Ibid.

207. Ibid., 251.

208. Fisher 43. Smith Kline Beecham.

209. Smith Kline Beecham.

210. Frederic Shaw, "Uproar over a Little-Known Preservative, Thimerosal, Jostles U.S. Hepatitis B Vaccine Policy," *Hepatitis Control Report* 4, no. 2 (summer 1999).

211. Ibid.

212. N. Linder, "Unexplained Fever in Neonates May Be Associated with Hepatitis B Vaccine," *Archives of Disease in Childhood: Fetal and Neonatal Edition* 81, no. 3 (November 1999): F206–7.

213. Ibid.

214. G. Vautier and J. E. Carty, "Acute Sero-Positive Rheumatoid Arthritis Occurring after Hepatitis Vaccination," *British Journal of Rheumatology* 33 (1994): 991. Eric Hachulla et al., "Reactive Arthritis after Hepatitis B Vaccination," *Journal of Rheumatology* 179 (1990): 1250–51. P. Poullin and B. Gabriel, "Thrombocytopenia Purpura after Recombinant Hepatitis B Vaccine," *Lancet* 344 (November 5, 1994): 1293.

215. Stratton et al., 223.

216. L. Herroelen et al., "Central-Nervous-System Demyelination after Immunisation with Recombinant Hepatitis B Vaccine," *Lancet* 338 (November 9, 1991): 1174.

217. E. Touze et al., "First Central Nervous System Demyelination and Hepatitis B Vaccination: A Pilot Case Control Study," *Revue Neurologique* (Paris) 156, no. 3 (2000): 242–46.

218. Jean Francis Maillefert et al., "Exacerbation of Systemic Lupus Erythematosus after Hepatitis B Vaccination," *Arthritis and Rheumatism* 43, no. 2 (February 2000): 468.

219. Daniel Battafarano et al., letter to the editor of *Arthritis and Rheumatism* 43, no. 2 (February 2000): 468–69.

220. J. Barthelow Classen, "Childhood Immunzation and Diabetes Mellitus," *New Zealand Journal of Medicine* 109, no. 1022 (May 24, 1996): 195.

221. Ibid.

222. Gary Freed et al., "Family Physician Acceptance of Universal Hepatitis B Immunization of Infants," *Journal of Family Practice* 36, no. 2 (February 1993): 153–57.

223. Gary Freed et al., "Reactions of Pediatricians to a New Centers for Disease Control Recommendation for Universal Immunization of Infants with Hepatitis B Vaccine, *Pediatrics* 91, no. 4 (April 1992): 699–702.

6. Personal Choices and Public Policies

1. M. M. Ipp et al., "Acetominophen Prophylaxis of Adverse Reactions Following Vaccination of Infants with Diphtheria–Pertussis–Tetanus Toxoids–Polio Vaccine," *Pediatric Infectious Disease Journal* 6 no. 8 (August 1987): 721–25.

2. M. M. Ipp et al., "Adverse Reactions to Diphtheria, Tetanus, Pertussis–Polio Vaccination at Eighteen Months of Age: Effect of Injection Site and Needle Length," *Pediatrics* 83, no. 5 (May 1989): 679–82.

3. L. J. Baraff et al., "DTP-Associated Reactions: An Analysis by Injection Site, Manufacturer, Prior Reactions, and Dose," *Pediatrics* 73, no. 1 (January 1984): 31–36.

4. Patty Brennan, *Vaccine Choices: Homeopathic Alternatives, and Parental Rights* (Ann Arbor, Mich.: Holistic Midwifery Institute, 1999).

5. Barbara Loe Fisher, *The Consumer's Guide to Childhood Vaccines* (Vienna, Va.: National Vaccine Information Center, 1997), 56.

6. Ibid., 58.

7. Ibid., 59.

8. Julius Landwirth, "Medical-Legal Aspects of Immunization," *Pediatric Clinics of North America* 37, no. 3 (June 1990) Pediatric Vaccinations: Update 1990 (special edition): 772.

9. Ibid.

10. Catherine J. M. Diodati, *Immunization: History, Ethics, Law, and Health* (Windsor, Ontario: Integral Aspects, 1999), 171.

11. Ibid.

12. Ibid., 172.

13. Fisher, 61.

14. Ibid., 60.

15. Brennan, 37. Fisher, 60.

16. V. J. Dietz et al., "Vaccination Practices, Policies, and Management Factors Associated with High Vaccination Coverage Levels in Georgia Public Clinics; Georgia Immunization Program Evaluation Team," *Archives of Pediatric and Adolescent Medicine* 154, no. 2 (February 2000): 184–89.

17. Richard Fried, "Health Consequences of Exemptions from Immunization Laws," *Journal of the American Medical Association* 283, no. 9 (March 1, 2000): 1140.

7. Natural Approaches to Health and Immunity

1. Walene James, *Immunization: The Reality behind the Myth* (Westport, Conn.: Bergin and Garvey, 1995), 109.

2. Richard Moskowitz, "Vaccination: A Sacrament of Modern Medicine" (presented at the annual conference of the Society of Homeopaths, Manchester, England, September 1991). Published in *Homeopath* 12 (March 1992): 137–44.

3. Vijendra Singh (presentation to the Committee on Government Reform, Hearings on Vaccination and Autism, June 4, 2000). Available at www.house.gov/reform/hearings/healthcare/00.06.04/singh.htm.

4. S. Chandra and R. K. Chandra, "Nutrition, Immune Response, and Outcome," *Progress in Food and Nutrition Science* 10, no. 1-2 (1986): 1–65.

5. James, 8.

6. Harold Buttram and John Chris Hoffman, "Bringing Vaccines into Perspective," *Mothering* (winter 1985): 31.

7. F. Wang and C. Shi, "Secretory Immunoglobulin A in Human Milk and Infants' Feces at One to Four Months after Delivery," *Chung Hua Fu Chan Ko Tsa Chih* 30, no. 10 (October 30, 1995): 588–90. C. P. Speer and H. Hein-Kreikenbaum, "Immunologic Importance of Breastmilk," *Monatasschiftr Kinderheilkunde* 141, no. 1 (January 1993): 10–20. A. Prentice, "Breast Feeding Increases Concentrations of IgA in Infants' Urine," *Archives of Disease in Childhood* 62, no. 8 (August 1987): 792–95.

8. Speer and Hein-Kreikenbaum, 10–20.

9. Ibid.

10. Ibid.

11. L. A. Hanson et al., "Breast Feeding: Overview and Breast Milk Immunology," *Acta Pediatrica* 36, no. 5 (October 1994): 557–61.

12. C. Barriga et al., "Effect of Serum from Breast- or Formula-Fed Infants on Polymorphonuclear Leukocyte Function," *Comparatuve Immunology, Microbiology, and Infectious Diseases* 20, no. 1 (January 1997): 21–27. C. Barriga et al., "Serum Hemolytic and Bactericidal Activity in Breast- and Formula-Fed Infants," *Revista Espanola de Fisiologia* 51, no. 4 (December 1995): 218–18.

13. L. A. Hanson, "Human Milk and Host Defense: Immediate and Long-term Effects," *Acta Pediatrica* 88, no. 4, supplement (August 30, 1999): 42–46.

14. Ibid.

15. J. S. Hawkes et al., "The Effect of Breastfeeding on Lymphocyte Subpopulations in Healthy Term Infants at Six Months of Age," *Pediatric Research* 45, no. 5 (May 1995), part 1: 648–51.

16. H. Hasselbalch, "Breast-feeding Influences Thymic Size in Late Infancy," *European Journal of Pediatrics* 158, no. 12 (December 1999): 964–67.

17. L. A. Hanson, "Breastfeeding Provides Passive and Likely Long-Lasting Active Immunity," *Annals of Allergy, Asthma, and Immunology* 82, no. 5 (May 1999): 478. Hanson et al., "Breast Feeding: Overview," 557–61. S. Villalpando and M. Hamosh, "Early and Late Effects of Breast-feeding: Does Breast-feeding Really Matter?" *Biology of the Neonate* 74, no. 2 (1998): 177–91.

18. Hanson, "Human Milk and Host Defense," 42–46. Hanson et al., "Breast Feeding: Overview," 557–61. K. M. Bernt and M. A. Walker, "Human Milk as a Carrier of Biochemical Messages," *Acta Pediatrica* 88, no. 430, supplement (August 1999): 27–41. D. Dai and W. A. Walker, "Protective Nutrients and Bacterial Colonization in the Immature Human Gut," *Advanced Pediatrics* 46 (1999): 353–82. M. B. Yellis, "Human Breast Milk and Facilitation of Gastrointestinal Development and Maturation, *Gastroenterologic Nursing* 18, no. 1 (January-February 1995): 11–15.

19. Joseph Bellanti, "Recurrent Respiratory Tract Infections in Pediatric Patients, *Drugs* 54, supplement 1 (1997): 1–4.

20. M. Xanthou et al., "Human Milk and Intestinal Host Defense in Newborns: An Update," *Advanced Pediatrics* 42 (1995): 171–208.

21. A. S. Goldman et al., "Immunologic Protection of the Premature Infant by Human Milk," *Seminars in Perinatology* 18, no. 6 (December 1994): 495–501.

22. S. Orlando, "The Immunologic Significance of Breast Milk," *Journal of Obstetric and Gynecologic Neonatal Nursing* 24, no. 7 (September 1995): 678–83.

23. M. K. Davis, "Review of the Evidence for an Association between Infant Feeding and Childhood Cancer," *International Journal of Cancer* 11, supplement (1998): 29–33.

24. Ibid.

25. P. B. Lawrence, "Breast Milk: Best Source of Nutrition for Term and Preterm Infants," *Pediatric Clinics of North America* 41, no. 5 (October 1994): 925–41. P. L. Engle et al., "Child Development: Vulnerability and Resilience," *Social Science and Medicine* 43, no. 5 (September 1996): 621–35.

26. L. A. Hanson, "The Mother-Offspring Dyad and the Immune System," *Acta Pediatrica* 89, no. 3 (March 2000): 252–58.

27. A. G. Cummings and F. M. Thompson, "Postnatal Changes in Mucosal Immune Response: A Physiological Perspective of Breast Feeding and Weaning," *Immunology and Cell Biology* 75, no. 5 (October 1997): 419–29.

28. N. B. Duerbeck, "Breast-feeding: What You Should Know So You Can Talk to Your Patients," *Comprehensive Therapy* 24, no. 6-7 (June-July 1998): 310–18.

29. V. Y. Yu, "The Role of Dietary Nucleotides in Neonatal and Infant Nutrition," *Singapore Medical Journal* 39, no. 4 (April 1998): 145–50.

30. A. E. Gordon et al., "The Protective Effect of Breastfeeding in Relation to Sudden Infant Death Syndrome (SIDS): The Effect of Human Milk and Infant Formula Preparations on Binding of Clostridium Perfringens to Epithelial Cells," *FEMS Immunology and Medical Microbiology* 25, no. 1-2 (August 1999): 167–73.

31. Chandra and Chandra, "Nutrition, Immune Response, and Outcome," 1–65.

32. J. P. Revillard and G. Cozon, "Experimental Models and Mechanisms of Immune Deficiencies of Nutritional Origin," *Food Additives and Contaminants* 1, supplement (1990): S82–86.

33. R. K. Chandra, "Nutrition and the Immune System: An Introduction," *American Journal of Clinical Nutrition* 66, no. 2 (August 1997): 460–63S.

34. R. K. Chandra, "Nutrition and Immunology: From the Clinic to Cellular Biology and Back Again," *Proceedings of the Nutrition Society* 58, no. 3 (August 1999): 681–83.

35. R. K. Chandra, "Nutrition and Immunoregulation: Significance for Host Resistance to Tumors and Infectious Diseases in Humans and Rodents," *Journal of Nutrition* 122, no. 3, supplement (March 1992): 754–57.

36. Chandra, "Nutrition and Immunology," 681–83.

37. R. K. Chandra, "Interactions between Early Nutrition and the Immune System," *Ciba Foundation Symposium* 156 (1991): 77–89.

38. Chandra, "Interactions," 77–89. R. K. Chandra, "Nutritional Regulation of Immunity and Risk of Illness," *Indian Journal of Pediatrics* 56, no. 5 (September-October 1989): 607–11.

39. G. Zuin and N. Principi, "Trace Elements and Vitamins in Immunomodulation in Infancy and Childhood," *European Journal of Cancer Prevention* 6, supplement 1 (March 1997): S69–77.

40. D. A. Hughes, "Effects of Dietary Antioxidants on the Immune Function of Middle-aged Adults, *Proceedings of the Nutrition Society* 58 (February 1999): 79–84. This article also focuses on antioxidant vitamins and their effects on the immune systems of young subjects.

41. A. Bendich, "Vitamin E and Immune Function," *Basic Life Science* 49 (1988): 615–20.

42. M. Del Rio et al., "Improvement by Several Antioxidants of Macrophage Function In Vitro," *Life Sciences* 63, no. 10 (1998): 871–81.

43. Y. Elitsur et al., "Vitamin A and Retinoic Acids in Immunomodulation on Human Gut Lymphocytes," *Immunopharmacology* 35, no. 3 (January 1997): 247–53.

44. R. D. Semba, "Vitamin A and Immunity to Viral, Bacterial, and Protozoal Infections," *Proceedings of the Nutrition Society* 58, no. 3 (August 1999): 719–27.

45. Ibid.

46. L. S. Harbige, "Nutrition and Immunity with Emphasis on Infection and Autoimmune Disease," *Nutrition and Health* 10, no. 4 (1996): 285–312.

47. M. M. Rahman et al., "Effects of Early Vitamin A Supplementation on Cell-Mediated Immunity in Infants Younger Than Six Months," *American Journal of Clinical Nutrition* 65, no. 1 (January 1997): 144–48.

48. D. I. Thurnham, "Micronutrients and Immune Function: Some Recent Developments," *Journal of Clinical Pathology* 50, no. 11 (November 1997): 887–91. S. Moriguchi, "Cellular Immunity and Vitamins," *Nippon Rinsho* [Japanese Journal of Clinical Medicine] 57, no. 10 (October 1999): 2313–18.

49. M. M. Rahman et al., "Simultaneous Vitamin A Administration at Routine Immunzation Contact Enhances Antibody Response to Diphtheria Vaccine in Infants Younger Than Six Months," *Journal of Nutrition* 129, no. 12 (December 1999): 2192–95. R Bahl et al., "Vitamin A Administration with Measles Vaccine to Nine-Month-Old Infants Does Not Reduce Immunogenicity," *Journal of Nutrition* 129, no. 8 (August 1999): 1569–73. C. S. Benn et al., "Randomised Trial of Effect of Vitamin A Supplementation on Antibody Response to Measles Vaccine in Guinea-Bissau, West Africa," *Lancet* 12, 350, no. 9071 (July 1997): 101–5.

50. Bendich, 615–20.

51. Harbige, 285–312.

52. Ibid.

53. Bendich, 615–20.

54. Thurnham, 887–91.

55. Ibid.

56. R. A. Good and E. Lorenz, "Nutrition and Cellular Immunity," *International Journal of Immunopharmacology* 14, no. 3 (April 1992): 361–66. Chandra and Chandra, "Nutrition, Immune Response, and Outcome," 1–65. Chandra, "Nutrition and the Immune System," 460–63S.

57. Chandra, "Nutritional Regulation of Immunity," 607–11.

58. Harbige, 285–312.

59. R. K. Chandra, "Interactions of Nutrition, Infection, and Immune Response," *Acta Pediatrica Scandinavia* 68, no. 1 (January 1979): 137–44.

60. K. S. Kubena and D. N. McMurray, "Nutrition and the Immune System: A Review of Nutrient-Nutrient Interactions," *Journal of the American Dietetic Association* 11 (November 1996): 1156–64.

61. Chandra, "Nutrition and the Immune System," 460–63S. Chandra and Chandra, "Nutrition, Immune Response, and Outcome," 1–65. Revillard and Cozon, S82–86. Good and Lorenz, 361–66.

62. Revillard and Cozon, S82–86. Good and Lorenz, 361–66.

63. Lori Smolin and Mary Grosvenor, *Nutrition: Science and Applications* (New York: Harcourt Brace, 1997).

64. Mary Bove, *An Encyclopedia of Natural Healing for Infants and Children* (New Canaan, Conn.: Keats, 1996).

65. A. Sanchez et al., "Role of Sugars in Human Neutrophilic Phagocytosis," *American Journal of Clinical Nutrition* 26 (1973): 1180–84. J. Bernstein et al., "Depression of Lymphocyte Transformation Following Oral Glucose Ingestion," *American Journal of Clinical Nutrition* 30 (1977): 613.

66. James, 54–55.

8. Herbal Medicines and Childhood Diseases

1. Xy Li, "Immunomodulating Chinese Herbal Medicines," *Memórias de Instituto Oswaldo Cruz* 86, no. l2, supplement (1991): 150–64. Y. Yoshida et al., "Immunomodulating Activity of Chinese Medicinal Herbs and *Oldenlandia diffusa* in Particular," *International Journal of Immunopharmacology* 19, no. 7 (July 1997): 359–70.

2. Li, 150–64. Stephen Buhner, *Herbal Antibiotics* (Pownal, Vt.: Storey Books, 1999), 71–72.

3. H. Wagner et al., "Immunostimulating Action of Polysaccharides (Heteroglycans) from Higher Plants," *Arzeimittelforschung* 35, no. 7 (1985): 1069–75.

4. Wagner et al., 1069–75. B. S. Uteshev at al., "The Immunomodulating Activity of the Heteropolysaccharides from German Chamomile during Air Immersion and Cooling," *Eksperimental'naia i Klinicheskaia Farmakologiia* 62, no. 6 (November-December 1999): 52–55.

5. V. R. Bauer et al., "Immunologic In Vivo and In Vitro Studies on Echinacea Extracts," *Arzeimittekforschung* 38, no. 2 (February 1988): 276–81. E. G. Coeugniet and E. Elek, "Immunomodulation with *Viscum album* and *Echinacea purpurea*," *Onkologie* 10, no. 3, supplement (June 1987): 27–33. Wagner et al., 1069–75. D. M. See et al., "In Vitro Effects of Echinacea and Ginseng on Natural Killer and Antibody-Dependent Cell Toxicity in Healthy Subjects and Chronic Fatigue Syndrome or Acquired Immunodeficiency Syndrome Patients," *Immunopharmacology* 35, no. 3 (January 1997): 229–35. J. Rehman et al., "Increased Production of Antigen-Specific Immunoglobulins G and M Following In Vivo Treatment with the Medicinal Plants *Echinacea angustifolia* and *Hydrastis canadensis*," *Immunol Lett* 1; 68, no. 2-3 (June 1999): 391–95. L. Z. Sun et al., "The American Coneflower: A Prophylactic Role Involving Nonspecfic Immunity," *Journal of Alternative and Complementary Medicine* 5, no. 5 (October 1999): 437–46.

6. A. I. Sow et al., "Antibacterial Activity of Essential Oils from Mint in Senegal," *Dakar Medical Journal* 40, no. 2 (1995): 193–95.

7. J. Dankert et al., "Antimicrobial Activity of Crude Juices of *Allium ascalonicum, Allium cepa,* and *Allium sativum,*" *Zentralblatt fur Bakteriologie* 245, no. 1-2 (October 1979): 229–39. B. H. Lau et al., "Garlic Compounds Modulate Macrophage and T-Lymphocyte Functions," *Molecular Biotherapy* 3, no. 2 (June 1991): 103–7. H. Salman et al., "Effects of a Garlic Derivative (Alliin) on Peripheral Blood Cell Immune Responses," *International Journal of Immunopharmacology* 21, no. 9 (September 1999): 589–97.

8. S. Nakajima, "The Effects of Ginseng radix rubra on Human Vascular Endothelial Cells," *American Journal of Chinese Medicine* 26, no. 3-4 (1998): 365–73. F. Scaglione et al., "Efficacy and Safety of the Standardized Ginseng Extract G115 for Potentiating Vaccination against the Influenza Syndrome and Protection against the Common Cold," *Drugs under Experimenal and Clinical Research* 22, no. 2 (1996): 65–72. C. Klein et al., "From Food to Nutritional Support to Specific Nutraceuticals: A Journey across Time in the Treatment of Disease," *Journal of Gastroenterology* 35, no. 12, supplement (2000): 1–6.

9. Wagner et al., 1069–75.

10. S. Szolomicki et al., "The Influence of Active Components of *Eleutherococcus senticosus* on Cellular Defense and Physical Fitness in Man," *Phytotherapy Research* 14, no. 1 (February 2000): 30–35.

11. N. Mascolo et al., "Ethnopharmacologic Investigation of Ginger *(Zingiber officinale),*" *Journal of Ethnopharmacology* 27, no. 1-2 (November 1989): 129–40.

12. M. Nose et al., "Activation of Macrophages by Crude Polysaccharide Fractions Obtained from Shoots of *Glycyrrhiza glabra* and Hairy Roots of *Glycyrrhiza uralensis* In Vitro," *Biological Pharmacology Bulletin* 21, no. 10 (October 1998): 1110–12.

10. Late-Breaking News

1. Anon. "Public health dispatch: certification of poliomyelitis eradication—Western Pacific region, October 2000," *Morbidity and Mortality Weekly Report,* 50, no. 1 (2001): 1–3.

2. J. T. John, "The final stages of the global eradication of polio," *New England Journal of Medicine,* 343 (2000): 806–7.

3. Anon. "FDA advisory panel urges agency not to approve GlaxoSmithKline vaccine," *Reuters Medical News,* 7 March 2001.

4. Marcia Buck, "2001 Pediatric Vaccine Update," *Pediatric Pharmacotherapy,* 7, no. 3 (2001): 703–10.

5. American Academy of Family Physicians, American Academy of Pediatrics, Advisory Committee on Immunization Practices, United States Public Health Service. Joint statement concerning removal of thimerosol from vaccines at www.cdc.gov/nip/vacsafe/con.../thimerosol/joint_statement00.htm (as of 3/20/01).

Glossary

adjuvant. A substance, such as aluminum phosphate or aluminum hydroxide, that when added to a vaccination increases the antigenic response.

anaphylaxis. An acute, often dramatic, life-threatening systemic reaction characterized by generalized itching, hives, respiratory distress, and vascular collapse, and sometimes by seizures, vomiting, cramps, and incontinence; immediate medical treatment with antihistamines is essential.

antigen. A substance that stimulates the production of antibodies that interact specifically with that substance.

arthralgia. Joint pain.

arthritis. Joint inflammation with pain, swelling, and redness.

aseptic meningitis. Inflammation of the meninges, with increased white blood cell count but no bacteria detectable upon culture and examination.

attenuated. Describing a substance with decreased virulence; this is often accomplished by exposing the substance to conditions such as extreme heat or other circumstances adverse to the substance (in the case of vaccines, microorganisms).

autism. A developmental disorder characterized by an inability to communicate and interact normally, with a tendency toward inaccessibility, highly repetitive play, rages, and language disturbances.

Bell's palsy. Sudden facial paralysis due to nerve inflammation; may be temporary or permanent; cause unknown but thought to be viral infection or immune system dysfunction.

complement. A series of enzymatic proteins in serum that are sensitized to destroy bacteria and other cells and that are involved in a large number of immune responses.

convulsions. Series of involuntary muscular contraction and relaxation caused by disturbed brain wave patterns as a result of high fever, head trauma, infection, or other insult.

Crohn's disease. Inflammation of the ileum of the bowel leading to ulceration, narrowing, and thickening; causes pain and severe digestive difficulty with alternating constipation and diarrhea, and sometimes vomiting.

cyanosis. Bluish or grayish discoloration of the skin due to deficiency of oxygen and excess carbon dioxide; can be caused by certain drugs or anything that interferes with breathing.

demyelination. Destruction of the myelin sheath, the outer protective coating of the nerves that assists in the transmission of nerve impulses; can be temporary but is often severely debilitating and fatal.

encephalitis. An inflammation of the brain, often accompanied by fever and changes in white blood cells in the cerebrospinal fluid.

encephalopathy. A condition in which the brain is affected, leading to changes in consciousness, and may include stupor, seizures, and coma.

endemic. A continuously occurring disease in a given population, often referring to a disease with low mortality.

epidemic. An infectious disease that attacks many people at the same time and in the same geographic location.

erythema multiforme. A skin eruption with dark red, circular, fluid-filled vesicles, usually on the extremities, usually causing no discomfort; can be caused by infections and drug reactions. Stevens-Johnson syndrome is a severe and potentially deadly form, with large blistering lesions.

Guillain-Barré syndrome (GBS). Also referred to as postinfectious neuritis or acute inflammatory demyelinating polyneuritis; the symptoms are acute, with rapid onset of extreme muscle weakness, paralysis, loss of tendon reflexes, and demyelination of the peripheral nerves. Symptoms may occur as long as four weeks following an infection or vaccination. Can be fatal owing to respiratory failure.

hemiparesis. Paralysis of one side of the body.

hypotonic-hyporesponsive episodes (HHE). Shock and collapse; characterized by loss of consciousness, pallor, limpness, cyanosis, and shallow respiration; there may be fever but the child can feel cold to the touch. DPT vaccine can cause HHE; long-term effects of such episodes are unknown.

immunogenicity. The ability of a substance to stimulate antibody formation.

inoculate. To inject microorganisms, serums, or toxic materials into the body.

insulin-dependent diabetes mellitus. Also known as juvenile diabetes or type I diabetes; an autoimmune disease characterized by low or absent levels of the insulin naturally circulating in the body.

lupus erythematosus. A chronic inflammatory autoimmune disorder primarily affecting young women, characterized by a butterfly-shaped rash over the cheekbones and across the bridge of the nose, fever, joint pain, malaise, disk-shaped skin lesions, hair loss, sensitivity to light, arthritis without deformity, and a number of other clinical symptoms and laboratory findings. Can be fatal in severe cases owing to damaging effects on various organ systems.

multiple sclerosis. A chronic demyelination of the central nervous system, occurring more frequently in men than in women, and causing symptoms of vision loss in one eye, eye pain, pain, numbness, tingling, burning, or twitching on the face or extremities, and eventual degeneration with vision loss, paralysis, slurred speech, bladder and bowel dysfunction, and seizures. It may be mild, go into remission, or lead to severe physical deterioration.

oophoritis. Inflammation of the ovaries.

optic neuritis. A demyelinating disease of the optic nerve; may be an initial sign of multiple sclerosis.

orchitis. Inflammation of the testicles.

prodromal. The initial stages of disease.

residual seizure disorder. Recurrent seizures in the absence of fever; also referred to as epilepsy.

Reye's syndrome. An acute and sometimes fatal encephalopathy syndrome of childhood in which there is degeneration of the liver and significant brain swelling with changes in consciousness; associated with viral infections and with the use of aspirin during viral infections; occurs only in those younger than eighteen years old.

sensorineural deafness. Hearing loss due to damage in the end organ structures within the cochlea of the ear, or in the nerve connections in the cochlea.

subacute sclerosing panencephalitis (SSPE). A rare form of encephalitis that can affect the white and gray matter of the brain; it is an insidious disease that appears up to several years after the initiating event and causes progressively worsening cerebral dysfunction that is frequently fatal.

thrombocytopenia. A significant decrease in platelet count, resulting in disorders in blood clotting.

thrombocytopenia purpura. A severe form of thrombocytopenia that leads to bleeding into the skin and mucous membranes; usually evident as scattered bruises, especially on the lower legs; in children it is often the result of a viral infection and it is generally self-limiting, though it may take many weeks or months for full recovery; severe cases can be fatal.

transverse myelitis. Acute spinal cord disease associated with lesions of the spinal cord resulting in sudden lower back pain that is followed by pain and weakness of the lower extremities, possible bowel and bladder paralysis, and frequently permanent disabilities.

trivalent. Containing three components, as in the diphtheria-pertussis-tetanus (DPT) vaccine.

viremia. The presence of viruses in the blood.

Recommended Reading

Throughout this book you will find numerous references to articles from the medical literature. Almost all such materials referenced in this book are available through on-line library sources (for example, Medline, which can be accessed through PubMed; use your favorite search engine) or from major medical libraries. Because of the extensive nature of the references and the ease of access to them as endnotes, I have chosen not to list the medical journal articles in this recommended reading list. The materials in this section represent the books used in my research. While I do not agree with the opinions of all vaccine critics, nor can I attest to the veracity of all their information, I highly encourage you to read and research this topic extensively. I have therefore included a variety of what I consider to be the best or most widely referenced vaccine literature. You will also find a number of books on alternative medicine and natural healing for children. A home reference library can be a valuable asset for all parents and is particularly important for pediatric health concerns.

Vaccine Literature

Buttram, Harold, and John Chris Hoffman. *Vaccinations and Immune Malfunction*. Quakertown, Pa.: Randolph Society, 1985.

Chaitow, Leon. *Vaccination and Immunisation: Dangers, Delusions, and Alternatives*. Somerset, England: C. W. Daniel, 1994.

Coulter, Harris. *Divided Legacy: Twentieth-Century Medicine: The Bacteriological Era*. Berkeley, Calif.: North Atlantic Books, 1994.

Coulter, Harris, and Barbara Loe Fisher. *DPT: A Shot in the Dark*. New York: Warner Books, 1985.

Diodati, Catherine J. M. *Immunization: History, Ethics, Law, and Health*. Windsor, Ontario: Integral Aspects, 1999.

Fisher, Barbara Loe. *The Consumer's Guide to Childhood Vaccines*. Vienna, Va.: National Vaccine Information Center, 1997.

James, Walene. *Immunization: The Reality behind the Myth*. Westport, Conn.: Bergin and Garvey, 1995.

Miller, Neil. *Immunization: Theory vs. Reality*. Santa Fe, N. Mex.: New Atlantean Press, 1999.

———. *Vaccines: Are They Really Safe and Effective?* Santa Fe, N. Mex.: New Atlantean Press, 1999.

Mothering Magazine. *Immunizations*. Albuquerque, N. Mex.: Mothering Publications, 1984.

Neustaedter, Randall. *The Immunization Decision*. Berkeley, Calif.: North Atlantic Books, 1990.

Plotkin, Stanley, and Edward Mortimer. *Vaccines*. Philadelphia: W. B. Saunders, 1988.

Stratton, Kathleen, et al. *Adverse Events Associated with Childhood Vaccines: Evidence Bearing on Causality*. Washington, D.C.: National Academy Press, 1994.

Medical Microbiology

Levinson, Warren, and Ernest Jawetz. *Medical Microbiology and Immunology*. Stamford, Conn.: Appleton and Lange, 1996.

Mims, Cedric, et al. *Medical Microbiology*. Boston, Md.: Mosby, 1993.

Natural Medicine, Herbs, and Nutrition

Bensky, Dan, and Randall Barolet. *Chinese Herbal Medicines: Formulas and Strategies*. Seattle, Wash.: Eastland Press, 1990.

Bove, Mary. *An Encyclopedia of Natural Healing for Infants and Children*. New Canaan, Conn.: Keats, 1996.

Brennan, Patty. *Vaccine Choices: Homeopathic Alternatives and Parental Rights*. Ann Arbor, Mich.: Holistic Midwifery Institute, 1999.

Brinker, Frances. *Herb Contraindications and Drug Interactions*. Sandy, Ore.: Eclectic Medical Publications, 1998.

Buhner, Stephen. *Herbal Antibiotics*. Pownal, Vt.: Storey Books, 1999.

Cummings, Stephen, and Dana Ullman. *Everybody's Guide to Homeopathic Medicines*. Los Angeles: Jeremy Tarcher, 1984.

Flaws, Bob. *A Handbook of TCM Pediatrics*. Boulder, Colo.: Blue Poppy Press, 1997.

———. *Turtle Tail and Other Tender Mercies*. Boulder, Colo.: Blue Poppy Press, 1985.

Galland, Leo. *SuperImmunity for Kids*. New York: Dell Publishing, 1988.

McGuffin, Michael, et al. *Botanical Safety Handbook*. Boca Raton, Fla.: CRC Press, 1997.

Mendelsohn, Robert. *How to Raise a Healthy Child in Spite of Your Doctor*. New York: Ballantine, 1984.

Mills, Simon, and Kerry Bone. *Principles and Practice of Phytotherapy*. New York: Churchill Livingstone, 2000.

Murray, Michael. *Encyclopedia of Nutritional Supplements*. Rocklin, Calif.: Prima, 1996.

Romm, Aviva Jill. *Natural Healing for Babies and Children*. Freedom, Calif.: Crossing Press, 1996.

———. *Naturally Healthy Babies and Children*. Pownal, Vt.: Storey Books, 2000.

Romm, Aviva Jill, and Tracy Romm. *ADHD Alternatives*. Pownal, Vt.: Storey Books, 2000.

Smolin, Lori, and Mary Grosvenor. *Nutrition: Science and Applications*. New York: Harcourt Brace, 1997.

Zand, Janet, et al. *Smart Medicine for a Healthier Child*. Garden City, N.Y.: Avery, 1994.

Index